# Radiographic Positioning and Related Anatomy

## Workbook and Laboratory Manual

### VOLUME ONE

Chapters 1-13

## Sixth Edition

# Radiographic Positioning and Related Anatomy

## Workbook and Laboratory Manual

### VOLUME ONE

#### Chapters 1-13

## Kenneth L. Bontrager, MA, RT(R)
## John P. Lampignano, MEd, RT(R)(CT)

ELSEVIER
MOSBY

ELSEVIER
MOSBY

11830 Westline Industrial Drive
St. Louis, Missouri 63146

RADIOGRAPHIC POSITIONING AND
RELATED ANATOMY: WORKBOOK AND LABORATORY MANUAL,
6TH EDITION, VOLUME 1

ISBN 0-323-02504-8

**Copyright © 2005, 2001, 1997 by Mosby, Inc.**

---

### NOTICE

Radiography is an ever-changing field. Standard safety precautions must be followed, but as new research and clinical experience broaden our knowledge, changes in treatment and drug therapy may become necessary or appropriate. Readers are advised to check the most current product information provided by the manufacturer of each drug to be administered to verify the recommended dose, the method and duration of administration, and contraindications. It is the responsibility of the licensed prescriber, relying on experience and knowledge of the patient, to determine dosages and the best treatment for each individual patient. Neither the publisher nor the author assumes any liability for any injury and/or damage to persons or property arising from this publication.

---

*Executive Editor:* Jeanne Wilke
*Developmental Editor:* Becky Swisher
*Editorial Assistant:* Christina Pryor
*Publishing Services Manager:* Pat Joiner
*Senior Project Manager:* Karen M. Rehwinkel
*Senior Designer:* Kathi Gosche

Printed in the United States of America

Last digit is the print number: 9  8  7  6  5  4  3  2  1

# Acknowledgments

I am pleased to acknowledge and recognize those persons who have made significant contributions to the sixth edition of this student workbook and laboratory manual.

I first want to thank **John Lampignano,** who as co-author expanded the objectives and content of each chapter by submitting first drafts of additional questions for the new sections of the textbook. John is a very qualified and effective educator and has put a lot of effort and energy into this project. Thank you, John, for your excellent contributions.

I also thank **Jeanne Wilke, Karen Rehwinkel,** and **Rebecca Swisher** of the Mosby/Elsevier staff for their help and support in the preparation of this manuscript.

Last and most important, I want to thank my expanding family for their continued love, support, and encouragement and for bringing much joy and happiness into my life. I love each of you very much. Thanks **Mary Lou, Neil, Troy, Kim, Robyn, Hallie, Alexis, Ashton,** and **Jonathan**.

*KLB*

I would like to thank **Ken Bontrager** for his patience and mentorship in developing my skills as a writer. I've been honored to work with him over the past three editions. Ken has poured his heart and expertise into this text. Through his hard work and vision he has created a tremendous resource for students. **Mary Lou Bontrager** continues to provide the energy, technical support, and encouragement behind the scenes. Thank you, Mary Lou, for being there for both of us.

**Ms. Rebecca Swisher,** our associate editor, deserves praise for her dedication and vision in coordinating this project. She kept us on task and focused but always with a smile and a gentle word. Special thanks also to **Jeanne Wilke** for being a great editor and friend.

I would like to thank the diagnostic medical imaging faculty and clinical instructors at Gateway Community College who provide a shining example of excellence each and every day for our students and community. To my students—past, present, and future—you have made teaching a rewarding experience! Without your energy, laughter, and enthusiasm, teaching and writing this text would have been a burden rather than a joy. Finally, to my close friend, **Jerry Olson,** who taught me everything about radiography and many things about life—you have made my life richer and more worthwhile.

My family—**Deborah, Daniel,** and **Molly**—provide me with the greatest joy of all. I look at each of you and realize that I'm the luckiest person alive. Thank you for your love and support for the past 27 years. This book is dedicated to each of you.

*JPL*

# Preface

The success of the first five editions of this workbook and laboratory manual and the accompanying textbook, along with the associated ancillary materials, is demonstrated by the many schools of radiologic technology throughout the United States, Canada, and other countries that have been using all or parts of these instructional media for more than 30 years.

## New to This Edition

New illustrations and **expanded questions** have been added to reflect all the new content added to the sixth edition of *Textbook of Radiographic Positioning and Related Anatomy*. The use of visuals in these review exercises not only increases comprehension but also increases retention, because most individuals retain information most effectively through visual images.

The **detailed laboratory activities** have been updated, and the positioning question and answer exercises have been expanded, with less emphasis on rote memory recall. More **situational questions** involving **clinical applications** have been added. These questions aid in the understanding of positioning principles and of which anatomical structures are best demonstrated on which projections. The clinical situational questions added to each chapter require students to think through and understand how application of this positioning information relates to specific clinical examples.

Pathology questions have been expanded that will help students understand why they are performing specific exams and how exposure factors or positioning may be affected.

As in the textbook, entirely new sections added to the workbook include **digital radiography** and **surgical radiography**. The **bone densitometry** section has also been expanded, introductions to **nuclear medicine, PET radiation oncology, ultrasound imaging,** and **MRI** have also been revised and/or expanded.

## How to Work with the Textbook and the Workbook and Laboratory Manuals

This sixth edition of the student workbook and laboratory manual is organized to be in complete agreement with the sixth edition of the *Textbook of Radiographic Positioning and Related Anatomy*. Each chapter in the textbook has a corresponding chapter in the workbook/manual to reinforce and supplement the information presented in the main text.

The most effective way to use this workbook/manual is for the student to complete the workbook chapter exercises immediately after reading and studying corresponding chapters in the textbook. To use both the student's and the instructor's time most effectively, this study should be done **before** the classroom presentation. The instructor can therefore spend more time in both the classroom and laboratory on problem areas and answering questions and less time on the fundamentals of anatomy and positioning, which students should already have learned.

## Information for Faculty

### ELECTRONIC ANCILLARIES (INSTRUCTORS ELECTRONIC RESOURCE CD)

These electronic resources are available on CD and consist of the following three components:

- **Computerized Test Bank (CTB) in Exam View**: This test bank features more than 2000 questions divided into the 24 chapters. It has been updated, expanded, and revised into more registry-level questions that can be used as final evaluation exams for each chapter. They can be used to produce paper-based exams, or they can be migrated into web-based course-authoring systems such as BlackBoard or WebCT, or test-authoring systems such as Respondus. Answer keys are provided for each examination.
- **Electronic Image Collection (EIC)**: Also available is an updated and expanded electronic image collection of images from all 24 chapters of the 6th edition of the textbook. These nonannotated images can be used by instructors for custom applications such as BlackBoard, Respondus, etc.
- **Electronic Instructional Presentation (EIP) in PowerPoint**: Now included is a new updated and epanded electronic image PowerPoint program that is fully coordinated with all 24 chapters of the 6th edition textbook and workbooks. These electronic images include text slides, some of which contain embedded anatomy and positioning images, resulting in a visually led instructional narrative. This can then be used as a complete chapter-by-chapter pre-programmed PowerPoint lecture guide. Sections from the more advanced chapters can also be used for in-service training or with post-graduate presentations.

# Student Instructions

The following information will show you how to correctly use this workbook/laboratory manual and the accompanying textbook to help you master radiographic anatomy and positioning.

This course becomes the core of all your studies and your work as a radiologic technologist. **This is one course that you must master.** You cannot become a proficient technologist by marginally passing this course. Therefore please read these instructions carefully **before** beginning Chapter 1.

## Objectives

Study the list of objectives carefully so that you will understand what you must know and be able to do after you complete each chapter.

## Textbook and Workbook

**Chapters 1** and **2** include a comprehensive introduction that prepares you for the remaining chapters of this positioning course. Your instructor may assign all or specific sections of these chapters at various times during your study of radiographic positioning and/or procedures.

**Chapters 3-17** are specific positioning chapters that include the anatomy, positioning, and related procedures for all parts of the body.

**Chapters 18-24** are more specialized procedures and modalities that are commonly studied later in a medical radiography program.

## Learning Exercises

These exercises are the focal point of this workbook/laboratory manual. Using them correctly will help you learn and remember the important information presented in each chapter of the textbook. To maximize the benefits from each exercise, **follow the correct six-step order of activities** as outlined below.

### ANATOMY ACTIVITIES

**Step 1.** (Textbook): Carefully read and learn the **radiographic anatomy** section of each of these chapters. Include the anatomic reviews on labeled radiographs provided in the textbook. Pay particular attention to those items in **bold type** and to the **summary review boxes,** where provided.

**Step 2.** (Workbook, Part I): Complete Part I of the review exercises on **radiographic anatomy.** Do **not** look up the answers in the textbook or look at the answer sheet until you have answered as many of the questions as you can. Then refer to the textbook and/or the answer sheet and correct or complete those questions you missed. Reread those sections of the textbook in which you could not answer questions. Textbook page numbers are provided next to each review exercise in this workbook.

### POSITIONING ACTIVITIES

**Step 3.** (Textbook): Carefully read and study Part II on all of the parts on **radiographic positioning.** Note the general **positioning considerations, alternate modalities,** and **pathologic indications** for each chapter. Information from these sections will be seen on workbook review exercises, self-tests, and chapter evaluations. This is followed by the specific positioning pages, which include **pathology demonstrated, technical factors,** and the **dose ranges** of skin, midline, and specific organ doses, where provided. Pay particular attention to dose comparisons between different techniques, or anteroposterior (AP) versus posteroanterior (PA) projections. Learn the **specific positioning steps,** the **central ray location and angle,** and the four-part **radiographic criteria** for each projection or position.

**Step 4.** (Workbook, Part II): Complete Part II of the review exercises, which include **technical considerations and positioning.** Also included is a section on **problem solving for technical and positioning errors.** As before, complete as many of the questions as you can before looking up the answers in the textbook or checking the answers on the answer sheet.

The last review exercise in each positioning chapter covers **radiographic critique questions** in the workbook. This challenging section is based on the critique radiographs at the end of chapters in the textbook. These important exercises will help you make the transition from factual knowledge to application and will help you prepare for clinical experience. **Compare each critique radiograph that demonstrates errors with the correctly positioned radiographs in that chapter of the textbook** and see if you can determine which radiographic criteria points could be improved and which are repeatable errors. With digital images you will learn that in some cases postprocessing adjustments can be made to improve the exposures and the diagnostic value of the images rather than repeating the exam. Positioning errors, however, would still need to be repeated the same as with film-screen imaging and processing. Students who complete these exercises successfully will be ahead of those students who don't attempt them before coming to the classroom. The instructor will then explain and clarify those repeatable and nonrepeatable errors on each radiograph.

## LABORATORY ACTIVITY

**Step 5.** (Workbook, Part III—Laboratory Activity): These exercises must be performed in a radiographic laboratory using a phantom and/or a student (without making exposure) with an energized radiographic unit and illuminators for viewing radiographs, and/or monitors for viewing digital images. Arrange for a time when you can use your radiographic laboratory or a diagnostic radiographic room in a clinic setting.

**This is one of the most important aspects of this learning series and should not be neglected or underemphasized.** Students frequently have difficulty transferring the information they have learned about positioning to effective use in a clinical setting. Therefore you must carry out the laboratory activities as described in each chapter. Your instructors and/or lab assistants will assist you as needed in these exercises.

Each radiograph taken of the phantom and/or other radiographs provided by your instructor should be evaluated as described in your lab manual. Critique and evaluate each radiograph for errors of less-than-optimal positioning or exposure factors based on radiographic criteria provided in the textbook. Also, with the help of your instructor, learn how to discriminate between less-than-optimal, but passable radiographs, and those that need to be repeated. This generally requires additional experience and practice before you can make these judgments without assistance from a supervising technologist or radiologist.

## SELF-TEST

**Step 6.** You should **take the self-test only after you have completed all of the preceding steps.** Treat the self-test like an actual exam. After you have completed it, compare your answers with the answer sheet at the end of this workbook. If your score is less than 90% to 95%, you should go back and review the textbook again; pay special attention to the areas you missed before you take the final chapter evaluation exam provided by your instructor.

**Warning:** Statistics prove that students who diligently complete all the exercises described in this section will invariably get higher grades in their positioning courses and will perform better in the clinical setting than those who don't. **Avoid the temptation of taking shortcuts.** If you bypass some of these exercises or just fill in the answers from the answer sheets, your instructors will know by your grade and by your clinical performance that you have taken these shortcuts. Most importantly, you will know that you are not doing your best and you will have difficulty competing with better prepared technologists in the job market when you graduate.

**Go to it** and enjoy the feeling of satisfaction and success that only comes when you know you're doing your best!

# Contents

**Volume 2**

# Radiographic Positioning and Related Anatomy

## Workbook and Laboratory Manual

### VOLUME ONE

Chapters 1-13

# General Anatomy, Terminology, and Positioning Principles

## CHAPTER OBJECTIVES

After you have successfully completed the activities in this chapter, you will be able to:

### A. General, Systemic, and Skeletal Anatomy and Arthrology

_____  1.  List the four basic types of tissues.

_____  2.  List the ten systems of the body.

_____  3.  Match specific bodily functions to their correct anatomic system.

_____  4.  List the four general classifications of bone.

_____  5.  Identify specific characteristics and aspects of bone.

_____  6.  Classify specific joints by their structure and function.

_____  7.  Classify specific synovial joints by their movement.

### B. Positioning Terminology

_____  1.  Define general radiographic and anatomic relational terminology.

_____  2.  Define the imaginary planes, sections, and surfaces of the body used to describe central ray angles or relationships among body parts.

_____  3.  Distinguish among a radiographic projection, position, and view.

_____  4.  Given various hypothetical situations, identify the correct radiographic projection.

_____  5.  Given various hypothetical situations, identify the correct radiographic position.

_____  6.  List the antonyms (terms with opposite meanings) of specific terms related to movement.

### C. Positioning Principles

_____  1.  Given a hypothetical clinical situation, identify the response as required in the professional code of ethics.

_____  2.  Identify the correct sequence of steps taken to perform a routine radiographic procedure.

_____  3.  Given a set of circumstances, apply the two general rules of radiography concerning the minimal number of projections required for specific regions of the body.

_____  4.  Match the correct vertebral level to specific topographical landmarks.

_____  5.  List the four types of body habitus.

_____  6.  Identify the correct way to view a conventional radiograph, computed tomography (CT) image, and magnetic resonance (MR) image.

## Learning Activity Exercises

The following review exercises should be completed only after careful study of the associated pages in the textbook as indicated by each exercise. Because certain topics may be too advanced for the entry-level student, the review exercises for Chapter 1 are divided into sections A through C. You can complete specific sections of review exercises, as directed by your instructor, to best meet your learning needs.

   After completing each of these individual exercises, check your answers with the answers provided at the end of the review exercises.

**REVIEW EXERCISE A:** General, Systemic, and Skeletal Anatomy and Arthrology (see textbook pp. 2-13)

1. The lowest level of the structural organization of the human body is the _____ .

2. List the four basic types of tissues of the body:

   A. _____    C. _____

   B. _____    D. _____

3. List the ten systems of the human body:

   A. _____    F. _____

   B. _____    G. _____

   C. _____    H. _____

   D. _____    I. _____

   E. _____    J. _____

4. Match the following functions to the correct body system:

   _____  1. Eliminates solid waste from the body                          A. Skeletal system

   _____  2. Regulates fluid and electrolyte balance and volume            B. Circulatory system

   _____  3. Maintains posture                                             C. Digestive system

   _____  4. Regulates body activities with electrical impulses            D. Respiratory system

   _____  5. Regulates bodily activities through various hormones          E. Urinary system

   _____  6. Eliminates carbon dioxide from blood                          F. Reproductive system

   _____  7. Receives stimuli such as temperature, pressure, and pain      G. Nervous system

   _____  8. Reproduces the organism                                       H. Muscular system

   _____  9. Helps regulate body temperature                              I. Endocrine system

   _____ 10. Stores calcium                                                J. Integumentary system

5. True/False: One of the six functions of the circulatory system is to protect against disease.

6. List the two divisions of the human skeletal system:

   A. _____    B. _____

7.  True/False: The adult skeleton system contains 256 separate bones.

8.  True/False: The scapula is part of the axial skeleton.

9.  True/False: The skull is part of the axial skeleton.

10. True/False: The pelvis is part of the appendicular skeleton.

11. List the four classifications of bones:

    A. _____    C. _____

    B. _____    D. _____

12. The outer covering of a long bone, which is composed of a dense, fibrous membrane, is called what?

    A.  Spongy or cancellous bone       C.  Medullary aspect

    B.  Compact bone                    D.  Periosteum

13. Which aspect of long bones is responsible for the production of red blood cells?

    A.  Spongy or cancellous bone       C.  Medullary aspect

    B.  Compact bone                    D.  Periosteum

14. Which aspect of the long bone is essential for bone growth, repair, and nutrition?

    A.  Medullary aspect       C.  Periosteum

    B.  Compact bone           D.  Articular cartilage

15. Identify the primary and secondary growth centers for long bones:

    A.  Primary growth center: _____

    B.  Secondary growth center: _____

16. True/False: Epiphyseal fusion of the long bones is complete by the age of 16 years.

17. The study of joints or articulations is called _____ .

18. List the three *functional* classifications of joints:

    A. _____

    B. _____

    C. _____

19. List the three *structural* classifications of joints:

    A. _____

    B. _____

    C. _____

20. Match the following joints to the correct structural classification:

    _____ 1. First carpometacarpal of thumb     A. Fibrous joint

    _____ 2. Roots around teeth     B. Cartilaginous joint

    _____ 3. Proximal radioulnar joint     C. Synovial joint

    _____ 4. Skull sutures

    _____ 5. Epiphyses

    _____ 6. Interphalangeal joints

    _____ 7. Distal tibiofibular joint

    _____ 8. Intervertebral disk space

    _____ 9. Symphysis pubis

    _____ 10. Hip joint

21. List the six types of movement for synovial joints (give both the preferred terms and the synonyms):

    A. _____     D. _____

    B. _____     E. _____

    C. _____     F. _____

22. Match the following synovial joints to the correct type of movement:

    _____ 1. First carpometacarpal joint     A. Plane

    _____ 2. Elbow joint     B. Ginglymus

    _____ 3. Shoulder joint     C. Trochoid

    _____ 4. Intercarpal joint     D. Ellipsoid

    _____ 5. Wrist joint     E. Sellar

    _____ 6. Third metacarpophalangeal joint     F. Spheroid

    _____ 7. First and second cervical vertebra joint

    _____ 8. Second interphalangeal joint

    _____ 9. Distal radioulnar joint

    _____ 10. Ankle joint

**REVIEW EXERCISE B:** Positioning Terminology (see textbook pp. 14-29)  *1-28*

1. A ___Radiography___ is an x-ray IR or other base material containing an image of an anatomic part of a patient.  *pg 29*

2. An upright position with the arms abducted, palms forward, and head and feet directed straight ahead describes the

   ___Anatomic___ position. *pg 14*

3. The vertical plane that divides the body into equal right and left parts is the ___midsagittal___ plane. *pg 15*

4. The vertical plane that divides the body into equal anterior and posterior parts is the ___midcoronal___ *pg 15* plane.

5. A plane taken at right angles along any point of the longitudinal axis of the body is the

   ___axial/transverse___ plane. *pg 15*

6. (True)/False: The *base plane of the skull* is a plane located between the infraorbital margin of the orbit and the *Pg 16* superior margin of the external auditory meatus.

7. (True)/False: The *Frankfort horizontal plane* is also referred to as *the anthropological plane.* *pg 16 = base plan of skull*

8. The direction or path of the central ray of the x-ray beam defines the following positioning term: *p 29*

   (A.) Projection    C.  Position

   B.  View        D.  Perspective

9. The positioning term that describes the general and specific body position is: *pg 18*

   A.  Projection    (C.)  Position

   B.  View        D.  Perspective

10. (True)/False: Oblique and lateral positions are described according to the side of the body closest to image receptor. *pg 19*

11. (True)/False: Decubitus positions always utilize a horizontal x-ray beam. *pg 20*

12. What is the name of the position in which the body is turned 90° from a true anteroposterior (AP) or

    posteroanterior (PA) projection? ___lateral position___ *pg 19*

13. **Situation:** A patient is erect with the back to the image receptor. The left side of the body is turned 45° toward the

    image receptor. What is this position? ___LPO___

14. **Situation:** A patient is recumbent facing the image receptor. The right side of the body is turned 15° toward the

    image receptor. What is this position? ___Recumbent RAO___

15. **Situation:** The patient is lying on the back. The x-ray beam is directed horizontally and enters the right side of the *pg 20* body. An image receptor is placed against the left side of the patient. Which specific position has been used?

    ___Dorsal decubitus Left lateral___

16. **Situation:** The patient is erect with the right side of the body against the image receptor. The x-ray beam enters the *pg 19*

    left side of the body. Which specific position has been used? ___Erect Right lateral___

17. **Situation:** A patient is lying on the left side on a cart. The x-ray beam is directed horizontally and enters the posterior aspect of the body. The image receptor is against the anterior surface. Which specific position has been *pg 20*

    used? ___Left lateral Decubitus PA___

18. Match the following definitions to the correct term (using each term only once):

   H   1.  Palm of the hand                                    A.  Posterior

   G   2.  Lying on the back facing upward                      B.  Anterior

   F   3.  An upright position                                  C.  Plantar

   I   4.  Lying down in any position                           D.  Dorsum pedis

   B   5.  Front half of the patient                            E.  Trendelenburg

   D   6.  Top or anterior surface of the foot                  F.  Erect

   J   7.  Position in which head is higher than the feet       G.  Supine

   C   8.  Posterior aspect of foot                             H.  Palmar

   E   9.  Position in which head is lower than feet            I.  Recumbent

   A   10. Back half of the patient                             J.  Fowler

19. What is the name of the projection in which the central ray enters the anterior surface and exits the posterior

   surface?  AP  Antero posterior

20. A projection directed parallel to or at an angle along the long axis of the body or a part is called a/an

   Axial  projection.  pg 21

21. The specific position that demonstrates the apices of the lungs, without superimposition of the clavicles, is called

   a/an  Lordotic Position  pg 21

22. True/False: The radiographic view is the radiographic image seen from the vantage point of the image receptor.  pg 29

23. True/False: The term *varus* describes the bending of a part outward.  inward  outward  P26  VARUS  Valgus

24. Match the following. (Indicate whether the following terms describe a position or projection.)  pg 29

   B   1.  Anteroposterior                                      A.  Position

   A   2.  Lying on abdomen                                     B.  Projection

   A   3.  Trendelenburg

   A   4.  Left posterior oblique

   A   5.  Left lateral chest

   B   6.  Mediolateral ankle

   B   7.  Apical AP

   A   8.  Lordotic  pg 21

   B   9.  Transthoracic

   A   10. Left lateral decubitus

25. For each of the following terms, list the term that has the **opposite** meaning: pg 29

    A. Flexion: _Extension_

    B. Ulnar deviation: _radial deviation_

    C. Dorsiflexion: _plantar flexion_

    D. Eversion: _Inversion_

    E. Lateral (external) rotation: _medial rotation_

    F. Abduction: _Adduction_

    G. Supination: _pronation_

    H. Retraction: _Protraction_

    I. Depression: _Elevation_

26. Match the following relationship terms to the correct definition (using each term only once):

| | | |
|---|---|---|
| _F_ 1. Near the source or beginning | A. Caudad or inferior | |
| D _E_ 2. On the opposite side | B. Deep | |
| _G_ 3. Toward the center | C. Distal | |
| _E_ 4. Toward the head end of the body | D. Contralateral | |
| _C_ 5. Away from the source or beginning | E. Cephalad or superior | |
| _J_ 6. Outside or outward | F. Proximal | |
| I _D_ 7. On the same side | G. Medial | |
| _H_ 8. Near the skin surface | H. Superficial | |
| _A_ 9. Away from the head end | I. Ipsilateral | |
| _B_ 10. Farther from the skin surface | J. Exterior | |

27. Moving or thrusting the jaw forward from the normal position is an example of _Protraction_ .

28. To turn or bend the wrist toward the radius side is called _Radial Deviation_ .

STOP

**REVIEW EXERCISE C:** Positioning Principles (see textbook pp. 30-40)    18 - 21

1. True/**False**: Technologists have the right to refuse to perform an examination on a patient whom they find offensive.

2. **True**/False: Technologists are responsible for the professional decisions they make during the care of the patient.

3. **True**/False: The technologist has the responsibility of communicating with the patient to obtain pertinent clinical information.

4. True/**False**: The technologist is expected to provide a preliminary interpretation of radiographic findings to the referring physician.

5.  True/False: The technologist may reveal confidential information pertaining to a patient who is less than 18 years of age to the patient or guardian.

6.  A *PBL* collimator refers to:

    A.  Positive beam limiting          C.  Patient-based life-saving

    B.  Power beam limiting             D.  Penumbra biased limiting

7.  True/False: PBL collimators are required for all x-rays units manufactured after 1995.

8.  Which one of the following steps should be performed *first* during a positioning routine?

    A.  Image receptor centering                  C.  Placing anatomic side markers on cassette

    B.  Placing gonadal shielding as needed       D.  Patient and part positioning

9.  What is the final step taken before making the exposure during a positioning routine?

    A.  Image receptor centering                  C.  Collimation

    B.  Placing anatomic markers on cassette      D.  Ensuring correct gonadal shield placement

10. List the two rules or principles for determining positioning routines as they relate to the maximum number of projections required in a basic routine: Pg 36

    A.  __Minimum two positions__          B.  __at 90° from each other__

11. Indicate the minimum number of projections required for each of the following anatomic regions:

    A.  Foot _____               F.  Fifth toe _____

    B.  Chest _____              G.  Postreduction of wrist (image of wrist in cast) _____

    C.  Wrist _____              H.  Left hip _____

    D.  Tibia/fibula _____       I.  Knee _____

    E.  Humerus _____

12. **Situation:** A young child enters the emergency room with a fractured forearm. After one projection is completed, which confirms a fracture, the child refuses to move the forearm for any additional projections.

    A.  What is the minimum number of projections that should be taken for this forearm study?

        (a)  One          (c)  Three

        (b)  Four         (d)  Two

    B.  If additional projections are required for a routine forearm series, what should the technologist do with the young patient described in this situation?

        (a)  Because only one projection is required for      (c)  Rather than move the forearm for a second
             a fractured forearm, the technologist is not          projection, place the cassette and x-ray tube as
             required to take additional projections.              needed for a second projection 90° from
                                                                   the first projection.

        (b)  With the help of a parent or guardian, gently   (d)  Ask the emergency room physician to move
             but firmly move the forearm for each                 the forearm for a second projection. This
             additional projection required.                      eliminates any liability for the technologist in case
                                                                   the patient is injured further.

13. Match the following metric measurements for image receptor sizes to the nearest equivalent traditional size:

| METRIC | TRADITIONAL (ENGLISH) |
|---|---|
| _D_ 1. 24 × 30 cm | A. 14 × 17 inches |
| _E_ 2. 18 × 24 cm | B. 14 × 36 inches |
| _A_ 3. 35 × 43 cm | C. 12 × 14 inches |
| _C_ 4. 30 × 35 cm | D. 10 × 12 inches |
| _F_ 5. 24 × 24 cm | E. 8 × 10 inches |
| _B_ 6. 35 × 90 cm | F. 8 × 8 inches |

14. Match the following topographical landmarks to the corresponding vertebral level:

| | |
|---|---|
| _C_ 1. Sternal angle | A. T9-10 |
| _D_ 2. Anterior superior iliac spine | B. L2-3 |
| _A_ 3. Xiphoid process | C. T4-5 |
| _F_ 4. Iliac crest | D. S1-2 |
| _E_ 5. Jugular notch | E. T2-3 |
| _B_ 6. Inferior costal margin | F. L4-5 |

15. The physical localization of bony landmarks on a patient is called _Palpation_ .
    _pg 38_

16. The greater trochanter is located on the:
    A. Proximal femur     B. Cervical spine     C. Sternum     D. Lower pelvis

17. The ischial tuberosity corresponds with the vertebral level of:
    A. T9-10              C. S1-2
    B. L4-5 interspace     D. 1 to 2 inches inferior to distal coccyx

18. List the four types of body habitus: _pg 39_
    A. _HypersThenic  5%_       C. _Hypo sThenic  35%_
    B. _Sthenic     50%_         D. _AsThenic  10%_

19. Which type of body habitus is described as being "average"? _Sthenic_

20. What percentage of the population has this "average" body type? _50%_

*Questions 21 to 24 refer to Fig. 1-1, A and B:*

21. Which body habitus type is represented by Fig. 1-1, A?

    <u>HyperSThenic</u>

22. Which body habitus type is represented by Fig. 1-1, B?

    <u>AsTenic</u>

23. What percentage of the population has the body habitus type in Fig. 1-1, A?

    <u>        5%        </u>

24. What percentage of the population has the body habitus type in Fig. 1-1, B?

    <u>        10%        </u>

25. True/False: Always place a radiograph for viewing as the x-ray tube "sees" the patient. (The patient's left is to the viewer's left on PA projections.)

26. True/False: CT images are viewed so that the patient's right is to the viewer's left.

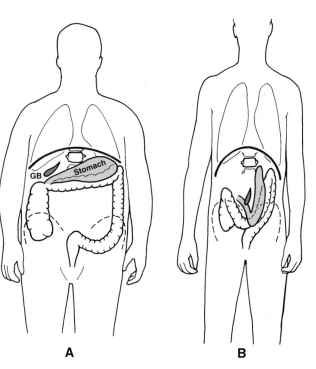

A                                                  B

**Fig. 1-1.**

# Answers to Review Exercises

## Review Exercise A: General, Systemic, and Skeletal Anatomy and Arthrology

1. Chemical level
2. A. Epithelial
   B. Connective
   C. Muscular
   D. Nervous
3. A. Skeletal
   B. Circulatory
   C. Digestive
   D. Respiratory
   E. Urinary
   F. Reproductive
   G. Nervous
   H. Muscular
   I. Endocrine
   J. Integumentary
4. 1. C
   2. E
   3. H
   4. G
   5. I
   6. D
   7. J
   8. F
   9. B
   10. A
5. True
6. A. Axial skeleton
   B. Appendicular skeleton
7. False (206)
8. False (part of appendicular)
9. True
10. True
11. A. Long bones
    B. Short bones
    C. Flat bones
    D. Irregular bones
12. D. Periosteum
13. C. Medullary aspect
14. C. Periosteum
15. A. Body (diaphysis)
    B. Epiphyses
16. False
17. Arthrology
18. A. Synarthrosis
    B. Amphiarthrosis
    C. Diarthrosis
19. A. Fibrous
    B. Cartilaginous
    C. Synovial
20. 1. C
    2. A
    3. C
    4. A
    5. B
    6. C
    7. A

8. B
9. B
10. C
21. A. Plane (gliding)
    B. Ginglymus (hinge)
    C. Trochoid (pivot)
    D. Ellipsoidal (condyloid)
    E. Sellar (saddle)
    F. Spheroid (ball and socket)
22. 1. E
    2. B
    3. F
    4. A
    5. D
    6. D
    7. C
    8. B
    9. C
    10. B

## Review Exercise B: Positioning Terminology

1. Radiograph
2. Anatomic
3. Median or midsagittal
4. Midcoronal
5. Transverse or axial
6. True
7. True
8. A. Projection
9. C. Position
10. True
11. True
12. Lateral position
13. Left posterior oblique (LPO)
14. Right anterior oblique (RAO)
15. Dorsal decubitus (left lateral)
16. Right lateral
17. Left lateral decubitus (PA)
18. 1. H
    2. G
    3. F
    4. I
    5. B
    6. D
    7. J
    8. C
    9. E
    10. A
19. Anteroposterior (AP)
20. Axial
21. Lordotic position
22. True
23. False (inward, toward midline)
24. 1. B
    2. A
    3. A
    4. A
    5. A

6. B
7. B
8. A
9. B
10. A
25. A. Extension
    B. Radial deviation
    C. Plantar flexion
    D. Inversion
    E. Medial (internal) rotation
    F. Adduction
    G. Pronation
    H. Protraction
    I. Elevation
26. 1. F
    2. D
    3. G
    4. E
    5. C
    6. J
    7. I
    8. H
    9. A
    10. B
27. Protraction
28. Radial deviation

## Review Exercise C: Positioning Principles

1. False
2. True
3. True
4. False
5. False
6. A. Positive beam limiting
7. False
8. D. Patient and part positioning
9. D. Ensuring correct gonadal shielding
10. A. A minimum of two projections 90° from each other
    B. A minimum of three projections when joints are in the prime interest area
11. A. 3
    B. 2
    C. 3
    D. 2
    E. 2
    F. 3
    G. 2
    H. 2
    I. 3
12. A. (d) Two
    B. (c) Rather than move the forearm for additional projections, place the cassette and x-ray tube as needed.

13. 1. D
    2. E
    3. A
    4. C
    5. F
    6. B
14. 1. C
    2. D
    3. A
    4. F

    5. E
    6. B
15. Palpation
16. A. Proximal femur
17. D. 1 to 2 inches inferior to distal coccyx
18. A. Hypersthenic
    B. Sthenic
    C. Hyposthenic
    D. Asthenic

19. Sthenic
20. 50%
21. Hypersthenic
22. Asthenic
23. 5%
24. 10%
25. False (Place as if technologist were facing the patient; patient's right to technologist's left.)
26. True

# SELF-TEST

My Score = _____ %

This series of self-tests should be taken only after completing all of the readings, review exercises, and laboratory activities for a particular section. This self-test is divided into three sections. The purpose of this test is not only to provide a good learning exercise but also to serve as a strong indicator of what your final evaluation exam will cover. It is strongly suggested that if you do not get at least a 90% to 95% grade on each self-test, you review those areas in which you missed questions before going to your instructor for the final evaluation exam. There are 102 questions or blanks—each is worth 0.98 (almost 1) point.

**SELF-TEST A:** General, Systemic, and Skeletal Anatomy and Arthrology

1. Which of the following is (are) **not** one of the four basic types of tissue in the human body? (More than one answer is possible.)

   A.  Integumentary      D.  Osseous

   B.  Connective         E.  Muscular

   C.  Nervous            F.  Epithelial

2. How many separate bones are found in the adult human body?

   A.  180      C.  206

   B.  243      D.  257

3. Which one of the following systems distributes oxygen and nutrients to the cells of the body?

   A.  Digestive      C.  Skeletal

   B.  Circulatory    D.  Urinary

4. Which one of the following systems maintains the acid-base balance in the body?

   A.  Digestive      C.  Reproductive

   B.  Urinary        D.  Circulatory

5. Which one of the following systems involves the skin and all structures derived from the skin?

   A.  Muscular      C.  Skeletal

   B.  Endocrine     D.  Integumentary

6. The two divisions of the human skeleton are:

   A.  Bony and cartilaginous      C.  Vertebral and extremities

   B.  Axial and appendicular      D.  Integumentary and appendicular

7. Which portion of the long bones is responsible for the production of red blood cells?

   A.  Spongy or cancellous      C.  Hyaline

   B.  Periosteum                D.  Compact aspect

8. What type of tissue covers the ends of the long bones?

   A.  Spongy or cancellous      C.  Hyaline or articular cartilage

   B.  Periosteum                D.  Compact aspect

9. The narrow space between the inner and outer table of the flat bones in the cranium is called the:

   A. Calvarium        C. Medullary portion

   B. Periosteum       D. Diploe

10. What is the primary center for endochondral ossification in long bones?

    A. Diaphysis (shaft)        C. Epiphyses

    B. Epiphyseal plate         D. Medulla

11. What is the name of secondary growth centers of endochondral ossification found in long bones?

    A. Diaphysis (shaft)        C. Epiphyses

    B. Epiphyseal plate         D. Medulla

12. A skull suture has the structural classification of a ——— joint.

    A. Fibrous              C. Synovial

    B. Cartilaginous        D. Diarthrosis

13. The symphysis pubis has the structural classification of a ——— joint.

    A. Fibrous              C. Synovial

    B. Cartilaginous        D. Synarthrosis

14. Which specific joint(s) is(are) the only true syndesmosis, amphiarthrodial, fibrous joint(s)?

    A. Joints between the roots of teeth and adjoining bone        C. Distal tibiofibular joint

    B. First carpometacarpal joint        D. Proximal and distal radioulnar joints

15. Match the following bones to their correct classification:

    ——— 1. Sternum        A. Long bone

    ——— 2. Femur          B. Short bone

    ——— 3. Tarsal bones   C. Flat bone

    ——— 4. Pelvic bones   D. Irregular bone

    ——— 5. Scapulae

    ——— 6. Humerus

    ——— 7. Vertebrae

    ——— 8. Calvarium

16. The three structural classifications of joints are synovial, cartilaginous, and:

    A. Amphiarthrodial        C. Diarthrodial

    B. Ellipsoid              D. Fibrous

17. Classify the following synovial joints based on their type of movement:

     _____ 1. First carpometacarpal joint          A. Plane (gliding)

     _____ 2. Intercarpal joint                    B. Ginglymus (hinge)

     _____ 3. Hip joint                            C. Trochoid (pivot)

     _____ 4. Proximal radioulnar joint         D. Ellipsoid (condyloid)

     _____ 5. Interphalangeal joint              E. Sellar (saddle)

     _____ 6. Fourth metacarpophalangeal joint    F. Spheroid (ball and socket)

     _____ 7. Knee joint

     _____ 8. Wrist joint

     _____ 9. Atlantoaxial joint (between C1 and C2)

## SELF-TEST B: Positioning Terminology

1. Which plane divides the body into equal anterior and posterior parts?

    A. Midsagittal      B. Transverse      (C.) Midcoronal      D. Longitudinal

2. True/False: The terms *radiograph* and *x-ray IR* refer to the same thing.

3. A longitudinal plane that divides the body into right and left parts is the:

    A. Coronal plane      (C.) Sagittal plane

    B. Horizontal plane      D. Oblique plane

4. Match the following definitions to the correct term:

    __E__ 1. Near the source or beginning               A. Eversion

    __I__ 2. Away from head end of the body          B. Circumduction

    __G__ 3. Nearer to the center                    C. Pronation

    __J__ 4. Increasing the angle of a joint           D. Contralateral

    __A__ 5. Outward stress of the foot               E. Proximal

    __K__ 6. Movement of an extremity away from the midline      F. Medial

    __C__ 7. Turning palm downward                 G. Interior

    __H__ 8. A backward movement                H. Retraction

    __B__ 9. To move around in the form of a circle      I. Caudad

    __F__ 10. Toward the center                    J. Extension

    __L__ 11. Away from the source or beginning       K. Abduction

    __D__ 12. On the opposite side of the body         L. Distal

5. Match the following definitions to the correct term:

_L_ 1. Lying down in any position

_G_ 2. Head lower than the feet position

_F_ 3. Upright position, palms forward

_J_ 4. Top of the foot

_A_ 5. Frankfort horizontal plane

_H_ 6. A plane at right angles to sagittal or coronal planes

_D_ 7. Head higher than feet position

_C_ 8. Palm of hand

_B_ 9. Sole of foot

_K_ 10. Front half of body

_I_ 11. A plane that divides body into anterior and posterior halves

_E_ 12. A recumbent position with knees and hips flexed with support for legs

A. Base plane of skull

B. Plantar

C. Palmar

D. Fowler's position

E. Lithotomy position

F. Anatomic position

G. Trendelenburg position

H. Horizontal plane

I. Midcoronal plane

J. Dorsum pedis

K. Anterior

L. Recumbent

6. The direction or path of the central ray of the x-ray beam defines the positioning term:

A. Position   C. Perspective

B. View   (D.) Projection

7. **Situation:** A patient is placed in a recumbent position facing downward. The left side of the body is turned 30° toward the image receptor. Which specific position has been performed?

A. LAO         (C.) LPO

B. Left lateral decubitus     D. RAO

8. **Situation:** A patient is placed into a recumbent position facing downward. The x-ray tube is directed horizontally and enters the left side of the body. An image receptor is placed against the right side of the patient. Which position has been performed?

A. Dorsal decubitus     C. Ventral decubitus

(B.) Left lateral decubitus     D. Right lateral decubitus

9. **Situation:** A patient is erect with the back to the image receptor. The central ray enters the anterior aspect and exits the posterior aspect of the body. Which projection has been performed?

A. Posteroanterior     C. Ventral decubitus

B. Tangential     (D) Anteroposterior

10. **Situation:** A patient is lying down facing upward with the posterior surface of the body against the image receptor. The right side of the body turned 45° toward the image receptor. The x-ray tube is directed vertically and enters the anterior surface of the body. Which position has been performed?

A. LPO     C. RPO

(B.) RAO     D. LAO

5. Indicate the minimum number of projections required for the following structures:

   \_\_\_\_ 1. Knee                 A. Two

   \_\_\_\_ 2. Fourth finger        B. Three

   \_\_\_\_ 3. Humerus

   \_\_\_\_ 4. Sternum

   \_\_\_\_ 5. Ankle

   \_\_\_\_ 6. Tibia/fibula

   \_\_\_\_ 7. Chest

   \_\_\_\_ 8. Hand

   \_\_\_\_ 9. Hip (proximal femur)

   \_\_\_\_ 10. Forearm

6. **Situation:** A patient enters the emergency room with a fractured forearm. The fracture is set, or *reduced*. The orthopedic physician orders a postreduction series. How many projections are required?

   A. One       C. Two

   B. Three     D. Four

7. A 24 × 30 cm imaging plate is equivalent to a(n) \_\_\_\_ inch imaging plate.

   A. 8 × 10        C. 11 × 14

   B. 10 × 12      D. 14 × 17

8. A 40-inch SID is equivalent to a(n) \_\_\_\_ -cm SID.

   A. 80       C. 100

   B. 110     D. 180

9. Which topographical landmark can be palpated to locate the L4-5 vertebral interspace?

   (A.) Iliac crest             C. ASIS

   B. Inferior costal margin     D. Xiphoid process

10. Which topographical landmark can be palpated to locate T2-3?

   A. Vertebra prominens     C. Sternal angle

   (B.) Jugular notch            D. Inferior costal margin

11. The xiphoid process corresponds to the \_\_\_\_ vertebral level.

   (A.) T9-10     B. T4-5     C. L2-3     D. T2-3

12. A "stocky," massive body build describes a/an \_\_\_\_ body habitus.

   A. Asthenic       C. Sthenic

   B. Hyposthenic     (D.) Hypersthenic

# Image Quality, Digital Technology, and Radiation Protection

After you have successfully completed the activities in this chapter, you will be able to:

## A. Image Quality in Film-Screen Imaging

_____ 1. Describe the major exposure factors that influence the diagnostic quality of the radiograph.

_____ 2. List the four image quality factors and their impact on a radiograph.

_____ 3. Define *radiographic density* and identify its controlling factors.

_____ 4. Given a hypothetical situation, select the correct factor to improve radiographic density.

_____ 5. Describe the correlation between radiographic density and the *anode heel effect*.

_____ 6. Explain the purpose and use of *compensating filters*.

_____ 7. Define *radiographic contrast* and identify its controlling factors.

_____ 8. Distinguish between long- and short-scale radiographic contrast.

_____ 9. Given a hypothetical situation, select the correct factor to improve radiographic contrast.

_____ 10. Define *resolution* and identify its controlling factors.

_____ 11. List the three geometric factors that influence image sharpness.

_____ 12. Identify the best ways of controlling voluntary and involuntary motion.

_____ 13. Given a hypothetical situation, select the correct factor to improve radiographic detail.

_____ 14. Define *radiographic distortion* and identify its controlling factors.

_____ 15. Given a hypothetical situation, select the correct factor to minimize radiographic distortion.

## B. Image Quality in Digital Radiography

_____ 1. List the six image quality factors specific to digital imaging.

_____ 2. Define *brightness* and identify its controlling factors in the digital image.

_____ 3. Define *contrast* and identify its controlling factors in the digital image.

_____ 4. List the two types of pixel sizes.

_____ 5. Define *resolution* and identify its controlling factors in the digital image.

_____ 6. Define *distortion* and identify its controlling factors in the digital image.

_____ 7. Define *exposure index* and describe its relationship to the amount of radiation striking the image receptor (IR).

_____ 8. Explain the concept of the signal-to-noise ratio (SNR).

_____ 9. Define specific terms related to the post-processing of the digital image.

## C. Applications of Digital Technology

_____    1.   List the differences between computed tomography (CT) and conventional radiography.

_____    2.   List and briefly describe the two types of digital fluoroscopy systems.

_____    3.   Identify the major components of a digital fluoroscopy system.

_____    4.   List the major components of a computed radiography (CR) system.

_____    5.   Describe briefly how an image is recorded, processed, and viewed with a CR system.

_____    6.   Explain the importance of correct centering, collimation, use of lead masking, and use of grids to the overall quality of the CR image.

_____    7.   Identify specific differences and similarities between CR and digital radiography (DR).

_____    8.   List advantages and disadvantages of digital mammography.

_____    9.   Define the acronyms *PACS, RIS, HIS,* and *IHE.*

_____   10.   Define the terms *telemedicine* and *teleradiology* and list the benefits and applications for each.

_____   11.   List the benefits of *computer-assisted detection* (CAD).

_____   12.   List, in proper sequence, the steps in producing the IR-based CR and DR images.

_____   13.   Define specific imaging terms and acronyms.

## D. Radiation Protection

_____    1.   List and define the traditional units and International System of Units (SI units) of radiation measurement and the conversion factors used to convert between systems.

_____    2.   List the specific annual dose limiting recommendations of *whole body effective dose* for the general population and occupationally exposed workers.

_____    3.   Define *ALARA.*

_____    4.   Apply the principles of ALARA to any given hypothetical situation.

_____    5.   Define *skin entrance exposure (SEE)* and *effective dose (ED).*

_____    6.   Identify specific methods to reduce exposure to the technologist during fluoroscopic and radiographic procedures.

_____    7.   Identify specific methods to reduce exposure to the patient during radiographic procedures.

_____    8.   Identify the major types of area and gonadal shields and the minimum lead equivalent thickness requirements of these shields.

_____    9.   Define the *10-day rule* and describe its limitations.

_____   10.   Define patient dose terminology for specific regions of the body.

## Learning Exercises

The following review exercises should be completed only after careful study of the associated pages in the textbook as indicated by each exercise. The review exercises for Chapter 2 are divided into four sections. You can complete specific sections of review exercises, as directed by your instructor, to best meet your learning needs.

   After completing each of these individual exercises, check your work with the answers provided at the end of the review exercises.

**REVIEW EXERCISE A:** Image Quality in Film-Screen Imaging (see textbook pp. 42-49) *1-11 16-21*

*Start* 1. The radiographic film image is composed of metallic ___*silver*___ on a polyester base. *P42*

2. List the four image quality factors of a radiograph: *p43-47*

A. ___Density (blackness) ↑ mAs - 25-30% ↑ mAs___ C. ___Resolution (sharpness)___

                               *15% ↑ kV*

B. ___Contrast (shades of gray, diff in density) ↓ mAs___ D. ___Distortion (size, shape)___

3. Which specific exposure factor controls the quality or penetrating ability of the x-ray beam?

___$KV_p$___ *P47*

              *P42*

4. Exposure time is usually expressed in units of ___*milliseconds*___.

5. The amount of blackness seen on a processed radiograph is called ___*Density*___.

6. The primary controlling factor for the overall blackness on a radiograph is ___*mAs*___.

7. If the distance between the x-ray tube and image receptor is increased from 40 to 80 inches, what specific effect will it have on the radiographic density, if other factors are not changed? *P43*

A. Increase density to 50%     C. No effect on density     *SID doubles, density red. to ¼*

(B.) Decrease density to 25%     D. Decrease density to 50%

     *SID*

8. Which term is used to describe a radiograph that has too little density? ___*under exposed*___ *p44*

9. Doubling the mAs will result in ___*double*___ the density on the IR image. *p43*

      *mAs*

10. True/(False): kV must be altered to change radiographic density on the IR image. *p43*

11. When IR images, using manual technique settings, are under- or overexposed, a minimum change in mAs of

*Stop* ___*25% - 30%*___ is required to make a visible difference in the radiographic density. *p43*

A. 1% to 3%     (C.) 25% to 30%

B. 10% to 15%     D. 50% to 100%

12. According to the anode heel effect, the x-ray beam is less intense at the ___*anode*___ (**cathode** or *p44* **anode**) end of the x-ray tube.

13. To best utilize the anode heel effect, the thicker part of the anatomic structure should be placed under the *p44*

___*Cathode*___ (**cathode** or **anode**) end of the x-ray tube.

14. What device or method (other than the anode heel effect) may be used to compensate for anatomic part thickness

difference and produce an acceptable density on the IR image? ___*Compensating filters*___

15. **Situation:** A radiograph of the foot is produced using conventional film-screen cassettes. The resulting radiograph demonstrates too little density and must be repeated. The original exposure was 5 mAs. What mAs is needed to *P43* correct the density on this radiograph? (Hint: Density needs to be about doubled.)

A. 5 mAs     C. 30 mAs     *25% 6.3 mAs*

B. 17.5 mAs     (D.) 10 mAs

*start* 16.   The difference in density on adjacent areas of the radiograph defines _____ContrasT_____ . *p45*

17.   What is the primary controlling factor for radiographic contrast? _____KVp_____ *p45*

18.   List the two scales of radiographic contrast, and identify which is classified as high contrast and which is low
      contrast:

*110KV* A. _____long Scale - Low ConTrast_____   *50KV* B. _____ShorT Scale   high ConTrast_____

19.   Which scale of contrast is produced with a 110 kV technique? _____Long Scale ConTrast Low_____

20.   True/False: A 50 kV technique will produce a **high**-contrast image. *ShorT Scale*

21.   True/False: A **low**-contrast image demonstrates more shades of gray on the radiograph. *long Scale*

*stop* 22.   Which one of the following sets of exposure factors will result in the least patient exposure and produce long-scale
      contrast on a PA chest radiographic image?

      A.   50 kV, 800 mAs          C.   80 kV, 100 mAs          *↑ KV, lower contrast*

      B.   70 kV, 200 mAs          D.   110 kV, 10 mAs

23.   **Situation:** A radiograph of the hand is underexposed and must be repeated. The original technique used was
      55 kV with 2.5 mAs. The technologist decides to keep the mAs at the same level but change the kV to
      increase radiographic density. How much of an increase is needed in kilovoltage (kV) to double the density?

      A.   3 to 5 kV increase          C.   10 to 15 kV increase
      B.   8 to 10 kV increase          D.   15 to 20 kV increase            *8.25 KV*

24.   The recorded sharpness of structures or objects on the radiograph defines _____resolution_____ .

25.   The lack of visible sharpness is called _____blur or unsharpness_____ .

26.   List the three **geometric** factors that control or influence image resolution:

      A.   _____focal Spot Size_____

      B.   _____SID (Source image receptor distance) the distance of the x-ray source from the IR_____

      C.   _____OID (Object image receptor distance) closer the object is to IR, less magnification and shape distortion
           & better detail e resolution_____

27.   The term that describes the unsharp edges of the projected image is _____Penumbra_____ .

28.   True/False: The use of a small focal spot will *decrease* ~~entirely eliminate~~ the problem identified in the previous question.

29.   The greatest contributor to image unsharpness as related to positioning is _____motion_____ .

30.   What is the best mechanism to control involuntary motion during an exposure?

      A.   Use of a small focal spot          C.   Decrease object image receptor distance (OID)

      B.   Use of a grid          D.   Shorten exposure time

31.   Which one of the following changes will improve image resolution?

      A.   Decrease OID          C.   Use a large focal spot

      B.   Decrease source image receptor distance (SID)          D.   Use a higher kilovoltage

32. **Situation:** The technologist is performing an elbow series on a pediatric patient. Because of the nature of the injury, the technologist has been asked to produce radiographs that have the highest degree of recorded resolution possible. Which one of the following sets of factors will produce that level of detail? *Small focal spot / Increase in SID / Decrease in OID*

    A. 0.3-mm focal spot and 30-inch SID     C. 0.5-mm focal spot and 40-inch SID

    B. 1-mm focal spot and 45-inch SID     (D) 0.3-mm focal spot and 40-inch SID

33. The misrepresentation of an object size or shape projected onto a radiographic recording medium is called

    _____distortion_____ .

34. True/(False): Through careful selection and control of exposure and geometric factors, it is possible to eliminate all image distortion.

35. List the four primary controlling factors for distortion:

    A. _____SID_____     C. _____Object image receptor alignment_____

    B. _____OID_____     D. _____Central ray alignment/centering_____

36. True/False: A ~~decrease~~ *increase* in SID reduces distortion.

37. True/False: An ~~increase~~ *decrease* in OID reduces distortion.

38. (True)/False: Distortion is reduced when the central ray (CR) is kept perpendicular to the plane of the image receptor.

39. The SID for general radiographic procedures resulting in maximum recorded resolution is:

    A. 40 inches (100 cm)     (C.) 44 inches (110 cm)

    B. 72 inches (180 cm)     D. 48 inches (120 cm)

40. **Situation:** A chest x-ray on a patient with an enlarged heart has been requested. Which SID is recommended for this study?

    A. 40 inches (100 cm)     C. 44 inches (110 cm)

    (B.) 72 inches (180 cm)     D. 48 inches (120 cm)

41. (True)/False: Every radiographic image reflects some degree of penumbra or unsharpness, even if the smallest focal spot is used.

42. True/(False): As the distance of between the object and the image receptor is ~~increased~~ *decreased*, magnification is reduced.

43. (True)/False: Image distortion increases as the angle of divergence increases from the center of the x-ray beam to the outer edges.

44. (True)/False: The greater the angle of inclination of the object or the IR, the greater the amount of distortion.

45. True/(False): Central ray alignment has little impact on image distortion.

## REVIEW EXERCISE B: Image Quality in Digital Radiography (see textbook pp. 50-54)    1-31

1. True/(False): Digital imaging requires that images be chemically processed.

2. (True)/False: Digital images are a numeric representation of the x-ray intensities that are transmitted through the patient.

3. True/(False): Digital images viewed on a monitor are referred to as ~~hard~~ *soft*-copies.

4. Digital processing involves the systematic application of highly complex mathematical formulas called:

    A. Matrices     C. Analog-to-digital converters

    B. PACS     (D) Algorithms

5.  The range or level of image contrast in the digital image is primarily controlled by:

    A.  kV          (C.)  Digital processing  p 51

    B.  mAs          D.   Matrix size

6.  Exposure latitude with digital imaging is more ___wide___ (**narrow** or **wide**) when compared with film-screen imaging.  p 50/52

7.  List the six image quality factors specific to digital images: p51

    A.  __Brightness__ | CTL FACTOR software | Film Density          D. __Distortion__ | CTL FACTORS SID OID CR Alignment | Film Distortion

    B.  __Contrast__ | Algorithms matrix | System ability to distinguish between diff. Tissue    E. __Exposure Index__ | Intensity of radiation striking → dector | mAs object kV exposure dector AREA

    C.  __Resolution__ | Pixel Size matrix | Resolution          F. __Noise__ | random disturbance obscuring or reducing clarity

8.  In digital imaging, the term ___brightness___ replaces *density* as applied in IR-screen imaging.
    p51
    (A.)  Brightness          C.  Latitude

    B.  Signal          D.  Noise

9.  True/False: Changes in mAs will **not** have a primary controlling effect on digital image brightness.  p5

10.  True/False: Brightness cannot be altered in the digital image once it has been processed.

11.  A digital imaging system's ability to distinguish between similar tissues is termed:  p51

    A.  Brightness          C.  Signal

    B.  Image resolution     (D.)  Contrast resolution

12.  Radiographic contrast in the digital image is primarily affected by:

    A.  kV                          (C.)  Application of processing algorithms

    B.  Signal-to-noise ratio        D.  Matrix size

13.  The greater the bit depth of a digital imaging system, the greater the:

    A.  Size of the matrix          C.  Brightness

    (B.)  Contrast resolution        D.  Pixel size

14.  List the terms describing the two pixel sizes used in digital imaging:

    A.  __aquisition pixel size - minimum size that is inherent to the system__

    B.  __display pixel size - minimum size that can be displayed on monitor__

15.  Which one of the two pixel sizes listed above is most critical in maintaining high-resolution digital images?

    __aquisition pixel size__

16.  True/False: Focal spot size has no impact on the resolution of the digital image.  p52

17.  The current range of image resolution for digital general radiographic imaging is between:

    A.  1 to 5 microns          C.  50 to 75 microns

    B.  10 to 50 microns        (D.)  100 to 200 microns  p52

18. Resolution in the digital image is primarily dependent on: *p 52*

    A. kV                     C. SID

    *(B.)* Display capabilities of the monitor     D. Use of a grid

19. True/False: The factors that affect image distortion for the digital image are different from those that affect film-screen systems. *p 52*

20. A numeric value that is representative of the exposure the digital image receptor receives is termed the

    __Exposure Index__.

21. List the four factors that affect exposure index in the digital image: *p 52*

    A. __mAs__

    B. __kV__

    C. __Total detector area irradiated__

    D. __Objects exposed__

22. Another term for "S number," as used by several manufacturers of CR equipment, is

    __Sensitivity Number__

    *\*Large S number under exposure*
    *\*Small S number over exposure*

23. An "*S number*" is __inversely__ (**directly** or **indirectly**) proportional to the radiation exposing

    the patient; and an "*exposure index*" *number*, as used by other manufacturers, is __directly__

    *Large index ↑ over exposure*
    *Small index ↓ under exposure*

    (**directly** or **indirectly**) proportional.

24. If the recommended exposure index range for a well-exposed image is between 150 and 250, an "*S number*" of

    350 to 550 would indicate __Under exposure__ (**overexposure** or **underexposure**) of the image.

25. If the recommended exposure index value range is between 2.0 to 2.4, an *exposure index number* of 1.2 would

    indicate __Under exposure__ (**overexposure** or **underexposure**) of the image.

    *scatter radiation*

26. A random disturbance that obscures or reduces clarity is the definition for __Noise__ *electronic noise* *p 53*

    *HIGH SNR Less NOISE mAs↑*

27. SNR is the acronym for the __Signal To Noise ratio__ *LOW SNR More noise mAs↓*

28. When insufficient mAs is applied in the production of a digital image, it will produce a

    __Low SNR__ (**high-SNR** or **low-SNR**) image. *mAs— Signal / Noise*

29. Another term for image noise is:

    A. Variance       *(C.)* Mottle

    B. Static          D. Digital spam

30. Changing or enhancing the electronic image in order to improve its diagnostic quality is called

    __Post processing__. *p 54*

31. Identify the type of post-processing described by listing the correct term for the following definitions:

   A. Adding text to images: _Annotation_

   B. Increasing brightness along the edges of structures to increase the visibility of the edges:

   _edge enhancement_

   C. Reversing the dark and light pixel values of an image—the x-ray image reverses from a negative to a

   positive: _image reversal_

   D. Magnifying all or part of an image: _magnification_

   E. Adjusting brightness values of adjacent pixels closer together: _Smoothing_

   F. Removing background anatomy to allow visualization of contrast media–filled structures:

   _Subtraction_

## REVIEW EXERCISE C: Applications of Digital Technology (see textbook pp. 55-63) _1~36_

1. True/False: CT has been used since the late 1950s.
2. True/False: CT has superior contrast resolution when compared with film-screen radiography.
3. True/False: Tissues such as lungs produce low attenuation of the x-ray beam as compared with muscle during the CT scanning process
4. Which one of the following is not a distinct advantage of CT as compared with film-screen radiography?
   A. Anatomy viewed in alternative planes       C. Lower dose
   B. Higher contrast resolution                 D. Structures visualized without superimposition
5. List the two types of digital fluoroscopy being used:
   A. _Analog to digital_
   B. _Direct digital conversion_

6. True/False: Direct conversion to digital fluoroscopy does not require the use of an image intensifier or video system.

7. List the three components of a CR system:
   A. _Image plates (IP)_
   B. _IP reader_
   C. _Technologist workstation_

8. What material on the CR imaging plate captures the latent image? _photostimulable phosphors_

9. With CR, the imaging plate (IP):
   A. Must be kept in a light-tight cassette and replaced with recharged plates daily
   B. Must be used in conjunction with light-sensitive IR
   C. Must be used in conjunction with intensifying screens
   D. None of the above

10. When using a CR image plate, patient data can be linked to the image by use of a(an): _ps?_

    (A.) Bar code reader      C. Laser

    B. White light source      D. Ultraviolet light source

11. True/False: Once the CR image plate has had an image recorded on it, it must be discarded.

12. True/False: The latent image on a CR image plate is read line by line by a laser within the CR reader.

13. True/False: It takes approximately 20 seconds to process a CR image and reload the cassette with a clean imaging plate.

14. The latent image is erased on the CR image plate by applying:

    (A.) Bright light      C. Low-level radiation

    B. Heat      D. Microwaves

15. The process of transferring the CR image to a storage device is termed _archiving_ .

16. Which one of the following technical factors does **not** apply to CR (computed radiography)?

    A. Close collimation

    B. Accurate centering of part and IR

    C. Use of lead masks

    (D.) A minimum of 72 inches (183 cm) is required for all CR projections

17. When using CR, a minimum of _30_ % of the IR must be exposed for an accurate exposure index.

18. True/False: The use of grids is optional with CR since the IP is not as sensitive to scatter radiation as film-screen radiography.

19. Which of the following imaging components is **not** required with direct digital radiography (DR)?

    A. IP      C. Grid

    B. Image reader      (D.) Both A and B

20. True/False: Patient dose may be lower with DR as compared with film-screen radiography and CR.

21. True/False: When using DR for most nongrid procedures, one reason the grid is generally not removed is its fragile construction.

22. A common detector size for DR chest radiography units is:

    A. 27.9 × 35.6 cm      (C.) 43 × 43 cm

    B. 43 × 49 cm      D. 19 × 23 cm

23. True/False: An advantage of digital mammography is high-contrast resolution with potential reductions in patient dose.

24. True/False: The 30% collimation rule applies to direct digital radiography (DR).

25. Define the acronym *PACS:*

    P : _Picture_

    A : _Archiving_

    C : _Communication_

    S : _System_

26. True/False: A PACS automatically transports conventional x-ray IRs to the chemical processor after they have been exposed.

27. What do the following acronyms represent? (Write the complete term.) *p 61*

    A. DICOM: _Digital Imaging Communications Medicine_

    B. RIS: _Radiology Information System_

    C. HIS: _Hospital Information system_

    D. HL7: _Health Care level 7_

28. True/False: The use of telemedicine has lowered the cost of health care. *p 61*

29. The electronic transmission of diagnostic imaging studies is termed _Teleradiology_. *p 61*

30. True/False: Studies show that computer-assisted detection (CAD) may eventually replace the need for the radiologist to interpret mammogram images. *p 62*

31. True/False: Recent studies have shown that CAD can increase a radiologist's performance in interpreting images overall by approximately 50%. _10%_ *p 62*

32. True/False: Film-based mammograms must be digitized to utilize CAD. _62_

33. In addition to mammography, CAD is currently being used with:

    A. CT *p 62*      C. Chest radiography

    B. Ultrasound      D. Bone age studies

34. An electronic, comprehensive database of all patient records and data is referred to as

    _IHE Intregrated Healthcare Enterprise_. (Include the acronym.)

35. Provide the correct term for the following definitions:

    _Display Matrix_    A.   Series of "boxes" that gives form to the image

    _Exposure latitude_    B.   Range of exposure factors that will produce an acceptable image

    _Windowing_    C.   The user adjusting the window level and window width

    _Penumbra_    D.   Unsharp edges of the projected image

    _Exposure Index_    E.   Numeric value that is representative of the exposure the image receptor received in digital radiography

    _Bit Depth_    F.   Representative of the number of shades of gray that can be demonstrated by each pixel

    _Distortion_    G.   Misrepresentation of object size or shape as projected onto radiographic recording media

    _kV_    H.   The energy of the x-ray photon

    _Noise_    I.   Random disturbance that obscures or reduces clarity

    _Telemedicine_    J.   The delivery of health care services using telecommunications and computer technology

    _Post Processing_    K.   Changing or enhancing the electronic image in order to view it from a different perspective or improve its diagnostic quality

36. List the complete term for the following acronyms: p 64

    A. DQE: _Detection Quantum Efficency_

    B. IR: _Image Receptor_

    C. OID: _Object image receptor distance_

    D. DR: _Direct Digital Radiography_

    E. AEC: _Automatic Exposure Control_

    F. IMAC: _Image ? Information Managoment ; Communication_

**REVIEW EXERCISE D:** Radiation Protection (see textbook pp. 65-73)   1-19, 24-39

Start 1. Which traditional unit is used to measure radiation exposure in air? _R/Roentgen_

2. Which traditional unit of measurement is used to describe patient dose? _Rads_

3. What does the acronym *ED* stand for? _Effective Dose_

4. What is the **whole body effective** dose limit per year for a technologist (in traditional and International System

    [SI] units)? _5rem / 50mSv_          $5rem \left( \frac{1Sv}{100rem} \right) =$

5. What is the cumulative dose limit for a 35-year-old technologist (in traditional and SI units)?

    _35rem / 350 mSv_        $35rem \left( \frac{1 Sv}{100 rem} \right) =$

6. For each of the following traditional units, list the equivalent SI unit of radiation measurement and its symbol:

| Traditional Unit | SI Unit |
|---|---|
| A. Roentgen (R) <br>    measure in Air | C/Kg dAir p 65 |
| B. Radiation absorbed dose (rad) <br>    patient Dose | .01Gy Gray (Gy) |
| C. Radiation equivalent man (rem) <br>    Radiation protection | .01Sv seivert (SU) |

7. Convert the following doses, stated in traditional units, into the equivalent SI unit:

    A. 3 rad = _0.03 Gy_ $\left( \frac{Gy}{100 rad} \right)$ Gy       C. 38 rem = _0.38Sv_ $\left( \frac{Sv}{100rem} \right)$ Sv

    B. 448 mrad = _4.48Gy_ $\left( \frac{Gy}{100 rad} \right)$ mGy    D. 15 rem = _0.15Sv_       mSv

8. What is the maximum dose limit for a pregnant technologist?           p66

    A. Per month: _.5mSv/.05 rem_ rem

    B. For the entire gestational period: _5 mSv / .5 rem_

9. The acronym *ALARA* stands for _As low as reasonably achievable_ .

10.  **Situation:** A young child comes to the radiology department for a skull series. The child is combative and will not hold still for the procedure. Which one of the following individuals should be asked to restrain the patient?    *p 66*

   A.  A family member (if not pregnant)          C.  The oldest technologist

   B.  A student technologist                     D.  A nuclear medicine technologist

11.  True/False: With accurate and close collimation, area shields do not need to be used.

12.  True/False: Skin entrance exposure (SEE) has the highest numeric value of all patient doses.

13.  True/False: In radiography, SEE carries the least biological significance.

14.  True/False: ED describes gonadal dose levels only for each radiographic procedure.

15.  What is the best method of reducing scatter to a worker's eyes and neck during fluoroscopy?    *P68*

   _____

   *keep Image Intensifier tower as close as possible to the patient*

16.  Which of the following is the best place for a technologist to stand during fluoroscopy to reduce occupational exposure?

   A.  Head end of table          C.  Behind the radiologist

   B.  Foot end of table          D.  Next to the radiologist

17.  What is the federal set limit for exposure rates for intensified fluoroscopy units?

   A.  1 R/min          C.  3 to 4 R/min

   B.  6 to 8 R/min     D.  10 R/min

18.  With most modern fluoroscopy equipment, the average exposure rate is:

   A.  0.5 R/min        C.  1 R/min

   B.  3 to 4 R/min     D.  10 R/min

*STOP*  19.  What is one of the **primary** causes for repeat radiographs? (Select the *best* answer.)

   A.  Excessive kilovoltage        C.  Poor communication between technologist and patient    *pg 69*

   B.  Wrong IR selection           D.  Distortion caused by incorrect SID

20.  In addition to the primary cause identified in the previous question, what two other factors often lead to repeat exposures?

   A. _Incorrect exposure time_____

   B. _Carelessness in positioning, incorrect exposure factors_____

21. Refer to the Patient Dose chart on p. 67 of the textbook to answer the following questions (A through G):

    A. The _____AP_____ (**AP** or **PA**) chest projection provides the greatest ED for females.

    B. _____Male_____ (**Male** or **Female**) patients receive a greater ED for an AP hip, with or without gonadal shielding.

    C. List the gonadal dose for male and female patients for an AP abdomen projection using 70 kV:

        Male, shielded: _2_

        Male, unshielded: _6_

        Female, unshielded: _80_

    D. Which specific organ in each gender receives the greatest dose in AP, PA, and lateral upper GI projections: lungs, testes, ovaries, thyroid, marrow, or breast? _____lungs_____

    E. List the gonadal doses for an AP hip projection for the following patients:

        Male, unshielded (testes): _322_        Female, unshielded (ovaries): _59_

        Male shielded: _42_            Female shielded: _14_

    F. Which radiographic procedure listed on the Patient Dose chart provides the **least amount of SEE** for males and females? _lateral upper GI_ (Note the correlation among kilovoltage peak, milliampere seconds, and dose.)

    G. Which procedure on the Patient Dose chart provides the **greatest amount** of

        ED for a **male** patient? ___PA Chest___

        For a **female** patient? ___AP Thoracic Spine unshielded on 14×17___

22. If a technologist receives 3.3 to 6.7 mR/min standing 1 foot from a fluoroscopy unit, what will the dose be if the technologist moves to a distance of 4 feet? (See Exposure Levels chart on p. 68 of the textbook.)

    A. Less than 0.25 mR/min      C. 0.8 to 1.7 mR/min

    B. 0.4 to 0.8 mR/min        D. 1.7 to 3 mR /min

23. List the two major forms of filtration found in x-ray tubes that affect the quality of the primary x-ray beam:

    A. _Inherent - built-in filtration from the structures making up the x-ray tube itself_

    B. _Added - the amount of filtration added between the x-ray tube and the collimator and within the collimator itself_

24. What is the most common metal used in filters for diagnostic radiology equipment? ___Aluminum___

    START

25. List the two ways collimation will reduce patient exposure:

    A. _reduces the volume of tissue directly irradiated_

    B. _reduces the accompanying scatter radiation_

26. True/False: Safety standards require that collimators be accurate to within 10% of the selected SID. *(handwritten: 2% P 70)*

27. True/False: Positive beam limitation (PBL) collimators restrict the size of the exposure field to the size of the cassette in a Bucky tray.

28. True/False: PBL collimators became optional on new equipment manufactured after May 1993 because of a change in Food and Drug Administration (FDA) regulations.

29. List the two general types of area shields: *(handwritten: P71)*

    A. _Shadow Shields_

    B. _Gonadal Contact Shields_

30. The minimum thickness of a gonadal shield placed within the primary x-ray field should be:

    A. 0.1-mm lead equivalent     (C.) 1-mm lead equivalent

    B. 0.25-mm lead equivalent     D. 0.5-mm lead equivalent

31. If placed properly, gonadal shields absorb _____ of the primary beam in the 50 to 100 kV range.

    (A.) 95% to 99%     C. 70% to 80%

    B. 80% to 90%     D. 50% to 70%

32. An area shield should be used when radiation-sensitive tissues lie within _2_ inches (or _5_ cm) of the primary beam. *(handwritten: P72)*

33. According to the 10-day rule, when is the safest time for a female of childbearing age to have a radiographic examination of the lower abdomen and pelvis?

    A. 10 days before beginning of menses     C. First 10 days of each month

    (B.) 10 days after onset of menses     D. Last 10 days of each month

34. True/False: The 10-day rule is considered by the International Commission on Radiological Protection (ICRP) and the American College of Radiology to be obsolete and no longer valid.

35. **Situation:** A 20-year-old female enters the emergency room with a possible fracture of the pelvis. What should the technologist do in regard to gonadal shielding? *(handwritten: ?)*

    A. Use it for all projections     C. Ask the patient whether she is pregnant

    B. Use it for the AP projections only     (D.) Do not use shielding for initial pelvis projection

36. What is the disadvantage of using faster-speed screens for all IR-screen radiographic procedures?

    _loss of image definition or sharpness of detail_

37. List the complete term for each of the following abbreviations used in patient dose icon boxes (found in the positioning pages of the textbook):

    A. Sk: _Skin Dose_

    B. ML: _Midline Dose_

    C. Gon: _Gonadal Dose_

    D. NDC: _No Detectable Contribution_

38.   True/False: Area shields must be used for all radiographic procedures with all patients.

39.   What is the minimum lead equivalency recommended for a protective apron worn during fluoroscopy?

STOP

_____ .5mm _____        P68

40.   List the three cardinal rules for radiation protection:   P 66

A.   _____ Time _____

B.   _____ distance _____

C.   _____ Shielding _____

Energy absorbed by tissue

$50 \text{ rem} \left( .01 \text{ Sv} \right) = .5 \text{ Sv} = 500 \text{ mS}$

$50 \text{ rem} \Big($

patient dose 1 rad = .01 Gy

radiation protection  1 rem = .01 Sv

# Answers to Review Exercises

## Review Exercise A: Image Quality in Film-Screen Imaging

1. Silver
2. A. Density
   B. Contrast
   C. Resolution
   D. Distortion
3. Kilovoltage (kV)
4. Milliseconds
5. Density
6. Milliampere seconds (mAs)
7. B. Decrease density to 25%
8. Underexposed
9. Doubling
10. False
11. C. 25%-30%
12. Anode
13. Cathode
14. Compensating filters
15. D. 10 mAs
16. Radiographic contrast
17. Kilovoltage (kV)
18. A. Long-scale contrast (low contrast)
    B. Short-scale contrast (high contrast)
19. Long-scale contrast (low)
20. True
21. True
22. D. 110 kV, 10 mAs
23. B. 8 to 10 kV increase
24. Resolution or definition
25. Blur or unsharpness
26. A. Focal spot size
    B. Source image receptor distance (SID)
    C. Object image receptor distance (OID)
27. Penumbra
28. False
29. Motion
30. D. Shorten exposure time
31. A. Decrease OID
32. D. 0.3-mm focal spot and 40-inch SID
33. Distortion
34. False (There is always some magnification and distortion caused by OID and divergence of the x-ray beam.)
35. A. Source image receptor distance (SID)
    B. Object image receptor distance (OID)
    C. Object IR alignment
    D. Central ray placement
36. False (increase distortion)
37. False (decrease distortion)
38. True
39. C. 44 inches (110 cm)
40. B. 72 inches (180 cm)
41. True
42. False
43. True
44. True
45. False

## Review Exercise B: Image Quality in Digital Radiography

1. False
2. True
3. False
4. D. Algorithms
5. C. Digital processing
6. Wide
7. A. Brightness
   B. Contrast
   C. Resolution
   D. Distortion
   E. Exposure index
   F. Noise
8. A. Brightness
9. True
10. False
11. D. Contrast resolution
12. C. Application of processing algorithms
13. B. Contrast resolution
14. A. Acquisition pixel size
    B. Display pixel size
15. Acquisition pixel size
16. False
17. D. 100 to 200 microns
18. B. Display capabilities of the monitor
19. False
20. Exposure index
21. A. mAs
    B. kV
    C. Total detector area irradiated
    D. Objects exposed
22. Sensitivity number
23. Indirectly; directly
24. Underexposure
25. Underexposure
26. Noise
27. Signal-to-noise ratio
28. Low-SNR
29. C. Mottle
30. Post-processing
31. A. Annotation
    B. Edge enhancement
    C. Image reversal
    D. Magnification
    E. Smoothing
    F. Subtraction

## Review Exercise C: Applications of Digital Technology

1. False
2. True
3. True
4. C. Lower dose
5. A. Analog converted to digital type
   B. Direct digital conversion type, or flat detector based type
6. True
7. A. Image plates (IP)
   B. IP reader
   C. Technologist QC workstation
8. Photostimulable phosphor
9. D. None of the above
10. A. Bar code reader
11. False
12. True
13. True
14. A. Bright light
15. Archiving
16. D. A minimum of 72" (183 cm) required for all CR projections
17. 30
18. False
19. D. Both A and B
20. True
21. True
22. C. 43 × 43 cm
23. True
24. False
25. Picture
    Archiving
    Communication
    System
26. False
27. A. Digital Imaging Communications Medicine
    B. Radiology Information System
    C. Hospital Information System
    D. Healthcare Level 7
28. True
29. Teleradiology
30. False
31. False
32. True
33. C. Chest radiography
34. Integrated Healthcare Enterprise (IHE)
35. A. Display matrix
    B. Exposure latitude
    C. Windowing
    D. Penumbra
    E. Exposure index
    F. Bit depth
    G. Distortion
    H. Kilovoltage
    I. Noise
    J. Telemedicine
    K. Post-processing
36. A. Detection Quantum Efficiency
    B. Image Receptor
    C. Object Image Distance
    D. Digital Radiography
    E. Automatic Exposure Control

F. Image and Information Management and Communication

## Review Exercise D: Radiation Protection

1. Roentgen
2. Rad
3. Effective dose
4. 5 rem (50 mSv) per year
5. 35 rem (350 mSv)
6. A. Coulombs per kilogram (C/kg) of air
   B. Gray (Gy)
   C. Seivert (Sv)
7. A. 0.03 Gy
   B. 4.48 mGy
   C. 0.38 Sv
   D. 150 mSv
8. A. 0.05 rem (0.5 mSv)
   B. 0.5 rem (5 mSv)
9. As low as reasonably achievable
10. A. Family member (if not pregnant)
11. False (still need to be used)
12. True
13. True
14. False (considers dose levels to all organs)
15. Keep the image intensifier tower as close as possible to the patient.

16. C. Behind the radiologist
17. D. 10 R/min
18. B. 3 to 4 R/min
19. C. Poor communication between technologist and patient
20. A. Carelessness in positioning
    B. Selection of incorrect exposure factors
21. A. AP (more than double because of increased thyroid and breast doses)
    B. Male (from greater dose to gonads because of proximity of testes to primary beam)
    C. Male, shielded: 2 mrad
       Male, unshielded: 6 mrad
       Female, unshielded: 80 mrad
    D. Lungs
    E. Male, unshielded: 322 mrad
       Male, shielded: 42 mrad
       Female, unshielded: 59 mrad
       Female, shielded: 14 mrad
    F. PA chest
    G. Male: AP hip projection without shielding
       Female: AP T spine on 14 × 17
22. B. 0.4 to 0.8 mR/min
23. A. Inherent
    B. Added
24. Aluminum

25. A. Reduces the volume of tissue irradiated
    B. Reduces the accompanying scatter radiation, which adds to patient dose
26. False (2%, not 10%)
27. True
28. True
29. A. Shadow shields
    B. Contact shields
30. C. 1-mm lead equivalent
31. A. 95% to 99%
32. 2 inches; 5 cm
33. B. 10 days after onset of menses
34. True
35. D. Do not use shielding (for initial pelvis projection)
36. Results in some loss of recorded detail
37. A. Skin dose
    B. Midline dose
    C. Gonadal dose
    D. No detectable contribution
38. False (only if it doesn't cover pertinent anatomic parts for that exam)
39. 0.5-mm lead (Pb) equivalent
40. A. Distance
    B. Time
    C. Shielding

# SELF-TEST

My Score = _____ %

This series of self-tests should be taken only after completing all of the readings, review exercises, and laboratory activities for a particular section. This self-test is divided into four sections. The purpose of this test is not only to provide a good learning exercise but also to serve as a strong indicator of what your final evaluation exam will cover. It is strongly suggested that if you do not get at least a 90% to 95% grade on each self-test, you review those areas in which you missed questions before going to your instructor for the final evaluation exam. There are 80 questions or blanks—each is worth 1.25 points.

**SELF-TEST A:** Image Quality in Film-Screen Imaging

1. Which one of the following is **not** one of the four primary image quality factors?

    A. Density           D. Detail

    B. Contrast         E. Distortion

    C. Kilovoltage (kV)

2. The amount of blackness on a processed radiograph is called:

    A. Density                  C. Contrast

    B. Milliampere seconds (mAs)     D. Penumbra

3. Which of the following exposure factors primarily controls radiographic density?

    A. kV       C. Focal spot size

    B. mAs     D. Source image receptor distance (SID)

4. True/False: For an underexposed radiograph, the mAs must be increased by a factor of four to produce a visible change in radiographic density.

5. **Situation:** A radiograph of the knee reveals that it is overexposed and must be repeated. The original technique used 10 mAs. Which one of the following changes will improve the image during the repeat exposure?

    A. Increase to 15 mAs      C. Increase to 20 mAs

    B. Decrease to 5 mAs      D. Decrease to 2 mAs

6. The primary controlling factor for radiographic contrast is:

    A. mAs      C. Focal spot size

    B. kV       D. SID

7. **Situation:** Chest radiographs require long-scale contrast. Which set of exposure factors will produce this?

    A. 50 kV, 20 mAs     C. 110 kV, 2 mAs

    B. 65 kV, 15mAs      D. 80 kV, 5 mAs

8. Which one of the following sets of exposure factors will produce the highest radiographic contrast?

    A. 60 kV, 30 mAs     C. 96 kV, 5 mAs

    B. 80 kV, 20 mAs     D. 120 kV, 2 mAs

9. True/False: Kilovoltage is a secondary controlling factor for radiographic density.

10. True/False: A low kilovoltage technique (50 kV) produces a ~~long~~ *Short*-scale contrast image.

11. **Situation:** A radiograph of the elbow reveals that it is overexposed. The technologist wants to adjust kV rather than mAs for the repeat exposure. This is contrary to common practice. The original exposure factors were 70 kV and 5 mAs. Which one of the following kV settings would reduce radiographic density by one-half?

    A.  80 kV and 5 mAs      C.  60 kV and 5 mAs

    B.  66 kV and 5 mAs      D.  56 kV and 5 mAs

12. Which one of the following techniques will reduce the amount of scatter radiation striking the IR?

    A.  Collimation      C.  Grids

    B.  Lower kV         D.  All of the above

13. True/False: Recorded detail or image resolution is optimal with a ~~long~~ *Short* object image receptor distance (OID) and a ~~short~~ *long* SID.

2

14. Which one of the following factors best controls involuntary cardiac motion artifact?

    A.  Careful instructions given to the patient

    B.  High kV technique

    C.  Practicing with patient when to hold breath

    D.  Shortening the exposure time

15. **Situation:** The technologist is asked to produce a high-quality image of the carpal (wrist) bones. The emergency room physician suspects that the patient has a very small fracture of one of the bones. Which one of following sets of technical factors will produce an image with the highest degree of radiographic resolution?

    A.  1-mm focal spot and 30-inch SID

    B.  2-mm focal spot and 36-inch SID

    C.  0.5-mm focal spot and 40-inch SID

    D.  0.3-mm focal spot and 40-inch SID

16. Rather than rely on the anode heel effect, _____ can be used to equalize density of specific anatomy.

    A.  Inherent filtration      C.  Added filtration

    B.  A compensating filter    D.  A diaphragm

17. The misrepresentation of an object's size or shape projected on a radiograph is called:

    A.  Magnification      C.  Unsharpness

    B.  Blurring           D.  Distortion

18. Which one of the following sets of factors minimizes radiographic distortion to the greatest degree?

    A.  40-inch SID and 8-inch OID

    B.  44-inch SID and 6-inch OID

    C.  72-inch SID and 3-inch OID

    D.  60-inch SID and 4-inch OID

19. True/False: To best utilize the anode heel effect, the ~~thinner~~ *thicker* aspect of the anatomic part should be placed under the cathode aspect of the x-ray tube.

20. The best method to reduce distortion of the joints of the hand is to keep the fingers _____ to the IR.

   A. Perpendicular      C. 30° angle

   B. Parallel           D. Vertical

## SELF-TEST B: Image Quality in Digital Radiography

1. Each digital image is formed by two dimensional elements termed:

   A. Pixels       C. Voxels

   B. Matrix       D. Bytes

2. Highly complex mathematical formulas used in creating the digital image are termed:

   A. Digital reconstructions      C. Digital displays

   B. Bit processing matrices      D. Algorithms

3. True/False: Changes in kV have little impact on patient dose with digital imaging.

4. True/False: kV and mAs do not have the same direct effect on image quality with digital imaging as they do with IR-screen imaging.

5. True/False: A wide exposure latitude associated with digital imaging systems will lead to less repeat exposures.

6. The intensity of light that represents the individual pixels in the image on the monitor is termed:

   A. Latitude      C. Contrast

   B. Brightness    D. Resolution

7. The primary controlling factor of contrast in the digital image is:

   A. kV       C. Processing algorithms

   B. mAs      D. Use of a grid

8. The greater the bit depth of a digital system, the greater the:

   A. Contrast resolution      C. Resolution

   B. Brightness               D. Noise

9. Which one of the following terms describes the minimum pixel size that can be displayed by a monitor?

   A. Acquisition pixel size      C. Monitor latent pixel size

   B. Display pixel size          D. Reconstructed pixel size

10. True/False: OID and SID have little impact on resolution of the digital image

11. True/False: The current range of resolution for digital general radiographic imaging is between approximately 100 to 200 microns (2.5 to 5 line pairs per mm).

12. A numeric value that is representative of the exposure the image receptor received is termed:

   A. Algorithm      C. Spatial resolution

   B. Noise          D. Exposure index

13. Random disturbance that obscures or reduces clarity is the definition for:

   A. Noise       C. Digital fluctuation

   B. Signal      D. Signal variation

14. True/False: If an acceptable exposure index range is between 2.0 and 2.4, an exposure index number of 4.0 would indicate overexposure of the image.

15. True/False: A high SNR results when insufficient mAs is used in creating a digital image.

16. Which one of the following factors will result in an increase in noise?

    A. Excessive mAs          C. Excessive kV

    B. Scatter radiation       D. Decrease in pixel size

17. Changing or enhancing the electronic image in order to improve its diagnostic quality describes:

    A. Noise reduction         C. Post-processing

    B. Smoothing               D. Edge enhancement

18. _____ adjusts brightness values of adjacent pixels closer together.

    A. Smoothing               C. Brightness gain

    B. Edge enhancement        D. Magnification

19. Window width controls the _____ of the digital image.

    A. Edge enhancement        C. Smoothing

    B. Contrast                D. Brightness

20. True/False: Post-processing can correct for a low-SNR image.

## SELF-TEST C: Applications of Digital Technology

1. True/False: Computed radiography (CR) and digital radiography (DR) both require the use of an IR plate.

2. True/False: Direct digital fluoroscopy does not require the use of an image intensifier or video camera.

3. Patient information may be linked to the image on the CR imaging plate by:

    A. Light source            C. X-ray source

    B. Laser                   D. Bar code reader

4. The CR imaging plate is composed of:

    A. Calcium tungstate phosphor      C. Silicon phosphor

    B. Zinc cadmium sulfate phosphor   D. Photostimulable phosphor

5. The latent image recorded on the CR image plate is read by a:

    A. Laser                   C. Microwave source

    B. Bright light source     D. Ultraviolet light source

6. True/False: Close collimation must be avoided when acquiring an image on a CR IP.

7. A minimum of _____ % of the CR imaging plate must be exposed to produce an accurate

    exposure index.

    A. 10          C. 30

    B. 20          D. 50

8. True /False: Grids must not be used with a CR system.

9. True/False: Grids are often used for extremity exams when using DR.

10. True/False: The initial cost for digital mammography systems is much higher than conventional film-screen systems.

11. True/False: Close collimation should be avoided when using DR.

12. True/False: Direct digital chest systems permit post-processing of the image to change or modify image exposure.

13. True/False: PACS is a digital network that permits viewing and storage of both digital and film-screen produced images.

14. The acronym RIS stands for:

    A. Rapid imaging system        C. Radiology information system

    B. Radiology imaging system     D. Reusable imaging system

15. The acronym DICOM refers to:

    A. A set of standards to ensure communication        C. A digital image transmission system
       among digital imaging systems

    B. A new direct digital "flat plate" receptor system     D. A new-generation CR system

16. A digital transmission system for transferring radiographic images to remote locations by telephone, by satellite, or by the Web is:

    A. PACS        C. HIS

    B. Direct DR     D. Teleradiology

17. _____ is the unsharp edges of the projected image.

    A. Noise        C. Mottle

    B. Penumbra     D. Electronic noise

18. A series of "boxes" that give form to the image is the definition for:

    A. Pixels        C. Display matrices

    B. Voxels     D. Acquisition matrices

19. CAD is an acronym for:

    A. Computer-assisted detection

    B. Computed-aided delivery

    C. Central access detector

    D. Computed algorithmic diagnosis

20. DQE is an acronym for:

    A. Dose quotient equivalent

    B. Digital quality efficiency

    C. Diagnostic quality error

    D. Detection quantum efficiency

**SELF-TEST D:** Radiation Protection

1. What is the International System (SI) unit of radiation measurement for *absorbed dose?*

    A. Seivert
    C. Coulombs per kilogram of air

    B. Gray
    D. Roentgen

2. What traditional unit measures radiation exposure in air?

    A. Seivert
    C. Coulombs per kilogram of air

    B. Gray
    D. Roentgen

3. What is the annual whole body effective dose (ED) for a technologist?

    A. 10 rem, or 100 mSv
    C. 1 rem, or 10 mSv

    B. 0.1 rem, or 1 mSv
    D. 5 rem, or 50 mSv

4. What is the cumulative lifetime ED for a 25-year-old technologist?

    A. 250 mSv
    C. 500 mSv

    B. 25 mSv
    D. 2500 mSv

5. What is the annual ED limit for an individual younger than 18 years of age?

    A. 5 rem, or 50 mSv
    C. 1 rem, or 1 mSv

    B. 0.1 rem, or 1 mSv
    D. 10 rem, or 100 mSv

6. The federal set maximum limit on exposure rates for intensified fluoroscopy units is:

    A. 3 to 4 R/min
    C. 1 R/min

    B. 0.5 R/min
    D. 10 R/min

7. For most modern equipment, the average fluoroscopy rate is:

    A. 10 R/min
    C. 3 to 4 R/min

    B. 5 to 8 R/min
    D. 15 to 20 R/min

8. What is the primary purpose of x-ray tube filtration?

    A. Absorb lower energy x-rays

    B. Harden the x-ray beam

    C. Increase penetrability of the x-ray beam

    D. All of the above

9. Which of the following results in the highest ED for females (assuming no specific area shields are used)?

    A. Anteroposterior (AP) thoracic spine (7- × 17-inch collimation)

    B. AP thoracic spine (14- × 17-inch collimation)

    C. AP hip (10- × 12-inch collimation)

    D. AP chest (14- × 17-inch collimation)

10. The use of a gonadal shield reduces the gonadal dose by _____ if the gonads are within the primary x-ray field.

   A. 20% to 30%     C. 50% to 90%

   B. 40% to 50%     D. 100%

11. Which type of shield is ideal when the affected tissue is part of a sterile field?

   A. Contact shield     C. Shadow shield

   B. Lead masking     D. Gonadal shaped shield

12. True/False: Low kV and high mAs techniques greatly reduce patient dose compared with high kV and low mAs techniques.

13. True/False: The total ED for females on an AP chest projection is more than double that for a PA chest.

14. True/False: The use of a positive beam limiting (PBL) collimator is no longer required by the FDA for new x-ray equipment manufactured after 1994.

15. True/False: Collimators must be accurate within 2% of the selected SID.

16. Which one of the following is not one of the cardinal rules of radiation protection?

   A. Distance     C. Time

   B. Shielding     D. Collimation

17. Which one of the following changes will best reduce patient dose?

   A. Decrease kV and increase mAs     C. Increase kV and lower mAs

   B. Using a grid     D. Increase mAs and lower kV

18. Where is the safest place for the technologist to be during a fluoroscopic procedure?

   A. Head end of table

   B. Foot end of table

   C. On floor behind the fluoroscopic tower!

   D. Behind radiologist

19. Which one of the following protection devices must be employed during a fluoroscopic procedure?

   A. Bucky slot shield     C. Compensating filter

   B. Lead gloves     D. Restraining devices

20. The ED for a pregnant technologist per month is:

   A. 0.1 rem (1 mSv)     C. 500 mrem (5 mSv)

   B. 0.05 rem (0.5 mSv)     D. 5 rem (50 mSv)

## CHAPTER 3

# Chest

## CHAPTER OBJECTIVES

After you have successfully completed the activities in this chapter, you will be able to:

_____ 1. List the parts of the bony thorax.

_____ 2. List specific topographic positioning landmarks of the chest.

_____ 3. Identify the parts and function of specific structures of the respiratory system.

_____ 4. List the four organs of the mediastinum.

_____ 5. Identify specific structures of the chest on line drawings.

_____ 6. Identify specific structures of the chest on posteroanterior (PA) and lateral radiographs.

_____ 7. Identify specific structures of the chest on a computed tomography (CT), transverse image.

_____ 8. Identify the four types of body habitus and their impact on chest positioning.

_____ 9. Describe the methods to ensure proper degree of inspiration during chest radiography.

_____ 10. Describe the importance of using close collimation, gonadal shielding, and anatomic side markers during chest radiography.

_____ 11. Identify the correct exposure factors to be used during chest radiography.

_____ 12. Identify alterations in positioning routine and exposure factors specific to pediatric and geriatric patients.

_____ 13. List three reasons for taking chest radiographs with the patient in the erect position whenever possible.

_____ 14. Describe the three important positioning criteria that must be present on chest radiographs using erect PA and lateral positions.

_____ 15. Describe the advantages of the central ray placement method compared with the traditional method of centering for the PA and lateral chest positions.

_____ 16. Identify advantages and disadvantages in using CT, sonography, nuclear medicine, and magnetic resonance imaging (MRI) to demonstrate specific types of pathologic conditions in the chest.

_____ 17. Match various types of pathologic chest conditions to their correct definition.

_____ 18. For specific forms of pathologic chest conditions, indicate whether manual exposure factors need to be increased, decreased, or remain the same.

_____ 19. List the correct central ray placement, part position, and criteria for specific chest positions.

_____ 20. List the patient dose ranges for skin, midline, thyroid, and breast for specific projections of the chest and upper airway.

_____ 21. Given a hypothetical situation, identify the correct modifications of position, exposure factors, or both to improve the radiographic image.

_____ 22. Given a hypothetical situation, identify the correct position for a radiograph of specific pathologic conditions.

## Positioning and Radiographic Critique

_____  1. Using a peer, position the patient for posteroanterior (PA), anteroposterior (AP), and lateral chest projections.

_____  2. Using a chest phantom, use routine PA and lateral chest positions to produce satisfactory radiographs (if equipment is available).

_____  3. Determine whether rotation is present on PA and lateral chest radiographs.

_____  4. Critique and evaluate chest radiographs based on the four divisions of radiographic criteria: (1) structures shown, (2) position, (3) collimation and central ray, and (4) exposure criteria.

_____  5. Distinguish between acceptable and unacceptable chest radiographs based on exposure factors, motion, collimation, positioning, or other errors.

## Learning Exercises

Complete the following review exercises after reading the associated pages in Chapter 3 of the textbook as indicated by each exercise. Answers to each review exercise are given at the end of the review exercises and laboratory activities.

## Part I: Radiographic Anatomy   1-19

**REVIEW EXERCISE A:** Radiographic Anatomy of the Chest (see textbook pp. 76-83)

1. The bony thorax consists of (A) the single ___Sternum___ anteriorly, (B) two _p76_

   ___Clavicles___ , (C) two ___Scapulae___ , (D) twelve pairs of

   ___ribs___ , and (E) twelve ___thoracic vertebrae___ posteriorly.

2. The two important bony landmarks of the thorax that are used for locating the central ray on a posteroanterior (PA)

   and anteroposterior (AP) chest projection are the (A) ___Vertebra prominens___ and

   (B) ___jugular notch___ , respectively.

3. The four divisions of the respiratory system are:

   A. ___pharynx___              C. ___bronchi___

   B. ___trachea___              D. ___lungs___

4. Identify correct anatomic terms for the following structures: _p76, 77_

   A. Adam's apple ___Thyroid cartilage___     D. Shoulder blade ___Scapulae___

   B. Voice box ___larynx___                  E. Collar bone ___Clavicles___

   C. Breastbone ___Sternum___

5. List the three divisions of the structure located proximally to the larynx that serve as a common passageway for both food and air:

   A. ___nasopharynx___          C. ___laryngopharynx___

   B. ___oropharynx___

6.  What is the name of the structure that acts as a lid over the larynx to prevent foreign objects such as food particles from entering the respiratory system? __epiglottis__ _p77_

7.  The trachea is located __anteriorly__ (**anteriorly** or **posteriorly**) to the esophagus.

8.  The __hyoid__ bone is seen in the anterior portion of the neck and is found just below the tongue or floor of the mouth.

9.  If a person accidentally inhales a food particle, which bronchus is it most likely to enter, and why?

    A.  The __right primary__ bronchus

    B.  Why? __wider, more verticle Therefore less abrupt angle angle from verticle__

10. A.  What is the name of the prominence, or ridge, seen when looking down into the bronchus where it divides into the right and left bronchi? __Carina (kah-ri'nah)__

    B.  This prominence, or ridge, is approximately at the level of the __T5__ vertebra.

11. What is the term for the small air sacs located at the distal ends of the bronchioles, in which oxygen and carbon dioxide are exchanged in the blood? __alveoli__

12. A.  The delicate, double-walled sac or membrane containing the lungs is called the __pleura__.

    B.  The outer layer of this membrane adhering to the inner surface of the chest wall and diaphragm is the __parietal pleura__.

    C.  The inner layer adhering to the surface of the lungs is the __pulmonary__ or __visceral pleura__.

    D.  The potential space between these two layers (identified in *B* and *C*) is called the __pleura cavity__.

    E.  Air or gas that enters the space identified in *D* results in a condition called __pneumothorax__.

13. Fill in the correct terms for the following portions of the lungs:

    A.  Lower, concave portion: __Inferior Base__ _p82_

    B.  Central area in which bronchi and blood vessels enter the lungs: __hilum__

    C.  Upper, rounded portion above the level of the clavicles: __apex__

    D.  Extreme, outermost lower corner of the lungs: __Costophrenic angle__

14. Explain why the right lung is smaller than the left lung and the right hemidiaphragm is positioned higher than the left hemidiaphragm: __t liver on The Rt side__

15. List the four important structures located in the mediastinum:

    A.  __Thymus gland__                      C.  __trachea__

    B.  __heart, great vessels__              D.  __esophagus__

16.   Identify the following structures in Fig. 3-1:

A.   _Thymus_____ gland

B.   _Aortic arch_____

C.   _heart_____

D.   _Inferior vena cava_____

E.   _Superior vena cava_____

F.   _Thyroid_____ gland

G.   _Trachea_____

H.   _esophagus_____

**Fig. 3-1.** Structures within the mediastinum.

17.   The heart is enclosed in a double-walled membrane called the _pericardium_____ .

18.   The three parts of the aorta are the _accending_ , _arch_____ , and _decending_ .

19.   Identify the following labeled structures as seen on PA and lateral chest radiographs in Figs. 3-2 and 3-3:

A.   _apex of left lung_____

B.   _Trachea_____

C.   _carina_____

D.   _heart_____

E.   _left costophrenic angle_____

F.   _right hemidiaphragm / base_____

G.   _hilum_____

H.   _apex_____

I.   _hilum_____

J.   _Heart_____

K.   _right + left hemidiaphragm_____

L.   _Rt + Lt costophrenic angle_____

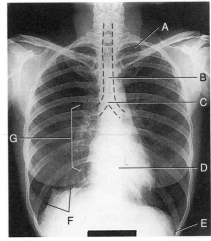

**Fig. 3-2.** Posteroanterior (PA) chest radiograph.

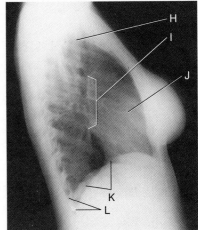

**Fig. 3-3.** Lateral chest radiograph.

**3**

20. Identify the labeled parts on this computed tomography (CT) image of a transverse section of the thorax at the level of T5, the fifth thoracic vertebra, which is also the level of the carina. (HINT: *B, G,* and *H* are major blood vessels.)

A. _____

B. _____

C. _____

D. _____

E. _____

F. _____

G. _____

H. _____

I. _____

**Fig. 3-4.** Computed tomography (CT) transverse section of the thorax at the level of T5.

## Part II: Radiographic Positioning

1-34

**REVIEW EXERCISE B:** Technical Considerations (see textbook pp. 84-91)

START  1. Which type of body habitus is associated with a broad and deep thorax? ___hypersthenic___

2. Which one of the following types of body habitus may cause the costophrenic angles to be cut off if careful vertical collimation is not used?

   A. Hypersthenic          C. Sthenic

   B. Hyposthenic          (D.) Hyposthenic and asthenic

3. What is the minimum number of ribs that should be demonstrated above the diaphragm on a PA radiograph of an

   average adult chest with full inspiration? ___10___

4. Which of the following objects should be removed (or moved) before chest radiography? (Choose all that apply.)

   (A.) Necklace                    D. Dentures          (F.) Hair fasteners

   (B.) Bra                         E. Pants             (G.) Oxygen lines

   (C.) Religious medallion around neck

5. True/False: Chest radiography is the most commonly repeated radiographic procedure because of poor positioning or exposure factor selection errors.

6. True/False: Generally, you do not need to use radiographic grids for adult patients for PA or lateral chest radiographs.

7. Chest radiography for the adult patient usually employs a kilovoltage peak of ___110___ to ___125___ kV.

8. Optimal technical factor selection ensures proper penetration of the:

   A. Heart                    D. Hilar region

   B. Great vessels           (E.) All of the above

   C. Lung regions

**3**

9.  Describe the way optimum density of the lungs and mediastinal structures can be determined on a PA chest

    radiograph. _faint outlines of the mid-3 upper vertebrae posterior ribs_
    _through the heart_

10. True/False: Because the heart is always located in the left thorax, the use of anatomic side markers on a PA chest projection may not be necessary.

*p 85* 11. Which one of the following devices should be used for the PA and lateral chest positions for a young pediatric patient?

    A.  Upright chest device       C.  Pigg-O-Stat

    B.  Supine table Bucky         D.  Plexiglas restraint board

*p 85* 12. Which one of the following sets of exposure factors is recommended for a chest examination of a young pediatric patient?

    A.  60 to 70 kV, short exposure time        C.  100 to 120 kV, short exposure time

    B.  90 to 100 kV, medium exposure time      D.  120 to 150 kV, long exposure time

*p 86* 13. True/False: Because they have shallower (superior-inferior dimension) lung fields, the central ray is often centered higher for geriatric patients.

14. To ensure better lung inspiration during chest radiography, exposure should be made during the _second full_ inspiration.

15. List four possible pathologic conditions that would suggest the need for both inspiration and expiration PA chest radiographs (five were given in the textbook):

    A.  _Small pneumo Thorax_                   C.  _present of foreign bodies_

    B.  _fixation or lack of normal movement_   D.  _to distinguish between opacity in_
        _of The diaphragm_                          _The ribs or in The lungs_

16. List and explain briefly the three reasons that chest radiographs should be taken with the patient in the erect position (when the patient's condition permits):

    A.  _Diaphragm moves down farTher_   C.  _Prevents Engorgment ; Hyperemia_

    B.  _Visualizes Possible Air : fluid levels in chest_   _of Pulmonary Vessels_

17. Explain the primary purpose and benefit of performing chest radiography using a 72-inch source image receptor

    distance (SID). _Magnifies The heart showdow less because The x-ray beam has_
    _less divergence,_

18. Why do the lungs tend to expand more with the patient in an erect position than in a supine position?

    _The diaphragm moves down farTher because abdominal organs drop_

*pg 79* 19. Respiratory distress syndrome (RDS) in adults, also known as hyaline membrane disease (HMD) in infants, is caused by:

    A.  Aspiration of foreign substances      C.  Alveoli collapse due to a lack of internal tension

    B.  Bacterial infection                   D.  Viral infection

20. Which one of the following anatomic structures is examined to determine rotation on a PA chest radiograph?

    A.  Appearance of ribs        C.  Symmetric appearance of sternoclavicular joints

    B.  Shape of heart            D.  Symmetric appearance of costophrenic angles

21. Which positioning tip will help you prevent the patient's chin from being superimposed over the upper airway and apices of the lungs for a PA chest radiograph? *Extend chin up*

*Sufficent extension of the patients neck will ensure that the chin and neck are not covering up or superimposing the upper lung region*

22. For patients with the following clinical histories, which lateral position would you perform—**right or left?**

    A. Patient with severe pains in left side of chest _____*Left*_____

    B. Patient with no chest pain but recent history of pneumonia in right lung _____*Right*_____

    C. Patient with no chest pain or history of heart trouble _____*left*_____

23. Why is it important to raise the patient's arms above the head for lateral chest projections?

    *To prevent superimposition on the upper portion of the chest*            *pg 88*

    _____

24. The traditional central ray centering technique for the chest is to place the top of the image receptor (cassette) *1½–2* inches (__*5*__ cm) above the shoulders. *p89*

25. A recommended central ray centering technique for a PA chest projection requires the technologist to palpate the _____*Vertebra prominens*_____ and measure down from that bony landmark __*8*__ inches (_*20*_ cm) for a male and __*7*__ inches (_*18*_ cm) for a female patient. *p89*

26. A. Should the 14- × 17-inch (35- × 43-cm) image receptor be aligned **lengthwise** or **crosswise** for a PA chest projection of a hypersthenic patient? _____*Crosswise*_____

    B. For a hyposthenic patient? _____*lengthwise*_____   *p90*

27. True/False: With most digital chest units, the question of IR placement into either vertical or crosswise positions is eliminated because of the larger IR.   *p90*

28. Which one of the following bony landmarks is palpated for centering of the AP chest position?

    A. Vertebra prominens        C. Thyroid cartilage   *p90*

    B. Jugular notch             D. Sternal angle

29. True/False: In general, for an average patient more collimation should be visible on the lower margin of the chest image than on the top for a PA or lateral chest projection.   *Should be equal*

30. True/False: For most patients, the central ray level for a PA chest projection is near the inferior angle of the scapula.

31. True/False: The height, or vertical dimension, of the average-to-large person's chest is greater than the width, or horizontal dimension.   *p90*

32. True/False: CT has replaced bronchography as the preferred imaging modality to study the bronchial tree. *p91*

33. True/False: Ultrasound is not an effective modality to detect pleural effusion. *p91*

34. True/False: Echocardiography and electrocardiography are basically the same procedure.

35.  Match each of the following descriptions of pathologic indicators to its correct term.

| | | | |
|---|---|---|---|
| _____ 1. | One of the most common inherited diseases | A. | Atelectasis |
| _____ 2. | Condition most frequently associated with congestive heart failure | B. | Bronchiectasis |
| _____ 3. | Coughing up blood | C. | Bronchitis |
| _____ 4. | Accumulation of air in pleural cavity | D. | Chronic obstructive pulmonary disease (COPD) |
| _____ 5. | Accumulation of pus in pleural cavity | | |
| _____ 6. | A form of pneumoconiosis | E. | Hemoptysis |
| _____ 7. | A contagious disease caused by an airborne bacterium | F. | Cystic fibrosis |
| _____ 8. | Irreversible dilation of bronchioles | G. | Empyema |
| _____ 9. | Most common form is emphysema | H. | Pleurisy |
| _____ 10. | Acute or chronic irritation of bronchi | I. | Pneumothorax |
| _____ 11. | Collapse of all or portion of lung | J. | Pulmonary edema |
| _____ 12. | Inflammation of pleura | K. | Tuberculosis |
| | | L. | Silicosis |

36.  For the following types of pathologic conditions, indicate whether manual exposure factors would be increased (+), decreased (−), or generally remain the same (0) as compared with standard chest exposure factors:

_____ Left lung atelectasis

_____ Lung neoplasm

_____ Severe pulmonary edema

_____ Respiratory distress syndrome (RDS) or adult respiratory distress syndrome (ARDS), known as hyaline membrane disease (HMD) in infants

_____ Secondary tuberculosis

_____ Advanced emphysema

_____ Large pneumothorax

_____ Pulmonary emboli

_____ Childhood tuberculosis

_____ Advanced asbestosis

**REVIEW EXERCISE C:** Positioning of the Chest (see textbook pp. 96-106)   1-8

1.  Why is a PA chest preferred to an AP projection?  Reduces magnification of the heart shadow p86

2.  The CR is placed at the level of the _____T7_____ vertebra for a PA chest projection. p89

3.  The shoulders need to be rolled forward for the PA projection to allow the ___scapulae___ to move laterally and to be clear of the lung fields.   p96

4.  When the automatic exposure control system (AEC) is being used for the PA projection, which ionization chambers should be activated?

    A.  Left chamber          C.  Right chamber

    B.  Center chamber       (D.) Left and right chambers  *p 96*

5.  What is the midline dose range for a PA projection of the chest for an average-size female?

    A.  10 to 100 mrad          (C.) Less than 10 mrad   *p 96*

    B.  Greater than 100 mrad       D.  0.5 to 1 rad

6.  (True)/False: The average breast dose and thyroid dose for a PA chest projection are approximately the same.

7.  The average female breast dose on an AP chest projection is approximately _____ times that for a PA chest dose.

    A.  1.5     (B.) 4     C.  10     D.  30   *p 96 3 100*

8.  How much separation of the posterior ribs on a lateral chest projection indicates excessive rotation from a true

    lateral position?  ___ *¼ - ½ inches* ___  (NOTE: Less separation than this is caused by the divergent x-rays.) *p 98*

9.  To prevent the clavicles from obscuring the apices on an AP projection of the chest, the central ray should be

    angled (A) _____ ((caudad) or **cephalad**) so that it is perpendicular to the

    (B) _*long axis of the sternum*_  *p 100*

*STOP*  10.  What is the name of the condition characterized by fluid entering the pleural cavity? _*Pleural Effusion*_

11.  Which specific position would be used if a patient were unable to stand but the physician suspected the patient had

     fluid in the left lung? _*Pleural effusion*_

12.  What is the name of the condition characterized by free air entering the pleural cavity? _____

13.  Which specific position would be used if the patient were unable to stand but the physician suspected the patient

     had free air in the left pleural cavity? _____

14.  What circumstances or clinical indications suggest that an apical lordotic projection should be ordered?

     _____

15.  What position/projection would be used for a patient who is too ill or weak to stand for an apical lordotic projection?

     _____

16.  A.  Which anterior oblique position would best demonstrate the left lung—right anterior oblique (**RAO**) or left

         anterior oblique (**LAO**)? _____

     B.  Which posterior oblique position would best demonstrate the left lung—**RPO** or **LPO**?

         _____

17.  For certain studies of the heart, the _____ (**right** or **left**) anterior oblique requires a rotation of _____ °.

18.  Which AEC ionization chamber(s) should be activated for an LAO chest projection? _____

**3**

19. Where is the central ray placed for a lateral projection of the upper airway? _____

20. Which one of the following tissues receives the greatest dose during an AP projection of the upper airway?

    A. Thyroid  C. Midline structures

    B. Breast  D. Gonads

## REVIEW EXERCISE D: Problem Solving for Technical and Positioning Errors (see textbook pp. 85-89) 1-15

The following radiographic problems involve technical and positioning errors that lead to substandard images. Other questions involve situations pertaining to various conditions and pathologic findings. As you analyze these problems and situations, use your textbook to help you find solutions to these questions.

1. A radiograph of a PA view of the chest reveals that the sternoclavicular (SC) joints are not the same distance from the spine. The right SC joint is closer to the midline than is the left SC joint. What is the positioning error?

   _____ RoTaTion RAO  Lt side out _____

2. A radiograph of a PA projection of the chest shows only seven posterior ribs above the diaphragm. What caused this problem, and how could it be prevented on the repeat exposures? _Little or No Inspiration_

   _____ Little or No Inspiration _____

3. A radiograph of a PA and left lateral view of the chest reveals that the mediastinum of the chest is underpenetrated. The technologist used the following factors for the radiograph: a 72-inch SID, an upright Bucky, a full-inspiration exposure, 75 kV and 600 mA, and a $\frac{1}{60}$-second exposure time.

   A. Which one of these factors is the most likely cause of the problem? Briefly explain. _____

   _____ KVp because Radiograph requires more penTraTion (110 - 125 KVp) _____

   B. How can the technologist improve the image when making the repeat exposure? _Increase KVp, reduce mAs_

4. A radiograph of a PA projection of the chest reveals that the top of the apices are cut off and a wide collimation border can be seen below the diaphragm. In what way can this be corrected during the repeat radiograph?

   _____ CR is NoT cxtredi correctly, Move higher to T7 _____

5. **Situation:** A patient with a clinical history of advanced emphysema comes to the radiology department for a chest x-ray. AEC will not be used. How should the technologist alter the manual exposure settings for this patient?

   A. Do not alter them. Use the standard exposure factors.

   B. Decrease the kV moderately (– –).

   C. Increase the kV slightly (+).

   D. Increase the kV moderately (+ +).

6. **Situation:** A patient with severe pleural effusion comes to the radiology department for a chest x-ray. AEC will not be used. How should the technologist alter the manual exposure settings for this patient?

   A. Do not alter them. Use the standard exposure factors.

   B. Decrease the kV moderately (– –).

   C. Increase the kV slightly (+).

   D. Increase the kV moderately (+ +).

7.  **Situation:** A patient comes to the radiology department for a presurgical chest examination. The clinical history indicates a possible situs inversus of the thorax (transposition of structures within the thorax). Which positioning step or action must be taken to perform a successful chest examination? <u>Rt side closes. To IR</u>

8.  A radiograph of a lateral projection of the chest reveals that the posterior ribs and costophrenic angles are separated more than ½ inch, or 1 cm, indicating excessive rotation. Describe a possible method of determining the direction *see Ans* of rotation: <u>Look for gastric air bubble in the Stomach or by inferior border of the heart Shadow both associated w/ Left hemisphere</u>

9.  **Situation:** A patient enters the emergency room with a possible hemothorax in the right lung caused by a motor vehicle accident (MVA). The patient is unable to stand or sit erect. Which specific position would best diagnose this condition, and why? <u>Lateral decub w/affected side down</u>      *p94*
    <u>                    PA projection                    </u>

10. **Situation:** A young child enters the emergency room with a foreign body in one of the bronchi of the lung. The foreign body, a peanut, cannot be seen on the PA and lateral projections of the chest projection.

    A.  Which additional projection(s) could the technologist perform to locate the foreign body?
    <u>Lat upper airway   Inspiration, expiration PA projection</u>

    B.  Which primary bronchi would most likely contain the peanut? <u>RT side More Vertical & larger Than Lt</u>

11. **Situation:** A routine chest study indicates a possible mass beneath a patient's right clavicle. The PA and lateral projections are inconclusive. Which additional projection(s) could the technologist take to diagnose this small tumor?
    <u>Due a AP which will make The object larger</u>
        AP apical lordotic

12. **Situation:** A patient has a possible small pneumothorax. Routine chest projections (PA and lateral) fail to reveal the pneumothorax conclusively. Which additional projections could be taken to rule out this condition?
    ② <u>Lat decub affected side up/PA</u> <sup>or AP</sup> <u>Inspiration/expiration</u> ①

13. **Situation:** A patient with a history of pleurisy comes to the radiology department. Which one of the following positioning routines should be used?

    A.  Soft tissue lateral of the upper airway      Ⓒ  Erect PA and lateral

    B.  Right and left lateral decubitus             D.  CT scan of the chest

14. **Situation:** A patient with a possible neoplasm in the right lung apex comes to the radiology department for a chest examination. The PA and lateral projections do not clearly demonstrate the neoplasm because of superimposition of the clavicle over the apex. The patient is unable to stand or sit erect. Which additional projection can be taken to clearly demonstrate the neoplasm and eliminate the superimposition of the clavicle and the left lung apex?
    <u>AP simiaxial lordotic proj: CR 15-20° Cephalad to project Clavicles</u>
        above apices & clearly show tumor

15. **Situation:** PA and left lateral projections demonstrate a suspicious region in the left lung. The radiologist orders an oblique that will best demonstrate or "elongate" the left lung. Which specific oblique projections will best elongate the left lung? (More than one oblique projection will accomplish this goal)
    *STOP*
    <u>        RAO or LPO        </u>

**REVIEW EXERCISE E:** Critique Radiographs of the Chest (see textbook p. 107)

The following questions relate to the radiographs found at the end of Chapter 3 in the textbook. Evaluate these radiographs for the radiographic criteria categories (*1* through *5*) that follow. Describe the corrections needed to improve the overall image. The major, or "repeatable," errors are specific errors that indicate the need for a repeat exposure, regardless of the nature of the other errors.

NOTE: The critique exercises and detection of positioning errors are challenging, but studying the radiographs and answering the questions will help prepare you for your instructor's classroom and/or lab presentation, which will include slides of the same radiographs alongside the improved images. These learning experiences and the laboratory positioning exercises that follow also include critiques of additional radiographs provided by your instructor to prepare you for evaluating and critiquing the radiographs you take to help you avoid making mistakes as you begin your clinical work.

A.  **PA chest, 43-year-old man (Fig. C3-91)**
    Description of possible error

    1.  Structures shown: _____

    2.  Part positioning: _____

    3.  Collimation and central ray: _____

    4.  Exposure criteria: _____

    5.  Markers: _____

    Repeatable error(s): _____

B.  **PA chest, 74-year-old man (Fig. C3-92)**
    Description of possible error

    1.  Structures shown: _____

    2.  Part positioning: _____

    3.  Collimation and central ray: _____

    4.  Exposure criteria: _____

    5.  Markers: _____

    Repeatable error(s): _____

C.  **Lateral chest, female (Fig. C3-93)**
    Description of possible error

    1.  Structures shown: _____

    2.  Part positioning: _____

    3.  Collimation and central ray: _____

    4.  Exposure criteria: _____

    5.  Markers: _____

    Repeatable error(s): _____

D.  **PA chest, 73-year-old female (Fig. C3-94)**
    Description of possible error

    1.  Structures shown: _____

    2.  Part positioning: _____

    3.  Collimation and central ray: _____

    4.  Exposure criteria: _____

    5.  Markers: _____

    Repeatable error(s): _____

E.  **Lateral chest, female in wheelchair (Fig. C3-95)**
    Description of possible error

    1.  Structures shown: _____

    2.  Part positioning: _____

    3.  Collimation and central ray: _____

    4.  Exposure criteria: _____

    5.  Markers: _____

    Repeatable error(s): _____

## Part III: Laboratory Activities (see textbook pp. 96-106)

You must gain experience in chest positioning before performing the following exams on actual patients. You can get experience in positioning and radiographic evaluation of these projections by performing exercises using radiographic phantoms and practicing on other students (although not taking actual exposures).

The following suggested activities assume that your teaching institution has an energized lab and radiographic phantoms. If not, perform only Laboratory Exercise B, the physical positioning activities. (Check off each step and projection as you complete it.)

### LABORATORY EXERCISE A: Energized Laboratory

1.  Using the chest radiographic phantom, produce radiographs using:

    _____ PA and AP views        _____ Lateral view

2.  Evaluate the radiographs you produced above, additional radiographs provided by your instructor, or both for the following criteria:

    _____ Rotation                      _____ Markers

    _____ Collimation                   _____ Proper exposure factors

    _____ Part and central ray centering    _____ Motion

## LABORATORY EXERCISE B: Physical Positioning

1. On another person, simulate taking all of the following basic and special projections of the chest. Follow the suggested positioning steps and sequence as listed below and as described in Chapter 1 of your textbook:

_____ PA chest          _____ AP supine or semisupine

_____ Anterior and posterior obliques          _____ Lateral decubitus

_____ Lateral chest          _____ AP lordotic

_____ AP and lateral upper airway

_Step 1. General Patient Positioning_

_____ Select the size and number of cassettes needed.

_____ Prepare the radiographic room. Check that tube is centered to the center of the IR holder (or the centerline of the table for Bucky exams).

_____ Correctly identify the patient and bring the patient into the room.

_____ Explain to the patient what you will be doing.

_____ Assist the patient to the proper place and position for the first radiograph.

_Step 2. Measuring Part Thickness_

_____ Measure the body part being radiographed and set correct exposure factors (technique). (If using an AEC system, select the correct chamber cells on the control panel.)

_Step 3. Part Positioning_

_____ Align and center the body part to the central ray or vice versa for chest positioning with the chest board. (For Bucky exams on a table, move the patient and table top together as needed [with floating-type table top]). (NOTE: In cases in which the correct central ray position is of primary importance, the central ray icon is included in the textbook on the appropriate positioning page.)

_Step 4. Image Receptor (IR) Centering_

_____ After the part has been centered to the central ray, the IR (cassette) is also centered to the central ray. (NOTE: This step can be omitted on most chest units where the x-ray tube and IR unit are attached and move together.)

_Additional Steps or Actions_

_____ 1. Collimate accurately to include only the area of interest.

_____ 2. Place the correct marker within the exposure field (so that you do not superimpose pertinent anatomic structures).

_____ 3. Restrain or provide support for the body part to prevent motion.

_____ 4. Use contact lead shielding as needed (e.g., gonadal, breast, thyroid).

_____ 5. Give clear breathing instructions and make the exposure while watching patient through window.

# Answers to Review Exercises

## Review Exercise A: Radiographic Anatomy of the Chest

1. A. Sternum
   B. Clavicles
   C. Scapulae
   D. Ribs
   E. Thoracic vertebrae
2. A. Vertebra prominens
   B. Jugular notch
3. A. Pharynx
   B. Trachea
   C. Bronchi
   D. Lungs
4. A. Thyroid cartilage
   B. Larynx
   C. Sternum
   D. Scapula
   E. Clavicle
5. A. Nasopharynx
   B. Oropharynx
   C. Laryngopharynx
6. Epiglottis
7. Anteriorly
8. Hyoid
9. A. Right
   B. It is larger in diameter and more vertical.
10. A. Carina
    B. T5
11. Alveoli
12. A. Pleura
    B. Parietal pleura
    C. Pulmonary or visceral pleura
    D. Pleural cavity
    E. Pneumothorax
13. A. Base
    B. Hilum (hilus)
    C. Apex (apices)
    D. Costophrenic angle
14. Presence of liver on right
15. A. Thymus gland
    B. Heart and great vessels
    C. Trachea
    D. Esophagus
16. A. Thymus
    B. Arch of aorta
    C. Heart
    D. Inferior vena cava
    E. Superior vena cava
    F. Thyroid
    G. Trachea
    H. Esophagus
17. Pericardial sac or pericardium
18. Ascending, arch, and descending aorta
19. A. Apex of left lung
    B. Trachea
    C. Carina
    D. Heart

E. Left costophrenic angle
F. Right hemidiaphragm (or base)
G. Hilum
H. Apex of lungs
I. Hilum
J. Heart
K. Right and left hemidiaphragm
L. Right and left costophrenic angles
20. A. Left main stem bronchus
    B. Descending aorta
    C. T5 (fifth thoracic vertebra)
    D. Esophagus
    E. Region of carina
    F. Right main stem bronchus
    G. Superior vena cava
    H. Ascending aorta
    I. Sternum

## Review Exercise B: Technical Considerations

1. Hypersthenic
2. D. Hyposthenic and asthenic
3. 10 ribs
4. A. Necklace
   B. Bra
   C. Religious medallion around neck
   F. Hair fasteners
   G. Oxygen lines
5. True
6. False
7. 110 to 125 kV
8. E. All of the above
9. Should be able to see faint outlines of at least middle and upper vertebrae and ribs through heart and other mediastinal structures
10. False (Situs inversus may be present.)
11. C. Pigg-O-Stat
12. A. 60 to 70 kV, short exposure time
13. True
14. Second
15. 1. Small pneumothorax
    2. Fixation or lack of normal diaphragm movement
    3. Presence of a foreign body
    4. Distinguishing between opacity in rib or lung.
    5. Possible atelectasis (incomplete expansion of the lungs)
16. A. To allow diaphragm to move down farther
    B. To show possible air and fluid levels in the chest
    C. To prevent engorgement and hyperemia of the pulmonary vessels
17. Reduces distortion and magnification of the heart and other chest structures

18. Erect position causes abdominal organs to drop, allowing the diaphragm to move farther down and the lungs to more fully aerate
19. C. Alveoli collapse due to a lack of internal tension
20. C. Symmetric appearance of sternoclavicular joints
21. Extend the chin upward
22. A. Left
    B. Right
    C. Left
23. Prevents upper arm soft tissue from being superimposed over upper chest fields
24. 1½ to 2 inches (5 cm)
25. Vertebra prominens, 8 inches (20 cm) for male, 7 inches (18 cm) for female
26. A. Crosswise
    B. Lengthwise
27. True
28. B. Jugular notch
29. False (should be equal)
30. True
31. False (greater width)
32. True
33. False
34. False
35. 1. F
    2. J
    3. E
    4. I
    5. G
    6. L
    7. K
    8. B
    9. D
    10. C
    11. A
    12. H
36. + Atelectasis
    + Lung cancer
    + Pulmonary edema
    + RDS or ARDS (HMD in infants)
    + Secondary tuberculosis
    − Emphysema
    − Pneumothorax
    0 Pulmonary emboli
    0 Childhood tuberculosis
    + Asbestosis

## Review Exercise C: Positioning of the Chest

1. Places the heart closer to the image receptor to reduce magnification of the heart
2. T7
3. Scapulae

4. D. Left and right chambers
5. C. Less than 10 mrad
6. True (Both are about 1 mrad.)
7. B. 4
8. Greater than 1 cm (½ to ¾ inch)
9. A. Caudad (±5°)
   B. Sternum
10. Pleural effusion
11. Left lateral decubitus
12. Pneumothorax
13. Right lateral decubitus (affected side up)
14. Rule out calcifications or masses beneath the clavicles
15. AP semiaxial projection, central ray 15° to 20° cephalad
16. A. RAO
    B. LPO
17. Left, 60°
18. Right upper chamber
19. Level of C6-C7, midway between thyroid cartilage and jugular notch
20. A. Thyroid

## Review Exercise D: Problem Solving for Technical and Positioning Errors

1. Rotation. The patient is rotated into a slight RAO position.
2. The lungs are underinflated. Explain to the patient the need for a deep inspiration, and take the exposure on the second deep inspiration.
3. A. The 75 kV is too low. The ideal kV range is 100 to 130.
   B. Increase the kV and reduce the mAs for the repeat exposure.
4. Center the central ray higher (to the level of T7, which will be found 7 to 8 inches below the vertebra prominens). Make sure the image receptor is centered to the central ray and the top collimation light border is at the vertebra prominens.
5. B. Decrease the kV moderately (– –).
6. C. Increase the kV slightly (+).
7. Ensure placement of the correct right or left anatomic side marker on the image receptor, because the heart and other thoracic structures may be transposed from right to left (see Chapter 1).
8. Determine which hemidiaphragm (right or left) is more posterior or more anterior. The left hemidiaphragm can frequently be identi-

fied by visualization of the gastric air bubble or the inferior heart shadow, both of which are associated with the left hemidiaphragm.
9. Right lateral decubitus; in a patient with hemothorax (fluid), the side of interest should be down.
10. A. Inspiration and expiration PA projections.
    B. The right bronchus is most likely to contain the foreign body because it is more vertical and larger in diameter.
11. AP apical lordotic.
12. Inspiration and expiration PA projections and/or a lateral decubitus AP chest with affected side up.
13. C. Erect PA and lateral
14. AP semiaxial lordotic projection; CR is angled 15 to 20 degrees cephalad to project the clavicles above the apices and clearly demonstrate the possible tumor.
15. Both the LPO and RAO oblique positions will best demonstrate or elongate the left lung.

## Review Exercise E: Critique Radiographs of the Chest (see textbook, p. 107)

A. PA chest (Fig. C3-91)
   1. Left costophrenic angle cut off (Cassette should have been placed crosswise.)
   2. Slight rotation into an RAO position (hips and lower thorax most rotated, spine shifted to right)
   3. Vertical centering correct; central ray centered to T7; tighter collimation desirable (to prevent excessive exposure to both neck and abdominal region)
   4. Acceptable
   5. Anatomic side marker present
   Repeatable error(s): 1
B. PA chest (Fig. C3-92)
   1. Additional left anatomic side marker obscuring portion of right lung
   2. Slight rotation into an LAO position
   3. Central ray centered slightly high (T6-T7 interspace); no evident collimation
   4. Acceptable
   5. Anatomic side marker present, but which one is truly correct?

This patient may have situs inversus.
Repeatable error(s): 1 and 5
C. Lateral chest (Fig. C3-93)
   1. All pertinent anatomy demonstrated (costophrenic angle nearly cut off)
   2. Excessive rotation (±1 inch or 2.5 cm); right side anterior (right diaphragm discernible because of association of gastric bubble with the higher [right] diaphragm)
   3. Central ray centered too high, (causing excessive exposure of neck and face); no upper collimation, as a result of poor central ray centering
   4. Acceptable
   5. No evident left side marker (may be present but is not visible here)
   Repeatable error(s): 2 and 5 (if not visible on radiograph)
D. PA chest (Fig. C3-94)
   1. Bra artifact in lung field; bra also creating increased breast shadow in lung field
   2. Some rotation into RAO position (right sternoclavicular joint closer to spine, and spine shifted to right, indicating entire thorax somewhat rotated)
   3. Central ray centered too high; collimation not evident on top because of high central ray centering; side collimation excellent
   4. Acceptable
   5. Left side marker evident
   Repeatable error(s): 1
E. Lateral chest (Fig. C3-95)
   1. All pertinent anatomy demonstrated
   2. Marginal rotation present; shoulders more rotated than hips (¾ inch or 2 cm measured along the posterior ribs); may or may not have to be repeated for this problem, depending on departmental protocol and other factors
   3. Central ray centering good (just slightly high); collimation excellent
   4. Motion present along the diaphragm and lower lung field (more visible on actual radiograph); shorter exposure time or better patient instruction needed
   5. Left side marker not visible
   Repeatable error(s): 2, 3, and 5

# SELF-TEST

This self-test should be taken only after completing all of the readings, review exercises, and laboratory activities for a particular section. The purpose of this test is not only to provide a good learning exercise but also to serve as a strong indicator of what your final unit evaluation exam will cover. It is strongly suggested that if you do not get at least a 90% to 95% grade on each self-test, you review those areas in which you missed questions before going to your instructor for the final unit evaluation exam. There are 50 questions or blanks—each is worth 2 points.

1. Match each of the following structures with its correct anatomic term:

   _____ 1. Breastbone            A. Clavicle

   _____ 2. Adam's apple          B. Larynx

   _____ 3. Shoulder blade        C. Thyroid cartilage

   _____ 4. Voice box             D. Scapula

   _____ 5. Collar bone           E. Sternum

2. The correct term for the seventh cervical vertebrae is:
   A. Xiphoid process       C. Axis
   B. Jugular notch         D. Vertebra prominens

3. A notch, or depression, located on the superior portion of the sternum is called the:
   A. Sternal notch         C. Jugular notch
   B. Xiphoid notch         D. Sternal angle

4. The trachea bifurcates and forms the:
   A. Right and left bronchi    C. Costophrenic angles
   B. Right and left hilum      D. Pulmonary arteries

5. A specific prominence, or ridge, found at the point where the internal distal trachea divides into the right and left bronchi is called the:
   A. Hilum        C. Epiglottis
   B. Carina       D. Alveoli

6. The area of each lung where the bronchi and blood vessels enter and leave is called the:
   A. Carina       C. Base
   B. Apex         D. Hilum

7. The structures within the lung where oxygen and carbon dioxide gas exchange occurs are called:
   A. Carina       C. Hilum
   B. Alveoli      D. Bronchi

8. Which of the following is *not* an aspect of the pleura?
   A. Parietal pleura       C. Pleural cavity
   B. Hilar pleura          D. Pulmonary pleura

3

9.  The condition in which blood fills the potential space between the layers of pleura is called:

    A.  Pneumothorax          C.  Atelectasis

    B.  Hemothorax            D.  Empyema

10. The extreme, outermost lower corner of each lung is called the:

    A.  Costophrenic angle     C.  Base

    B.  Apex                   D.  Hilar region

11. Which one of the following structures is *not* found in the mediastinum?

    A.  Thymus gland           C.  Epiglottis

    B.  Heart and great vessels     D.  Trachea

12. A narrow thorax that is shallow from the front to back but very long in the vertical dimension is characteristic of a

    _____ body habitus.

    A.  Hypersthenic          C.  Hyposthenic

    B.  Sthenic               D.  Asthenic

13. Identify the best technique for chest radiography from the following choices:

    A.  85 kV, 300 mA, ⅟₃₀ second, 40-inch SID

    B.  110 kV, 100 mA, ⅟₁₀ second, 40-inch SID

    C.  120 kV, 600 mA, ⅟₆₀ second, 60-inch SID

    D.  130 kV, 600 mA, ⅟₆₀ second, 72-inch SID

14. Match the correct answers for the structures labeled on this midsagittal section of the pharynx and upper airway:

    _____ A.          1.  Laryngopharynx

    _____ B.          2.  Uvula

    _____ C.          3.  Epiglottis

    _____ D.          4.  Esophagus

    _____ E.          5.  Spinal cord

    _____ F.          6.  Oral cavity

    _____ G.          7.  Hyoid bone

    _____ H.          8.  Nasopharynx

    _____ I.          9.  Thyroid gland

    _____ J.          10. Oropharynx

    _____ K.          11. Larynx

    _____ L.          12. Hard palate

    _____ M.          13. Thyroid cartilage

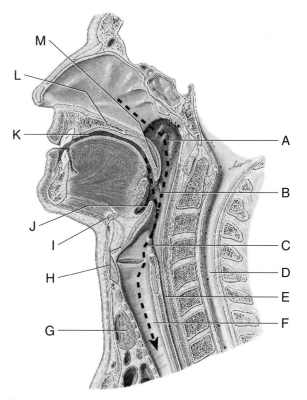

**Fig. 3-5.** Midsagittal section of the pharynx and upper airway.

15.  Identify the structures labeled on this computed tomography (CT) axial section of the thorax at the level of T3 (the third thoracic vertebra):

A.  _____

B.  _____

C.  _____

D.  _____

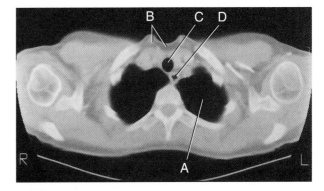

**Fig. 3-6.** Computed tomography (CT) axial section of the thorax at the level of T3.

16.  Identify the structures on this CT axial section of the thorax at the approximate level of T4-T5, 1 cm proximal to carina (HINT: B, E, and F are major blood vessels):

A.  _____

B.  _____

C.  _____

D.  _____

E.  _____

F.  _____

G.  _____

H.  _____

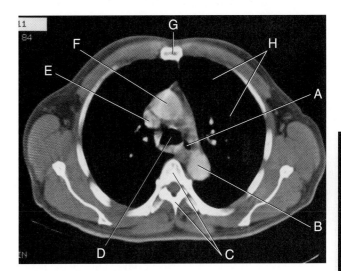

**Fig. 3-7.** Computed tomography (CT) axial section of the thorax at the approximate level of T4-T5.

17.  What is the name of the special immobilization device used for pediatric chest studies?

A.  Pigg-O-Stat            C.  Chest immobilizer

B.  Restraining chair      D.  Franklin unit

18.  Which one of the following exposure factors is recommended for a chest study of a young pediatric patient?

A.  110 kV, short exposure time      C.  65 kV, short exposure time

B.  90 kV, medium exposure time      D.  60 kV, long exposure time

19.  Which of the following is *not* a valid reason to perform chest projections with the patient in the erect position?

A.  To reduce patient dose

B.  To demonstrate air and fluid levels

C.  To allow the diaphragm to move down farther

D.  To prevent hyperemia of pulmonary vessels

20. Why are the shoulders pressed downward and toward the IR for a posteroanterior (PA) projection of the chest?

    A. To remove scapulae from lung fields

    B. To prevent hyperemia of pulmonary vessels

    C. To allow the diaphragm to move down farther

    D. To reduce chest rotation

21. Why are the shoulders rolled forward for a PA projection of the chest?

    A. To remove scapulae from lung fields

    B. To prevent hyperemia of pulmonary vessels

    C. To allow the diaphragm to move down farther

    D. To reduce chest rotation

22. Where is the central ray placed for an anteroposterior (AP) supine projection of the chest?

    A. 7 to 8 inches (18 to 20 cm) below vertebra prominens

    B. 1 to 2 inches (2.5 to 5 cm) below jugular notch

    C. 3 to 4 inches (8 to 10 cm) below jugular notch

    D. 3 to 4 inches (8 to 10 cm) below thyroid cartilage

23. True/False: CT is replacing bronchography for the study of bronchial tree conditions.

24. A condition in which all or a portion of the lung is collapsed is:

    A. Atelectasis          C. Pneumothorax

    B. Pleural effusion      D. Pneumoconiosis

25. A condition in which excess fluid builds in the lungs as a result of obstruction of the pulmonary circulation is termed:

    A. Pulmonary emboli      C. Pulmonary edema

    B. Pneumothorax          D. Bronchopneumonia

26. A sudden blockage of an artery in the lung is called:

    A. Pleurisy              C. Adult respiratory distress syndrome (ARDS)

    B. Pulmonary emboli      D. Chronic obstructive pulmonary disease (COPD)

27. Which one of the following is *not* a form of pneumoconiosis?

    A. Asbestosis      C. Anthracosis

    B. Silicosis       D. Tuberculosis

28. Manual exposure factors for a patient with a large pneumothorax should:

    A. Be reduced            C. Be increased

    B. Remain the same       D. Change from automatic exposure control (AEC) to manual technique

29. A PA chest radiograph reveals that the left sternoclavicular joint is superimposed over the spine (in comparison with the right joint). What specific positioning error is involved?

    A. Poor inspiration

    B. Rotation into a right anterior oblique (RAO) position

    C. Rotation into a left anterior oblique (LAO) position

    D. Tilting of the chest toward the left

30. A PA chest radiograph shows 10 posterior ribs above the diaphragm.

    Is this an acceptable radiograph? _____ Yes _____ No

31. A PA and lateral chest radiographic study has been completed. The PA projection reveals that the right costophrenic angle was collimated off, but both angles are included on the lateral projection.

    Would you repeat the PA projection? _____ Yes _____ No

32. A lateral chest radiograph demonstrates that the soft tissue of the upper limbs is superimposed over the apices of the lungs. How can this situation be prevented?
    A. Deeper inspiration        C. Slight rotation to the patient's left
    B. Extend chin               D. Raise upper limbs higher

33. A lateral chest radiograph reveals that the posterior ribs and costophrenic angles are separated by approximately ½

    inch (slightly less than 1 cm). Should the technologist repeat this projection? _____ Yes _____ No

34. **Situation:** A radiograph of an apical lordotic projection reveals that the clavicles are projected within the apices. The clinical instructor informs the student technologist that the study is unacceptable, but during the repeat exposure, the patient complains of being too unsteady to lean backward for another projection. What other options are available if the student wants to complete the study?
    A. Perform the PA lordotic projection        C. Perform both lateral decubitus projections
    B. Perform an AP semiaxial projection        D. Perform inspiration and expiration PA projections

35. **Situation:** An ambulatory patient with a clinical history of advanced emphysema enters the emergency room. The patient is having difficulty breathing and is receiving oxygen. The physician has ordered a PA and lateral chest study. Should the technologist alter the typical exposure factors for this patient?
    A. No. Use the standard exposure factors.
    B. Yes. Increase the exposure factors.
    C. Yes. Decrease the exposure factors.
    D. No. Increase the SID instead of changing the exposure factors.

36. **Situation:** A patient enters the ER with an injury to the chest. The ER physician suspects a pneumothorax may be present in the right lung. The patient is unable to stand or sit erect. Which specific position can be performed to confirm the presence of the pneumothorax?
    A. Left lateral decubitus        C. Right lateral decubitus
    B. Inspiration and expiration PA        D. AP lordotic

37. **Situation:** A PA and lateral chest study reveals a suspicious mass located near the heart in the right lung. The radiologist would like a radiograph of the patient in an anterior oblique position to delineate the mass from the heart. Which position should the technologist use to accomplish this objective?
    A. 45° LAO        C. 60° LAO
    B. 45° RAO        D. AP lordotic

38. **Situation:** A patient with a history of pulmonary edema comes to the radiology department and is unable to stand. The physician suspects fluid in the left lung. Which specific position should be used to confirm this diagnosis?
    A. Right lateral decubitus        C. AP lordotic
    B. AP semiaxial                   D. Left lateral decubitus

39.  For the following critique questions, refer to textbook p. 107 (Fig. C3-91) (PA chest).

    A.  Which positioning error(s) is(are) visible on this radiograph? (More than one answer may be selected.)

       (a)  All essential anatomic structures are not demonstrated.

       (b)  Central ray is incorrectly centered.

       (c)  Collimation is not evident.

       (d)  Exposure factors are incorrect.

       (e)  No anatomic side marker is visible.

       (f)  Rotation into the RAO position is evident. (The spine is shifted to the right.)

       (g)  Rotation into the LAO position is evident. (The spine is shifted to the left.)

       (h)  The chin is not elevated.

    B.  Which error(s) on this radiograph is(are) considered "repeatable"?

    C.  Which of the following modifications must be made during the repeat exposure? (More than one answer may be selected.)

       (a)  Increase closer collimation.

       (b)  Center CR correctly to T7.

       (c)  Decrease exposure factors.

       (d)  Increase exposure factors.

       (e)  Place anatomic side marker on IR prior to exposure.

       (f)  Correct for rotation of shoulders and hips.

       (g)  Place image receptor crosswise.

       (h)  Elevate chin higher.

40.  For the following critique questions, refer to Fig. C3-93 (Lateral chest)

    A.  What positioning error(s) is(are) seen on this radiograph? (More than one answer may be selected.)

       (a)  All essential anatomy is not demonstrated on the radiograph.

       (b)  CR centering is incorrect.

       (c)  Collimation is not evident.

       (d)  Exposure factors are incorrect.

       (e)  No anatomic side marker is seen on radiograph.

       (f)  Excessive rotation of the chest is demonstrated.

    B.  Which error(s) on this radiograph is(are) considered "repeatable"?

    C.  Which of the following modifications must be made during the repeat exposure? (More than one answer may be selected.)

       (a)  Center the central ray correctly—to T7.

       (b)  Decrease the exposure factors.

       (c)  Increase the exposure factors.

       (d)  Place an anatomic marker correctly on the IR before exposure.

       (e)  Ensure that the shoulders and hips are superimposed to eliminate rotation.

       (f)  Raise the upper limbs higher.

# Abdomen

## CHAPTER OBJECTIVES

After you have successfully completed the activities in this chapter, you will be able to:

_____ 1. List the location of the three muscles of the abdomen that are important in abdominal radiography.

_____ 2. List the major organs and structures of the digestive, biliary, and urinary systems.

_____ 3. Using drawings and radiographs, identify the principle structures of the digestive system, biliary system, urinary system, and accessory organs involved in digestion.

_____ 4. Identify whether select organs of the abdomen are intraperitoneal, retroperitoneal, or infraperitoneal.

_____ 5. Identify the correct quadrant or region of the abdomen where specific organs are located.

_____ 6. Identify specific bony topographic landmarks used for positioning of the abdomen.

_____ 7. Using drawings, radiographs, and computed tomography (CT) images, identify the major bony and soft tissue structures of the abdomen.

_____ 8. List specific types of pathologic findings that are clinical indications for an acute abdominal series.

_____ 9. List specific methods for controlling involuntary and voluntary motion during abdominal radiography.

_____ 10. Describe the factors that affect collimation and the use of gonadal shielding during abdominal radiography.

_____ 11. Identify the correct exposure factors to be used during abdominal radiography.

_____ 12. Identify alterations in positioning routine and exposure factors for pediatric and geriatric patients.

_____ 13. Identify the pathologic conditions and diseases of the abdomen that are best demonstrated with CT, sonography, nuclear medicine, and magnetic resonance imaging (MRI).

_____ 14. Match various types of abdominal pathologic findings to their correct definition.

_____ 15. Match specific types of abdominal pathologic findings to their correct radiographic appearance.

_____ 16. Describe variations in cassette and central ray placement that can be used to accommodate differences in body habitus.

_____ 17. List the dose ranges for skin, midline, and gonadal doses for the various projections of the abdomen on an average-size patient.

_____ 18. Identify the reason for the difference in female ovarian doses on an anteroposterior (AP) versus a posteroanterior (PA) abdomen projection with the same exposure factors.

_____ 19. List the correct central ray placement, part position, and radiographic criteria for specific abdomen positions.

_____ 20. List the pathologic indications for the acute abdominal series.

_____ 21. List the projections taken for the acute abdominal series and variations that can be used to accommodate specific patient conditions.

_____ 22. Given various hypothetical situations, identify the correct modification of position, exposure factors, or both to improve the radiographic image.

_____ 23. Given various hypothetical situations, identify the correct position for a specific pathologic feature or condition.

## Positioning and Radiographic Critique

_____ 1. Use another student as a model to practice putting a patient in supine, erect, and lateral decubitus abdominal positions.

_____ 2. Using an abdomen phantom, produce an AP projection of the abdomen that results in a satisfactory radiograph (if equipment is available).

_____ 3. Determine whether rotation, tilt, or both are present on a radiograph of an AP projection of the abdomen.

_____ 4. Critique and evaluate abdominal radiographs based on the four divisions of radiographic criteria: (1) structures shown, (2) position, (3) collimation and central ray, and (4) exposure criteria.

_____ 5. Distinguish between acceptable and unacceptable abdominal radiographs based on exposure factors, motion, collimation, positioning, or other errors.

_____ 6. Identify specific bony and soft tissue structures seen radiographically.

_____ 7. Discriminate among radiographs taken in supine, erect, or lateral decubitus positions.


## Learning Exercises

Complete the following review exercises after reading the associated pages in Chapter 4 of the textbook as indicated by each exercise. Answers to each review exercise are given at the end of the review exercises.


## Part I: Radiographic Anatomy

22-26

**REVIEW EXERCISE A:** Abdominopelvic Anatomy (see textbook pp. 110-115)

1. The two large muscles that are found in the posterior abdomen adjacent to the lumbar vertebra and are usually

   visible on an anteroposterior (AP) radiograph are called the _Rt & Lt Psoas (so'es)_ p110

2. The medical prefix for stomach is _Gastro_ . p111

3. List the three parts of the small intestine:

   A. _Duodenum 10"_        B. _Jejunun_ 2/5        C. _Ileum_ 3/5

4. Which portion of the small intestine is considered to be the longest? _Ileum_ .

5. The large intestine begins in the _Lower RT Quad_ quadrant with a saclike area called the

   _Cecum_ .

6. The sigmoid colon is located between the _Decending Colon_ and _RecTum_ of the large intestine.

7. List the three accessory digestive organs:              p112

   A. _pancreas_        B. _liver_        C. _gallblatter_

8. Circle the correct term. The pancreas is located **anteriorly** or **posteriorly** to the stomach.

9. Which one of the following organs is _not_ directly associated with the digestive system?

   A. Gallbladder        C. Jejunum

   B. Spleen             D. Pancreas

10.   Which one of the following organs is considered to be part of the lymphatic system?

    A.  Liver       C.  Pancreas

    B.  Spleen     D.  Gallbladder

11.   Why is the right kidney found in a more inferior position than the left kidney?

    _____

12.   Which endocrine glands are superomedial to each kidney?

    _____

13.   True/False: The correct term for the radiographic study of the urinary system is intravenous pyelogram (IVP).

14.   The double-walled membrane lining the abdominopelvic cavity is called the _____ .

15.   The organs located posteriorly to, or behind, the serous membrane lining of the abdominopelvic cavity are referred

    to as _____ .

16.   Which one of the following structures helps stabilize and support the small intestine?

    A.  Omentum      C.  Viscera

    B.  Peritoneum    D.  Mesentery

17.   Which one of the following structures is a double fold of peritoneum that connects the transverse colon to the greater curvature of the stomach?

    A.  Mesocolon      C.  Greater omentum

    B.  Lesser omentum   D.  Mesentery

18.   Match the following structures to the correct portion of the peritoneum:

    _____  1.  Liver               A.  Intraperitoneum

    _____  2.  Urinary bladder     B.  Retroperitoneum

    _____  3.  Kidneys          C.  Infraperitoneum

    _____  4.  Spleen

    _____  5.  Ovaries

    _____  6.  Duodenum

    _____  7.  Transverse colon

    _____  8.  Testes

    _____  9.  Adrenal glands

    _____  10.  Stomach

    _____  11.  Pancreas

    _____  12.  Ascending and descending colon

**4**

19. For each of the following organs, identify the correct abdominal quadrant in which the organ is found—left upper quadrant (LUQ), left lower quadrant (LLQ), right lower quadrant (RLQ), or right upper quadrant (RUQ):

A.   Liver _____

B.   Spleen _____

C.   Sigmoid colon _____

D.   Left colic flexure _____

E.   Stomach _____

F.   Appendix _____

G.   Two-thirds of jejunum _____

20. What is the correct name for the abdominal region found directly in the middle of the abdomen?

A.   Epigastric        C.   Umbilical

B.   Inguinal          D.   Pubic

21. Which one of the following abdominal regions contains the rectum?

A.   Pubic          D.   Epigastric

B.   Inguinal        E.   Hypochondriac

C.   Umbilical       F.   Lumbar

22. Identify the bony landmarks in Fig. 4-1:

A.   ___Ischial  tuberosity_____

B.   ___Greater trochanter_____

C.   ___Iliac Crest_____

D.   ___ASIS (Anterior Superior Iliac Spine)___

E.   ___Symphysis  pubis_____

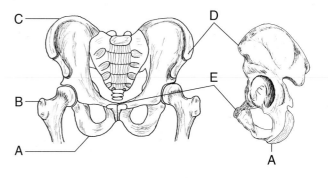

**Fig. 4-1.** Osteology of the pelvis.

23. The superior margin of the greater trochanter is about __1-1½__ inches ( __3-4__ cm) ___Superior_____

(**superior** or **inferior**) to the level of the symphysis pubis, and the ischial tuberosity is about __1½__ inches

( __3-4__ cm) ___Superior_____ (**superior** or **inferior**) to the superior aspect of the symphysis pubis.

24. Which topographic landmark corresponds to the inferior margin of the abdomen and is formed by the anterior

junction of the two pelvic bones? ___Symphysis pubis_____

25. Which topographic landmark is found at the level of L2-L3? ___Inferior costal rib margin___

26. The iliac crest is at the level of the ___L4-L5_____ vertebra.

27.  Identify the labeled parts of the digestive system (Fig. 4-2):

A.  _____

B.  _____

C.  _____

D.  _____ valve

E.  _____

F.  _____

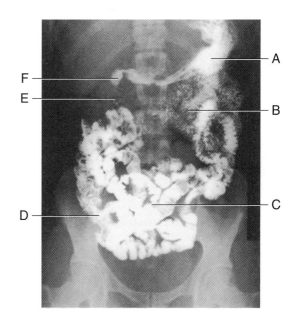

**Fig. 4-2.** Radiograph of the digestive tract.

28.  Identify the labeled structures present on the computed tomography (CT) image (Fig. 4-3):

A.  _____

B.  _____

C.  _____

D.  _____

E.  _____

F.  _____

G.  _____

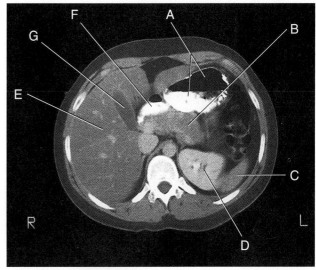

**Fig. 4-3.** Computed tomography (CT) cross-sectional image of abdomen at the level of L1 or L2.

## Part II: Radiographic Positioning and Other Patient Considerations

1-26

**REVIEW EXERCISE B:** Shielding, Patient Dose, Pathology, Exposure Factors, and Positioning (see textbook pp. 118-127)

START 1.  What are the two causes of voluntary motion?

A.  _Patient Moving during exam_          B.  _Patient Breathing Exam_   _p118_

2.  Voluntary motion can best be prevented by _Careful Breathing instructions_ to the patient.

3.  What is the primary cause for involuntary motion in the abdomen?

_Peristaltic motion in bowel_

4.   What is the best mechanism to control involuntary motion?

_____Use shortest time exposure possible p118_____

5.   True/False: Because the liver margin is visible in the right upper quadrant of the abdomen, it is not necessary to place a right or left IR marker on the cassette before exposure.

6.   Gonadal shielding should *not* be used during abdomen radiography if:

A.  It obscures essential anatomy          C.   The technologist does not elect to use it

B.   The patient requests that it not be used          D.   The patient is 40 years or older

7.   True/False: For an adult abdomen, a collimation margin must be visible on all four sides of the radiograph.

8.   Gonadal shielding for _____ may be impossible for studies of the lower abdominopelvic region.

A.  Males          C.   Both males and females

B.   Females          D.   Small children

9.   Gonadal shielding for females involves placing the top of the shield at or slightly above the level of the

_____ASIS_____ , with the bottom at the _____Lower border_____ of the symphysis

10.  Which one of the following exposure factors would be most ideal for an AP abdomen of a small- to average-size adult?

A.   110 kV, 200 mA, ¼ second, grid, 40-inch SID

B.   85 kV, 300 mA, ⅕ second, grid, 40-inch SID

C.   75 kV, 600 mA, ¹⁄₃₀ second, grid, 40-inch SID     70-80 kVp

D.   60 kV, 400 mA, ¹⁄₁₅ second, grid, 40-inch SID

11.  Which of the following technical factors is essential when performing abdomen studies on a young pediatric patient?

A.   Short exposure times          C.   High milliamperage

B.   High-speed image receptor          D.   All of the above

12.  True/False: A radiolucent pad should be placed underneath geriatric patients for added comfort.

13.  With the use of iodinated contrast media, _____CT_____ is able to distinguish between a simple

p119

cyst or tumor of the liver:

A.   Ultrasound          C.   CT

B.   Nuclear medicine          D.   MRI

14.  _____ is being used to evaluate patients with acute appendicitis:

A.   Ultrasound          C.   CT

B.   Nuclear medicine          D.   MRI

15.  The preferred imaging modality for examining the gallbladder quickly is:

A.   Ultrasound          C.   Barium enema study

B.   Nuclear medicine          D.   MRI

16. Match the following definitions to the correct pathologic indicator:

    ___E___ 1. Free air or gas in the peritoneal cavity                       A. Volvulus

    ___D___ 2. Inflammatory condition of the colon                     B. Paralytic ileus

    ___F___ 3. Telescoping of a section of bowel into another loop of bowel     C. Ascites

    ___C___ 4. Abnormal accumulation of fluid in the peritoneal cavity       D. Ulcerative colitis

    ___B___ 5. Bowel obstruction caused by a lack of intestinal peristalsis     E. Pneumoperitoneum

    ___A___ 6. A twisting of a loop of bowel creating an obstruction         F. Intussusception

    ___G___ 7. Chronic inflammation of the intestinal wall that may result in bowel obstruction     G. Crohn's disease

17. Match each of the following radiographic appearances of the abdomen to its corresponding type of pathologic condition:

    ___F___ 1. Distended loops of air-filled small intestine               A. Ascites

    ___E___ 2. Air-filled "coiled spring" appearance                  B. Volvulus

    ___A___ 3. General abdominal haziness                       C. Pneumoperitoneum

    ___C___ 4. Thin crest-shaped radiolucency underneath diaphragm     D. Ulcerative colitis

    ___D___ 5. Deep air-filled mucosal protrusions of colon wall        E. Intussusception

    ___B___ 6. Large amount of air trapped in sigmoid colon with a tapered narrowing at the site of obstruction     F. Crohn's disease

18. The central ray is centered to the level of the _Iliac Crest_ for a supine AP projection of the abdomen.

19. Exposure for an AP projection of the abdomen should be taken on _expiration_ (**inspiration or expiration**).

20. Rotation can be determined on a KUB radiograph by the loss of symmetric appearance of:

    A. _Iliac Wings_                               C. _Ischial Spine_

    B. _Obturator foramina_                        D. _Outer rib margins_

21. Which type of body habitus may require two lengthwise images to be taken if the entire abdomen is to be included?

    _Tall hyposthenic & asthenic_

22. **True/False**: A tall asthenic patient may require two 14- × 17-inch (35- × 43-cm) image receptors placed lengthwise if the entire abdomen is to be included.

23. Which of the following generates the largest gonadal dose?

    A. Female AP abdomen         C. Female posteroanterior (PA) abdomen

    B. Male lateral decubitus abdomen     D. Male erect AP abdomen

24. What is the gonadal dose range for an average-size female patient with an AP projection of the abdomen?

    A. 1 to 5 mrad         C. 35 to 75 mrad

    B. 5 to 10 mrad        D. 200 to 300 mrad

25. Which one of the following abdominal structures is not visible on a well-exposed KUB?

    A.  Kidneys                          C.  Pancreas

    B.  Margin of liver processes        D.  Lumbar transverse processes

26. Why may the PA projection of a KUB generally be less desirable than the AP projection?

    *If kidneys are of primary intrest because OID increase distortion*

27. Which decubitus position of the abdomen best demonstrates intraperitoneal air in the abdomen?

    _____

28. Why should a patient be placed in the decubitus position for a minimum of 5 minutes before exposure?

    _____

29. Which decubitus position best demonstrates possible aneurysms, calcifications of the aorta, or umbilical hernias?

    _____

30. Which position best demonstrates a possible aortic aneurysm in the prevertebral region of the abdomen?

    _____

31. List the projections commonly performed for an acute abdominal series or three-way abdomen series:

    A.  _____     B.  _____     C.  _____

32. Which position of the three-way acute abdominal series best demonstrates free air under the diaphragm?

    _____

33. Which positioning routine should be used for an acute abdominal series if the patient is too ill to stand?

    _____

34. To ensure that the diaphragm is included on an erect abdomen projection, the central ray should be at the level of

    _____ , which places the top of the 14- × 17-inch (35- × 43-cm) cassette at the level of the

    _____ .

35. Which one of the following projections involves a kV setting of 110 to 120?

    A.  Erect abdomen for ascites

    B.  Supine abdomen for intraabdominal mass

    C.  PA, erect chest for free air under diaphragm

    D.  Dorsal decubitus abdomen for calcified aorta

36. When using automatic exposure control (AEC) systems, which ionization chamber(s) should be activated for an average- to large-size patient when performing an AP projection of the abdomen?

    _____

37. True/False: A larger patient receives a greater amount of skin dose and midline dose as compared with a smaller patient during an AP projection of the abdomen.

1.5

**REVIEW EXERCISE C:** Problem Solving for Technical and Positioning Errors  1-4 , 7-12

The following radiographic problems involve technical and positioning errors that may lead to substandard images. As you analyze these problems, review your textbook to find solutions to these questions.

Other questions involve situations pertaining to various patient conditions and pathologic findings. If you need more information about a particular pathologic condition, review your textbook or a medical dictionary to learn more about it.

START

1. A KUB radiograph reveals that the symphysis pubis was cut off along the bottom of the image. Is this an acceptable radiograph? If it is not, how can this problem be prevented during the repeat exposure?

   No- Symphysis is required. Take Two KUB Images or
   realign CR because of possible alignment error

2. A radiograph of an AP projection of an average-size adult abdomen was produced using the following exposure factors: 90 kV, 400 mA, 1/10 second, grid, and 40-inch SID. The overall density of the radiograph was acceptable, but the soft tissue structures such as the psoas muscles and kidneys were not visible. Which adjustment to the technical factors will enhance the visibility of these structures on the repeat exposure?

   Reduce KVp To between 70 - 80 kVp

3. A radiograph image of an AP projection of the abdomen demonstrates motion. The following exposure factors were selected: 78 kV, 200 mA, 3/10 second, grid, and 40-inch SID. The technologist is sure that the patient didn't breathe or move during the exposure. What may have caused this blurriness? What can be done to correct this problem on the repeat exposure?

   involuntary movement perastalsis
   decrease exposure To 1 1/10 S or below

4. A radiograph of an AP abdomen reveals that the left iliac wing is more narrowed than the right. What specific positioning error caused this?

STOP

   Rt wing is higher than left wing or roTaTion

5. **Situation:** A patient with a possible **ileus** enters the emergency room. The patient is able to stand. The physician has ordered an acute abdominal series. What specific positioning routine should be used?

   AP Supine , AP Erect, PA Erect Chest

6. **Situation:** A patient with a possible perforated duodenal ulcer enters the emergency room. The ER physician is concerned about the presence of free air in the abdomen. The patient is in severe pain and **cannot** stand. What positioning routine should be used to diagnose this condition?

   AP Supine abdomen , left lateral decubitus

7. **Situation:** The ER physician suspects a patient has a kidney stone. The patient is sent to the radiology department to confirm the diagnosis. What specific positioning routine would be performed to rule out the presence of a kidney stone?

START

   AP Supine Abdomain (KUB)

**4**

8. **Situation:** A patient in intensive care may have developed intraabdominal bleeding. The patient is in critical condition and cannot go to the radiology department. The physician has ordered a portable study of the abdomen. Which specific position or projection can be used to determine the extent of the bleeding?

   *AP Supine      LAT Supine*

   *lateral decubitus for fluid levels*

9. **Situation:** A patient with a history of ascites comes to the radiology department. Which one of the following positions best demonstrates this condition?

   A. Erect AP abdomen    B. Erect PA chest    C. Supine KUB    D. Prone KUB

10. **Situation:** A KUB radiograph reveals that the gonadal shielding is superior to the upper margin of the symphysis pubis. The female patient has a history of kidney stones. What is the next step the technologist should take?

    A. Accept the radiograph because the kidneys were not obscured by the shielding.

    B. Repeat the exposure without using gonadal shielding.

    C. Repeat the exposure only if the patient complains of pain in the lower abdomen.

    D. Repeat the exposure with gonadal shielding, but position it below the symphysis pubis.

11. **Situation:** A hypersthenic patient comes to the radiology department for a KUB. The radiograph reveals that the symphysis pubis is included on the image, but the upper abdomen, including the kidneys, is cut off. What is the next step the technologist should take?

    A. Accept the radiograph.

    B. Repeat the exposure, but expose it during inspiration to force the kidneys lower into the abdomen.

    C. Ask the radiologist whether the upper abdomen really needs to be seen. Repeat only if requested.

    D. Repeat the exposure. Use two 14- × 17-inch (35- × 43-cm) cassettes crosswise to include the entire abdomen.

12. **Situation:** A patient comes from the ER with a large distended abdomen caused by an ileus. The physician suspects that the distention is caused by a large amount of bowel gas that is trapped in the small intestine. The standard technique for a KUB on an adult is 76 kV, 30 mAs. Should the technologist change any of these exposure factors for this patient? (AEC is not being used.)

    A. No. Use the standard exposure settings.

    B. Yes. Decrease the milliamperage seconds (mAs). *because air is easier than soft Tissue to penetrate*

    C. Yes. Increase the milliamperage seconds (mAs).

    D. Yes. Increase the kilovoltage (kV).

## REVIEW EXERCISE D: Critique Radiographs of the Abdomen (see textbook p. 128)

The following questions relate to the radiographs found at the end of Chapter 4 in the textbook. Evaluate these radiographs for the radiographic criteria categories (*1* through *5*) that follow. Describe the corrections needed to improve the overall image. The major, or "repeatable" errors, are specific errors that indicate the need for a repeat exposure, regardless of the nature of the other errors.

A. **Abdomen (left lateral decubitus) (Fig. C4-48)**
   Description of possible error:

   1. Structures shown: _____

   2. Part positioning: _____

3.  Collimation and central ray: _____

4.  Exposure criteria: _____

5.  Markers: _____

Repeatable error(s): _____

B.  **AP supine abdomen (KUB) (Fig. C4-49)**
    Description of possible error:

1.  Structures shown: _____

2.  Part positioning: _____

3.  Collimation and central ray: _____

4.  Exposure criteria: _____

5.  Markers: _____

Repeatable error(s): _____

C.  **AP supine abdomen (KUB) (Fig. C4-50)**
    Description of possible error:

1.  Structures shown: _____

2.  Part positioning: _____

3.  Collimation and central ray: _____

4.  Exposure criteria: _____

5.  Markers: _____

Repeatable error(s): _____

D.  **AP supine abdomen (KUB) (Fig. C4-51)**
    Description of possible error:

1.  Structures shown: _____

2.  Part positioning: _____

3.  Collimation and central ray: _____

4.  Exposure criteria: _____

5.  Markers: _____

Repeatable error(s): _____

4

## Part III: Laboratory Exercises (see textbook pp. 118-127)

You must gain experience in chest positioning before performing the following exams on actual patients. You can get experience in positioning and radiographic evaluation of these projections by performing exercises using radiographic phantoms and practicing on other students (although you will not be taking actual exposures).

    The following suggested activities assume that your teaching institution has an energized lab and radiographic phantoms. If not, perform only Laboratory Exercise B, the physical positioning activities. (Check off each step and projection as you complete it.)

### LABORATORY EXERCISE A: Energized Laboratory

1. Using the abdominal radiographic phantom, produce a radiograph of:

      _____ KUB

2. Evaluate the KUB radiograph, additional radiographs provided by your instructor, or both for the following criteria:

      _____ Rotation       _____ Part and central ray centering

      _____ Proper exposure factors       _____ Motion

      _____ Collimation       _____ Markers

### LABORATORY EXERCISE B: Physical Positioning

1. On another person, simulate taking all of the following basic and special projections of the chest. Follow the suggested positioning steps and sequence as listed below and as described in Chapter 1 of your textbook:

      _____ KUB of the abdomen       _____ Dorsal decubitus

      _____ Left lateral decubitus       _____ Acute abdominal series to include: AP supine, AP erect, PA chest

*Step 1. General Patient Positioning*

_____ Select the size and number of cassettes needed.

_____ Prepare the radiographic room. Check that tube is centered to the center of the IR holder (or the centerline of the table for Bucky exams).

_____ Correctly identify the patient and bring the patient into the room.

_____ Explain to the patient what you will be doing.

_____ Assist the patient to the proper place and position for the first radiograph.

*Step 2. Measuring Part Thickness*

_____ Measure the body part being radiographed and set correct exposure factors (technique). (If using an AEC system, select the correct chamber cells on the control panel.)

*Step 3. Part Positioning*

_____ Align and center the body part to the central ray or vice versa. For Bucky exams on a table, move the patient and table top together as needed (with floating-type table top). (NOTE: In cases in which the correct central ray position is of primary importance, the central ray icon is included in the textbook on the appropriate positioning page.)

*Step 4. IR Centering:*

_____    After the part has been centered to the central ray, the IR (cassette) is also centered to the central ray.

*Additional Steps or Actions*

_____    1.    Collimate accurately to include only the area of interest.

_____    2.    Place the correct marker within the exposure field (so that you do not superimpose pertinent anatomic structures).

_____    3.    Restrain or provide support for the body part to prevent motion.

_____    4.    Use contact lead shielding as needed.

_____    5.    Give clear breathing instructions and make the exposure while watching the patient through the window.

**4**

# Answers to Review Exercises

## Review Exercise A: Abdominopelvic Anatomy

1. Psoas muscles
2. Gastro-
3. A. Duodenum
   B. Jejunum
   C. Ileum
4. Ileum
5. Right Lower, cecum
6. Descending colon, rectum
7. A. Pancreas
   B. Liver
   C. Gallbladder
8. Posteriorly
9. B. Spleen
10. B. Spleen
11. Presence of liver on right
12. Suprarenals (adrenal)
13. False (intravenous urogram [IVU])
14. Peritoneum
15. Retroperitoneal
16. D. Mesentery
17. C. Greater omentum
18. 1. A
    2. C
    3. B
    4. A
    5. C
    6. B
    7. A
    8. C
    9. B
    10. A
    11. B
    12. B
19. A. RUQ
    B. LUQ
    C. LLQ
    D. LUQ
    E. LUQ
    F. RLQ
    G. LUQ
20. C. Umbilical
21. A. Pubic
22. A. Ischial tuberosity
    B. Greater trochanter
    C. Iliac crest or crest of ilium
    D. Anterior superior iliac spine (ASIS)
    E. Symphysis pubis
23. 1.5 (inches), 3 to 4 (cm), superior; 1.5 (inches), 3 to 4 (cm), inferior
24. Symphysis pubis
25. Inferior costal margin
26. Interspace between L4-5
27. A. Stomach
    B. Jejunum
    C. Ileum
    D. Region of ileocecal
    E. Duodenum
    F. Duodenal bulb
28. A. Stomach
    B. Pancreas
    C. Spleen
    D. Kidney (left)
    E. Liver
    F. Duodenum
    G. Gallbladder

## Review Exercise B: Shielding, Patient Dose, Pathology, Exposure Factors, and Positioning

1. A. Patient breathing
   B. Patient movement during exposure
2. Careful breathing instructions
3. Peristaltic action of the bowel
4. Use the shortest exposure time possible.
5. False
6. A. It obscures essential anatomy
7. False
8. B. Female
9. ASISs
   Symphysis pubis
10. C  (70 to 80 kV range)
11. D. All of the above
12. True
13. C. Computed tomography (CT)
14. A. Ultrasound
15. A. Ultrasound
16. 1. E
    2. D
    3. F
    4. C
    5. B
    6. A
    7. G
17. 1. F
    2. E
    3. A
    4. C
    5. D
    6. B
18. Iliac crest
19. Expiration
20. A. Iliac wings
    B. Obturator foramina (if visible)
    C. Ischial spines
    D. Outer rib margins
21. Tall hyposthenic or asthenic body type
22. True
23. A. (female AP abdomen)
24. C. (35 to 75 mrad)
25. C. Pancreas
26. Increased object image receptor distance (OID) of kidneys on PA
27. Left lateral decubitus (free air best visualized in upper right abdomen in area of liver)
28. To allow intraabdominal air to rise or abnormal fluids to accumulate
29. Dorsal decubitus (p. 125)
30. Lateral position
31. A. AP supine
    B. AP erect or lateral decubitus abdomen
    C. PA erect chest
32. PA chest
33. Two-way abdomen; AP supine abdomen, and left lateral decubitus
34. 2 inches (5 cm) above iliac crest; axilla
35. C. (chest technique)
36. Center and upper left chambers
37. True (p. 121)

## Review Exercise C: Problem Solving for Technical and Positioning Errors

1. No. A KUB must include the symphysis pubis on the radiograph to ensure that the bladder is seen. The positioning error involves centering of the central ray to the iliac crest. The technologist should also palpate the symphysis pubis or greater trochanter to ensure that it is above the bottom of the cassette.
2. The selected kilovoltage (90 kV) was too high. The technologist needs to lower the kilovoltage to between 70 and 80 kV. The milliamperage and exposure time can be altered to maintain the density.
3. The blurriness may be caused by involuntary motion. To control this motion, the technologist needs to increase the milliamperage and decrease the exposure time (e.g., 400 mA at ¹⁄₁₀ second).
4. Patient was rotated into a slight right posterior oblique (RPO) position. (The downside will appear wider.)
5. The three-way acute abdominal series, including the anteroposterior (AP) supine and erect abdomen and posteroanterior (PA) erect chest projections.
6. The two-way acute abdomen series: AP supine abdomen and left lateral decubitus

**4**

7. A KUB would be performed with the correct exposure factors to visualize the possible stone.

8. A bedside portable left lateral decubitus projection could be performed to demonstrate any fluid levels in the abdomen.

9. A. The erect AP abdomen position best demonstrates air/fluid levels. Ascites produces free fluid in the intraperitoneal cavity

10. B. Because the patient may have renal calculi in the distal ureters and urinary bladder, gonadal shielding cannot be used.

11. D. Repeat the exposure using two 14- × 17-inch cassettes placed crosswise. The hypersthenic patient often requires this type of IR placement for abdomen studies

12. B. Decrease the mAs. Because trapped air is easier to penetrate than soft tissue with x-rays, reducing the mAs will prevent overexposing the radiograph

## Review Exercise D: Critique Radiographs of the Abdomen

A. Left lateral decubitus abdomen (Fig. C4-48)
   1. Diaphragm cut off
   2. Slight rotation of pelvis evident by asymmetric appearance of pelvis
   3. Central ray centered too low (right upper quadrant cut off); collimation not evident
   4. Exposure factors acceptable
   5. Anatomic side marker missing
   Repeatable error(s): 1 and 3 (central ray centering)

B. AP supine abdomen (Fig. C4-49)
   1. Top of kidneys cut off
   2. Slight rotation toward right (RPO)—NOTE: Left obturator foramen wider than right; patient slightly off center to the right
   3. Central ray centered correctly to the iliac crest, but image receptor (IR) not centered to central ray—too low; unequal collimation because of centering error; too close side collimation
   4. Exposure factors acceptable
   5. Anatomic side marker present
   Repeatable error(s): 1 and 3 (central ray to image receptor [CR-to-IR] centering)

C. AP supine abdomen (Fig. C4-50)
   1. Upper abdomen cut off because central ray and IR centered too low
   2. No rotation evident; upper abdomen slightly off center toward left because of body tilt
   3. Central ray and IR centered too low; only lower collimation visible because of poor CR-to-IR centering
   4. Motion present; must use shorter exposure time or give more complete breathing instructions
   5. Anatomic side marker evident (over femur)
   Repeatable error(s): 1 (upper abdomen cut off), 3 (central ray centered too low), and 4 (motion present, general blurring of gas pattern margins—may be difficult to discern on this printed radiograph)

D. AP supine abdomen (Fig. C4-51)
   1. Region of bladder cut off
   2. No rotation
   3. Central ray and IR centered too high; excellent side-to-side collimation
   4. Exposure factors acceptable
   5. Anatomic side marker present (but difficult to see)
   Repeatable error(s): 1 and 3

**4**

# SELF-TEST

My Score = _____ %

This self-test should be taken only after completing all of the readings, review exercises, and laboratory activities for a particular section. The self-test is divided into six sections. The purpose of this test is not only to provide a good learning exercise but also to serve as a strong indicator of what your final unit evaluation exam will cover. It is strongly suggested that if you do not get at least a 90% to 95% grade on each self-test, you review those areas in which you missed questions before going to your instructor for the final unit evaluation exam. There are 96 questions or blanks—each is worth 1.04 (just over 1) point.

1.  The double-walled membrane lining the abdominal cavity is called the:

    A.  Greater omentum    C.  Lesser omentum

    B.  Mesentery          D.  Peritoneum

2.  Which of the following soft-tissue structures are seen on a well-exposed KUB?

    A.  Spleen      C.  Psoas muscles

    B.  Pancreas   D.  Stomach

3.  The first portion of the small intestine is called the:

    A.  Duodenum    C.  Jejunum

    B.  Ileum        D.  Pylorus

4.  At the junction of the small and large intestine is the:

    A.  Sigmoid colon    C.  Ileocecal valve

    B.  Rectum         D.  Ascending colon

5.  Match the correct answers to the structures labeled on Fig. 4-4:

    _____  1.    A.  Sigmoid colon

    _____  2.    B.  Liver

    _____  3.    C.  Jejunum

    _____  4.    D.  Oral cavity

    _____  5.    E.  Spleen

    _____  6.    F.  Stomach

    _____  7.    G.  Esophagus

    _____  8.    H.  Oropharynx

    _____  9.    I.  Pancreas

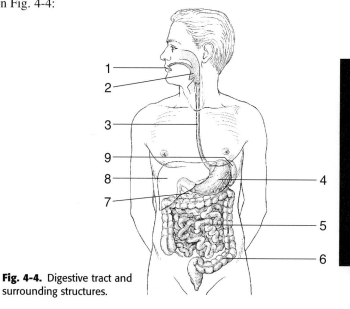

**Fig. 4-4.** Digestive tract and surrounding structures.

6.  Which one of the following is not an accessory organ of digestion?

    A.  Liver      C.  Pancreas

    B.  Spleen    D.  Kidney

7. The kidneys are connected to the bladder by way of the:

    A. Urethra      B.   Renal artery          C.  Ureter        D.  Renal vein

8. Which structure stores and releases bile?

    A. Liver        B.   Spleen      C.   Pancreas       D.   Gallbladder

9. Which one of the following structures connects the small intestine to the posterior abdominal wall?

    A. Greater omentum          C.   Lesser omentum

    B. Peritoneum                D.   Mesentery

10. For each of the following organs, identify the correct abdominal quadrant(s) in which the organ would be found on an average sthenic patient—left upper quadrant (LUQ), left lower quadrant (LLQ), right lower quadrant (RLQ), or right upper quadrant (RUQ) (NOTE: Some organs may be found in more than one quadrant):

    A. Cecum _____

    B. Liver _____

    C. Spleen _____

    D. Stomach _____

    E. Right colic flexure _____

    F. Sigmoid colon _____

    G. Appendix _____

    H. Pancreas _____

    I. Gallbladder _____

11. Which region of the abdomen would contain the T12 vertebra?

    A. Epigastric       C.  Hypochondriac

    B. Umbilical        D.  Pubic

12. Match the following structures to the correct compartment of the peritoneum:

    _____   1.   Cecum              A.   Intraperitoneum

    _____   2.   Jejunum            B.   Retroperitoneum

    _____   3.   Ascending colon    C.   Infraperitoneum

    _____   4.   Liver

    _____   5.   Adrenal glands

    _____   6.   Gallbladder

    _____   7.   Ovaries

    _____   8.   Duodenum

    _____   9.   Urinary bladder

    _____  10.   Pancreas

13.  The xiphoid process corresponds with which vertebral level?

  A.  T9-10        C.  L2-3

  B.  L4-5         D.  T4-5

14.  Identify the topographic positioning landmarks as labeled on Figs. 4-5 and 4-6:

  _____   1.  Iliac crest

  _____   2.  Ischial tuberosity

  _____   3.  Xiphoid process

  _____   4.  Symphysis pubis

  _____   5.  Greater trochanter

  _____   6.  Lower costal margin

  _____   7.  Anterior superior iliac spine (ASIS)

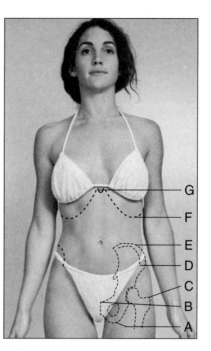

**Fig. 4-5.** Anterior surface landmarks.

**Fig. 4-6.** Lateral surface landmarks.

15.  To identify the **inferior margin** of the abdomen, the technologist can palpate the symphysis pubis or:

  A.  Iliac crest              C.  ASIS

  B.  Greater trochanter       D.  Ischial tuberosity

16.  The most important anatomic landmark that is commonly used to locate the center of the abdomen is the:

  A.  Iliac crest              C.  ASIS

  B.  Greater trochanter       D.  Ischial tuberosity

17.  Which one of the following factors best controls the involuntary motion of a pediatric patient during abdominal radiography?

  A.  Short exposure time

  B.  High kV (100 to 125)

  C.  Clear, concise breathing instructions

  D.  Use of compression band across abdomen

18.  An abnormal accumulation of fluid in the abdominal cavity is called:

  A.  Ileus                    C.  Volvulus

  B.  Ulcerative colitis       D.  Ascites

19.  The general term describing a nonmechanical bowel obstruction is:

  A.  Pneumoperitoneum         C.  Ascites

  B.  Ileus                    D.  Intussusception

**4**

20. The telescoping of a section of bowel into another loop is called:

    A. Intussusception        C. Volvulus

    B. Ascites                D. Ulcerative colitis

21. A chronic disease involving inflammation of the colon is:

    A. Ascites        C. Crohn's disease

    B. Volvulus       D. Ulcerative colitis

22. Free air or gas in the peritoneal cavity is:

    A. Pneumothorax        C. Pneumoperitoneum

    B. Ileus               D. Volvulus

23. Free air in the intraabdominal cavity rises to the level of the _____ in a patient who is in the erect position:

    A. Greater omentum        C. Intraperitoneal cavity

    B. Diaphragm              D. Liver

24. Which one of the following conditions is demonstrated radiographically as general abdominal haziness?

    A. Pneumoperitoneum        C. Ileus

    B. Ascites                 D. Volvulus

25. Which one of the following conditions is demonstrated radiographically as distended, air-filled loops of small bowel?

    A. Ascites                C. Pneumoperitoneum

    B. Ulcerative colitis     D. Ileus

26. Identify the structures labeled on this anteroposterior (AP) KUB radiograph (Fig. 4-7):

    A. _____

    B. _____

    C. _____

    D. _____

    E. _____

    F. _____

**Fig. 4-7.** Anteroposterior (AP) KUB radiograph.

27. Identify the organs or structures labeled on this computed tomography (CT) scan (Fig. 4-8) at the level of L1 or L2:

    A. _____

    B. _____

    C. _____

    D. _____

    E. _____

    F. _____

    G. _____

    H. _____

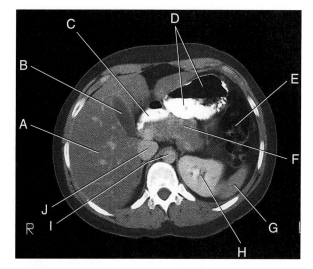

**Fig. 4-8.** Computed tomography (CT) cross-sectional image at the level of L1 or L2.

    Major blood vessels:

    I. _____

    J. _____

28. Which one of the following sets of exposure factors would be the best for abdominal radiography (for an average-size adult)?

    A. 110 kV, 400 mA, $\frac{1}{20}$ second, grid, 40-inch SID

    B. 78 kV, 600 mA, $\frac{1}{30}$ second, grid, 40-inch SID

    C. 78 kV, 200 mA, $\frac{1}{10}$ second, grid, 40-inch SID

    D. 65 kV, 600 mA, $\frac{1}{15}$ second, grid, 40-inch SID

29. A radiograph of an AP projection of the abdomen reveals that the right iliac wing is wider than the left. What type of positioning error was involved?

    A. Rotation toward the left        C. Rotation toward the right

    B. Tilt to the left                D. Tilt to the right

30. Most abdominal projections are taken during:

    A. Expiration          C. Inspiration

    B. Shallow breathing   D. Deep breathing

31. A KUB radiograph on a large hypersthenic patient reveals that the entire abdomen is not included on the 35 × 43 cm (14 × 17 inch) IR. What can be done to correct this on the repeat radiograph?

    A. Use two cassettes placed lengthwise.        C. Expose during deep inspiration.

    B. Use two cassettes placed crosswise.         D. Perform KUB with patient in erect position.

32. What is the **minimum** amount of time a patient should be upright before taking a projection to demonstrate intraabdominal free air?

    A. 20 minutes      C. 2 minutes

    B. 30 minutes      D. 5 minutes

4

33. If the posteroanterior (PA) chest projection is *not* performed for the acute abdomen series, centering for the erect abdomen projection **must** include the:

    A. Inferior liver margin     C. Entire kidneys

    B. Diaphragm     D. Bladder

34. Which specific decubitus position of the abdomen should be used in an acute abdomen series if the patient cannot stand?

    A. Left lateral decubitus     C. Right lateral decubitus

    B. Dorsal decubitus     D. Ventral decubitus

35. **Situation:** A patient with a possible **ileus** enters the emergency room. The physician orders an acute abdominal series. The patient can stand. Which specific position best demonstrates air/fluid levels in the abdomen?

    A. AP supine abdomen     C. Dorsal decubitus

    B. Right lateral decubitus     D. AP erect abdomen

36. **Situation:** A patient with a possible **perforated bowel** caused by trauma enters the ER. The patient is unable to stand. Which projection would best demonstrate any possible free air within the abdomen?

    A. Dorsal decubitus     C. AP supine abdomen

    B. Left lateral decubitus     D. Right lateral decubitus

37. **Situation:** A patient with a clinical history of a possible **umbilical hernia** comes to the radiology department. The KUB is inconclusive. Which additional projection can be taken to help confirm the diagnosis?

    A. AP erect abdomen     C. Dorsal decubitus

    B. Left lateral decubitus     D. Ventral decubitus

38. **Situation:** A patient comes to the radiology department with a clinical history of **pneumoperitoneum**. The patient is able to stand. Which one of the following projections will best demonstrate this condition?

    A. AP supine abdomen     C. Dorsal decubitus

    B. AP erect abdomen     D. Left lateral decubitus

39. **Situation:** A patient comes to the radiology department with a clinical history of **ascites.** The patient is unable to stand or sit erect. Which one of the following projections will best demonstrate this condition?

    A. AP supine abdomen     C. Dorsal decubitus

    B. Left lateral decubitus     D. AP supine chest

40. **Situation:** A patient comes in the ER with possible **gallstones.** The patient is in severe pain. Which of the following imaging modalities or projections would provide the quickest method for confirming the presence of gallstones?

    A. Sonography     C. MRI

    B. Acute abdomen series     D. KUB

41. Which one of the following alternative imaging modalities is most effectively used to evaluate **GI motility and reflux?**

    A. CT     C. Sonography

    B. MRI     D. Nuclear medicine

42. Which one of the following technical factors is essential when using computed radiography (CR) to ensure a high-quality image is produced?

    A.  Low kV                         C.  Large focal spot

    B.  72-in (180-cm) SID             D.  Close collimation

43. True/False: Identify whether each of the following statements concerning average-size patient doses for abdominal radiographs is true or false:

    _____ A.  The female ovarian dose on a PA abdomen is close to the midline dose (±10%).

    _____ B.  The skin dose for an average-size AP or PA abdomen is in the 50 to 75 mrad range.

    _____ C.  The female ovarian dose for an AP abdomen is about double that for a PA projection.

    _____ D.  The male testes dose is less than one-tenth that of the female ovarian dose with proper collimation.

44. For the following critique questions, refer to the textbook, p. 128 (Fig. C4-49) (AP supine abdomen):

    A.  Which positioning error(s) is(are) visible on this radiograph? (More than one answer may be selected.)

        (a)  All essential anatomic structures are not demonstrated.

        (b)  CR-to-IR centering is incorrect.

        (c)  CR-to-anatomy centering is incorrect.

        (d)  Collimation is not evident.

        (e)  Exposure factors are incorrect.

        (f)  No marker is seen on the radiograph.

        (g)  Rotation is toward the right.

        (h)  Rotation is toward the left.

    B.  Which error(s) on this radiograph is(are) considered "repeatable"?

        _____

    C.  Which of the following modifications must be made during the repeat exposure? (More than one answer may be selected.)

        (a)  Open up collimation.

        (b)  Center CR-to-IR correctly.

        (c)  Center CR-to-anatomy correctly.

        (d)  Decrease exposure factors.

        (e)  Increase exposure factors.

        (f)  Place marker on IR before exposure.

        (g)  Ensure that ASISs are equal distance from table top to eliminate rotation.

45. For the following critique questions, refer to Fig. C4-51 (AP supine abdomen) on p. 128 in your textbook.

    A.  Which positioning error(s) is(are) visible on this radiograph? (More than one answer may be selected.)

        (a)  All essential anatomic structures are not demonstrated.

        (b)  CR-to-IR centering is incorrect.

        (c)  Collimation is not evident.

(d)  Exposure factors are incorrect.

(e)  No marker is seen on the radiograph.

(f)  Rotation is toward the right.

(g)  Rotation is toward the left.

B.   Which error(s) on this radiograph is(are) considered "repeatable"?

_____

C.   Which of the following modifications must be made during the repeat exposure? More than one answer may be selected.

(a)  Open up collimation.

(b)  Center CR-to-IR correctly.

(c)  Decrease exposure factors.

(d)  Increase exposure factors.

(e)  Place marker on IR before exposure.

(f)  Ensure that ASISs are equal distance from table top to eliminate rotation.

## CHAPTER 5

# Upper Limb

After you have successfully completed the activities in this chapter, you will be able to:

_____ 1. List the total number of bones of the hand and wrist.

_____ 2. Identify specific aspects of the phalanges, metacarpals, and carpal bones.

_____ 3. On drawings and radiographs, identify specific anatomic structures of the hand and wrist.

_____ 4. List and describe the location, size, and shape of each carpal bone of the wrist.

_____ 5. Match specific joints of the hand and wrist according to classification and movement type.

_____ 6. List four specific ligaments of the wrist.

_____ 7. On drawings and radiographs, identify specific fat pads and stripes of the upper limb.

_____ 8. Distinguish between ulnar and radial deviation wrist movements.

_____ 9. Identify specific parts of the forearm, elbow, and distal humerus.

_____ 10. On drawings and radiographs, identify specific anatomic structures of the forearm, elbow, and distal humerus.

_____ 11. List the technical factors commonly used for upper limb radiography.

_____ 12. Match specific pathologic features of the upper limb to their correct definition.

_____ 13. Match specific pathologic features of the upper limb to their correct radiographic appearance.

_____ 14. For select pathologic conditions of the upper limb, indicate whether manual exposure factors should be increased or decreased or remain the same.

_____ 15. Identify the correct central ray placement, part position, and radiographic criteria for specific positions of the fingers, thumb, hand, wrist, forearm, and elbow.

_____ 16. Identify which structures are best seen with each basic and special projection of the upper limb.

_____ 17. Based on clinical situations, describe the preferred positioning routine to assist the physician with the diagnosis of a specific condition or disease process.

_____ 18. Identify and apply the exposure conversion chart for various sizes of plaster and fiberglass casts.

_____ 19. List the three radiographic criteria for a true lateral elbow position.

_____ 20. List the skin and midline dose ranges and the relative differences among these doses for each body part of the upper limb.

_____ 21. Given various hypothetical situations, identify the correct modification of a position, exposure factors, or both to improve the radiographic image.

_____ 22. Given various hypothetical situations, identify the correct position for a specific condition or pathologic feature.

_____ 23. Given radiographs of specific upper limb positions, identify specific positioning and exposure factor errors.

## Positioning and Radiographic Critique

_____ 1. Using another student as a model, practice basic and special projections of the upper limb.

_____ 2. Using a hand and elbow radiographic phantom, produce satisfactory radiographs of the hand, thumb, wrist, and elbow (if equipment is available).

_____ 3. Critique and evaluate upper limb radiographs based on the four divisions of radiographic criteria: (1) structures shown, (2) position, (3) collimation and central ray, and (4) exposure criteria.

_____ 4. Distinguish between acceptable and unacceptable upper limb radiographs based on exposure factors, motion, collimation, positioning, or other errors.

## Learning Exercises

Complete the following review exercises after reading the associated pages in the textbook as indicated by each exercise. Answers to each review exercise are given at the end of the review exercises.

## Part I: Radiographic Anatomy

**REVIEW EXERCISE A:** Anatomy of the Hand and Wrist (see textbook pp. 130-136)

1. Identify the number of bones for each of the following:

    A. Phalanges (fingers and thumb) _28_ (14)    C. Carpals (wrist) _16_ (8)

    B. Metacarpals (palm) _10_ (5)    D. Total _54_ (27)

2. The two portions of the thumb (first digit) are the:

    A. _proximal pha lange_    B. _Distal pha lange_

3. The three portions of each finger (second through fifth digits) are the:

    A. _proximal phalanges_

    B. _medial_   ''

    C. _distal_   ''

4. The three parts of each phalanx, starting distally, are the:

    A. _Head_    B. _body_    C. _base_

5. List the three parts of each metacarpal, starting proximally:

    A. _base_    B. _body_    C. _Head_

6. The name of the joint between the proximal and distal phalanges of the first digit is the _Inter phalangeal joint_

7. The joints between metacarpals and phalanges are the _Metacarpophalangeal joints_ .

8.  Fill in the names and parts of the following bones
    and parts of the following bones and joints of the right hand as labeled on Fig. 5-1.
    Include abbreviations for joints if applicable:

CMC  A.  5ᵗʰ carpo metacarple joint of 5ᵗʰ Digit

     B.  3ʳᵈ metacarpal

     C.  head of 5ᵗʰ metacarpal

MCP  D.  4ᵗʰ metacarpophalangeal joint of 4th Dig

     E.  Head of 5ᵗʰ proximal phalange

     F.  base of 4ᵗʰ medial phalange

     G.  4ᵗʰ Distal interphalanged joint

     H.  Body of 2ⁿᵈ medial phalange

IP   I.  2ⁿᵈ Proximal interphalangeal joint

     J.  Body of 1ˢᵗ Distal phalange

     K.  interphalangeal joint of first digit

     L.  1ˢᵗ metacarpiophalangeal joint of the 1st dig

     M.  head of 1ˢᵗ metacarpial

     N.  2ⁿᵈ carplometacarpal joint of the 2nd dig.

     O.  1ˢᵗ carplometacarpal joint of the 1st dig

**Fig. 5-1.** Posteroanterior (PA) right hand.

9.  Match each of the carpal bones labeled
    in Figs. 5-2 and 5-3 with its correct
    name:

    _8_  A.    1.  Lunate

    _1_  B.    2.  Hamate

    _5_  C.    3.  Trapezium

    _4_  D.    4.  Pisiform

    _3_  E.    5.  Triquetrum

    _6_  F.    6.  Trapezoid

    _7_  G.    7.  Capitate

    _2_  H.    8.  Scaphoid

**Fig. 5-2.** Posterior view of wrist.

**Fig. 5-3.** Posteroanterior (PA) wrist.

10.  Which is the largest of the carpal bones?  ___Capitate___

11.  What is the name of the hooklike process extending anteriorly from the hamate?  ___hamulus___
     ___hamular process___

12. Which is the most commonly fractured carpal bone? _scaphoid_

13. List one of the mnemonics given in the textbook that uses the first letter of each of the preferred terms of the eight carpal bones. _Steve left the party to take Carol home_

14. Match each of the structures labeled on Figs. 5-4 and 5-5 with its the correct term:

3 _3_ A.  1.  Capitate

9 _b_ B.  2.  Scaphoid

2 _7_ C.  3.  Base of first metacarpal

5 _3_ D.  4.  Pisiform      H C T T

1 _1_ E.  5.  Trapezoid     p + L s

8 _E_ F.  6.  Hamulus (hamular process)

6 _G_ G.  7.  Triquetrum

7 _H_ H.  8.  Hamate

4 _4_ I.  9.  Trapezium

J metacarpal of the 5th digit

**Fig. 5-4.** Carpal tunnel view.

**Fig. 5-5.** Carpal canal, inferosuperior projection.

15. Identify the carpals and other structures labeled on Fig. 5-6:

A. _1st metacarple body_

B. _1st carpo metacarple joint_

C. _trapezium_

D. _scaphoid_

E. _Lunate_

F. _radialcarple joint_

**Fig. 5-6.** Lateral wrist.

**REVIEW EXERCISE B:** Anatomy of the Forearm, Elbow, and Distal Humerus (see textbook pp. 134-139)

START 1.   A.   In the anatomic position, which of the bones of the forearm is located on the lateral (thumb) side?     *P134-135*

_Radius_

     B.   Which is on the medial side?   _ulna_

2.   Indicate whether the following structures are part of the radius (R), ulna (U), or distal humerus (H) by listing the appropriate letter next to the structure:

   _U_    A.   Trochlear notch      _U_    E.   Coronoid tubercle

   _U_    B.   Radial notch         _U_    F.   Coronoid process

   _H_    C.   Olecranon fossa       _U_    G.   Olecranon process

   _H_    D.   Trochlea            _H_    H.   Coronoid fossa

3.   Which two joints of the forearm allow it to rotate during pronation?

_proximal radioulnar joint ; distal radioulnar joint_

4.   A.   The articular portion of the medial aspect of the distal humerus is called the _Troclea_.

     B.   The similar structure found on the lateral aspect of the distal humerus is called the _Capitulum_.

5.   The deep depression located on the posterior aspect of the distal humerus is the _Olecranon fossa_.

6.   The criteria for evaluating a true lateral position of the elbow are the appearance of three concentric arcs (Fig. 5-7). These arcs include:

     A.   The first and smallest of the arcs: _trochlear sulcus_

     B.   The intermediate double arc, consisting of the outer ridges of:

         (a) The smaller arc: _Capitulum_

         (b) The larger arc: _trochlea -_

     C.   The third arc, which is part of the ulna: _Coronoid notch_

**Fig. 5-7.** True lateral elbow. Three concentric circles.   *P 136*

7.   Match the following articulations with the correct joint movement types:

   _1_    A.   Interphalangeal                 1.   Ginglymus (hinge) _flexion ; extension_

   _5_    B.   Carpometacarpal of first digit      2.   Ellipsoidal (condyloid) _flexion ; extension_ _circumduction_ _abduction ; adduction_

   _1_    C.   Elbow joint (humeroulnar and humeroradial)      3.   Trochoidal (pivot)

   _2_    D.   Metacarpophalangeal of second to fifth digits      4.   Plane (gliding)

   _2_    E.   Radiocarpal                  5.   Sellar (saddle) _flexion, extension_ _abduction, adduction_ _circumduction, opposition_ _a deg of rotation_

   _4_    F.   Intercarpal

   _1_    G.   Elbow joint

   _3_    H.   Proximal and distal radioulnar joint
   _4_    _CMC 2nd - 5th_

P137

8. Ellipsoidal or condyloid joints are classified as freely movable, or ___diarthrodial___, and allow

movement in ___fourical___ directions.

9. True/False: In addition to the ulnar and radial collateral ligaments, the following five additional ligaments are also important in stability of the wrist joint:

A. Dorsal radiocarpal              D. Scapulolunate

B. Palmar radiocarpal              E. Lunotriquetral

C. Triangular fibrocartilage complex (TFCC)

10. Which ligament of the wrist extends from the styloid process of the radius to the lateral aspect of the scaphoid and

trapezium bones? ___radial collateral ligament___

11. What is the name of the two special turning or bending positions of the hand and wrist that demonstrate medial and lateral aspects of the carpal region?

A. ___ulnar deviation___              B. ___radial deviation___

138

12. Of the two positions listed in the previous question, which one is most commonly performed to detect a fracture of

the scaphoid bone? ___ulnar deviation___

13. How does the forearm appear radiographically if pronated for a posteroanterior (PA) projection?
___The radial (proximal) crosses the ulnar___

P139

14. The two important fat stripes or bands around the wrist joint are the:

A. ___scaphoid fat strip___              B. ___pronator fat stripe___

15. The fat pads around the elbow joint are valuable diagnostic indicators if the following three technical/positioning requirements are met with the lateral position: ___The elbow must be___

A. ___flexed 90°___              C. ___optimum exposure technique___

B. ___true lateral position___

16. True/False: If the posterior fat pad of the elbow is not visible radiographically, it suggests that a nonobvious radial head or neck fracture is present. ___→ There is nothing wrong___

17. True/False: If the elbow is flexed correctly at 90°, the posterior fat pad is visible if pathologic elbow trauma is present.

18. True/False: Trauma or infection makes the anterior fat pad more difficult to see on a lateral elbow radiograph. ___visible___

19. Which projections best demonstrate the scaphoid fat pad? ___PA wrist or oblique wrist___

20. Which projection best demonstrates the pronator fat stripe? ___Lateral wrist___

21. Identify the parts labeled on Figs. 5-8 and 5-9:

A.   radial Tuberosity

B.   radial neck

C.   Capitulum

D.   lateral epicondyle

E.   olecranon fossa

F.   medial epicondyle

G.   trochlea

H.   coronoid tubercle

I.   olecranon process

J.   Superimposed humeral epicondyles

K.   radial head

L.   radial neck

M.   radial Tuberosity

N.*   Capitulum & trochlea outer ridges

O.*   Trochlear sulcus (groove)

P.*   trochlea notch

*HINT: These are concentric arcs as evidence of a true lateral position.

**Fig. 5-8.** Anteroposterior (AP) elbow.

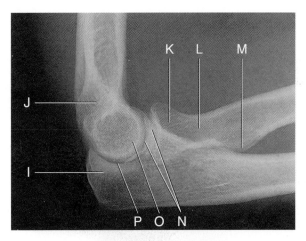

**Fig. 5-9.** Lateral elbow.

22. Identify the parts labeled on Figs. 5-10 and 5-11:

A.   Radial Tubercle

B.   Radial neck

C.   Radial head

D.   Capitulum

E.   lateral epicondyles

F.   Coronoid process

G.   Trochlea

H.   olecranon process

**Fig. 5-10.** Lateral (external) rotation of the elbow.

**Fig. 5-11.** Medial (internal) rotation of the elbow.

5

## Part II: Radiographic Positioning   1-39

**REVIEW EXERCISE C:** Positioning of the Fingers, Thumb, Hand, and Wrist (see textbook pp. 145-165)

START

1.  Identify the following technical factors most commonly used for upper limb radiography:

    A.  Kilovoltage (kV) range: ___50-60 KV___ Low-Med

    B.  Long or short exposure time? ___Short exposure___

    C.  Large or small focal spot? ___Small focal spot___

    D.  Most common minimum source image receptor distance (SID): ___40in___ 100 cm

    E.  Grids are used if the body part measures more than __10__ cm. 5"

    F.  Type of intensification screens most commonly used: ___Detail Screen?___

    G.  Small to medium dry plaster casts: Increase ___5-7___ kilovoltage. MAS 50%-60%

    H.  Large plaster casts: Increase ___8-10___ kilovoltage or

        ___100%___% milliamperage seconds.

    I.  Fiberglass casts: Increase ___3-4___ kilovoltage or ___25%-30%___%

        milliamperage seconds.

    J.  Correctly exposed radiographs: Visualize ___Soft Tissue___ margins as well as

        ___Tribecular-___ markings of all bones.

2.  The general rule for collimation for upper limb radiography states: ___Collimation borders should be visible___
    on all four sides if the IR is large enough to allow this w/o cutting off anatomy

3.  Circle all pertinent factors that help control distortion during upper limb radiography:

    A.  Kilovoltage (kV)

    (B.)  40 to 44 inches (100 to 110 CMC) SID

    C.  Milliamperage seconds (mAs)

    (D.)  Minimal object image receptor distance (OID)

    (E.)  Correct central ray placement  CR

    (F.)  Use of small focal spot  F Spot

4.  Gonadal shielding is especially important for upper limbs on all persons who are ___Child bearing age or___
    younger

5.  True/False: Guardians of young pediatric patients who are having upper limb studies can be asked to hold their
    child during the radiographic study.

6.  ___Arthrography___ is a radiographic procedure that uses contrast media injected into the joint capsule to

    visualize soft tissue pathology of the wrist, elbow, and shoulder joints.

7.  What is the basic positioning routine for the second through fifth digits of the hand? _____
    PA, PA Oblique, & Lateral

8.  How much of the metacarpals should be included for PA projection of the digits? _____

    _the Distal half of meTacarpels_

9.  List the two radiographic criteria used to determine whether rotation is present on the PA projection of the digits:

    A. _equal margins of soft Tissue on each side of phanlages_

    B. _symerTical concaves on both sides phanlages 3 disTal meTacarples_

10. Identify which positioning modification(s) may be used for a study of the second digit to improve definition for each of the following:

    A. PA oblique projection: _perform a medial oblique To decrease oid_   _Lateral oblique_

    B. Lateral position: _perform a Thumb down Lateral (medial o lateral proj) To decrease old_

11. Where is the central ray centered for a PA oblique projection of the second digit? _2nd Proximal interphanlageal (PIP) JoinT_

12. Why is it important to keep the affected digit parallel to the image receptor (IR) for the PA oblique and lateral projections?

    A.  To prevent distortion of the phalanx       C.  To demonstrate small, nondisplaced fractures near the joint

    B.  To prevent distortion of the joints        (D.)  All of the above

13. Why is the anteroposterior (AP) position of the thumb recommended instead of the PA? _AP posiTion_

    _decrease OID 3 increase resolution_

14. Which projection of the thumb is achieved naturally by placing the palmar surface of the hand in contact with the cassette? _PA Oblique_

15. Which IR size should be used for a thumb routine? _8 x 10"_

16. A sesamoid bone is frequently found adjacent to the _1st meTacarpo phanlangeal_ joint of the thumb.

17. (True)/False: The entire metacarpal and trapezium must be demonstrated on all projections of the thumb.

18. Where is the central ray centered for an AP projection of the thumb?

    A.  First interphalangeal (IP) joint          (C.)  First metacarpophalangeal (MCP) joint

    B.  Midaspect of proximal phalanx            D.  First proximal interphalangeal (PIP) joint

19. A Bennett's fracture involves:

    (A.)  Base of first metacarpal              C.  Scaphoid bone

    B.  Trapezium bone                        D.  Fracture extending through first IP joint

20. A.  Which special positioning method can be performed to demonstrate a Bennett's fracture? _____

       _Modified RoberTs Method_

    B.  Which central ray angulation is required for this projection? _15° proximal cTr on CMC Joint_

21. Where is the central ray centered for a PA projection of the hand?

    (A.)  Third MCP joint                      C.  Second MCP joint

    B.  Midaspect of third metacarpal          D.  Third PIP joint

22. A minimum of _____1_____ inch(es) (_____2.5_____ cm) of the forearm should be included radiographically for a PA projection of the hand.

23. True/False: Some superimposition of the distal third, fourth, and fifth metacarpals is expected with a well-positioned PA oblique projection of the hand.

24. Which preferred lateral position of the hand best demonstrates the phalanges without excessive superimposition?

    _____Lateral Fan_____

25. Which lateral projection of the hand best demonstrates a possible foreign body in the palm of the hand?

    _____lateral in Extension_____

26. What is the proper name for the position referred to as the "ball-catcher's position?" _AP Oblique Bilateral Norgaard_

27. The "ball-catcher's position" is commonly used to evaluate for early signs of:

    A. Osteoporosis        C. Osteopetrosis

    B. Osteomyelitis       D. Rheumatoid arthritis        p157

28. The elbow generally should be flexed _____90_____° for the basic positions of the wrist.

29. How much rotation is required for an oblique projection of the wrist? _____45°_____

30. Which alternative projection to the routine PA wrist best demonstrates the intercarpal joint spaces and wrist joint?

    _____AP projection w/a slight arch_____

31. Which positioning error is involved if significant aspects of the third, fourth, and fifth metacarpals are

    superimposed in an oblique wrist projection? _Excessive lateral rotation from PA_

32. Which one of the following fractures is not demonstrated in a wrist routine?

    A. Barton's        C. Smith's

    B. Pott's          D. Colles'

33. During the PA scaphoid projection with central ray angle and ulnar flexion, the central ray must be

    angled _____10°-15°_____° _proximal_ (distally or proximally).

34. How much are the hand and wrist elevated from the IR for the modified Stecher method?

    A. None        C. 20°        p162

    B. 10°         D. 15°

35. How much central ray angulation to the long axis of the hand is required for the carpal canal (tunnel) projection?

    _____25°-30°_____

36. Which special projection of the wrist best demonstrates the interspaces on the ulnar side of the wrist between the lunate, triquetrum, pisiform, and hamate bones?

    _____PA Proj Radial Deviation wrist_____

37. Which special projection of the wrist helps rule out abnormal calcifications in the carpal sulcus?

    _____Carpal Canal_____

38.  How much central ray angulation from the long axis of the forearm is required for the carpal bridge projection?

_____ 45° _____

39.  What is the approximate difference in mrad between skin and midline doses for the hand and wrist?

STOP _____ None _____

**REVIEW EXERCISE D:** Pathologic Features of the Fingers, Thumb, Hand, and Wrist (see textbook p. 142)

1.  List the correct pathology term for each of the following definitions:

A.  _____ Fracture and dislocation of the posterior lip of the distal radius

B.  _____ Most common type of primary malignant tumor occurring in bone

C.  _____ Reduction in the quantity of bone or atrophy of skeletal tissue

D.  _____ Accumulated fluid in the joint cavity

E.  _____ An abnormality of the cartilage affecting long bones

F.  _____ Transverse fracture extending through the distal aspect of the fifth metacarpal

G.  _____ Hereditary condition marked by abnormally dense bone

H.  _____ Transverse fracture of the distal radius with posterior displacement of the distal fragment

2.  Match the pathologic condition or disease to its radiographic appearance:

_____  A.  Narrowing of joint space with periosteal growths on the joint margins       1.  Achondroplasia

_____  B.  Fluid-filled joint space with possible calcification                        2.  Bursitis

_____  C.  Possible calcification in the carpal sulcus                                 3.  Carpal tunnel syndrome

_____  D.  Underdeveloped arms with trumpeting of the shafts of the long bones         4.  Osteoarthritis

_____  E.  Mixed areas of sclerotic and cortical thickening along with radiolucent lesions    5.  Osteopetrosis

3.  For the following types of pathologic conditions, indicate whether the manual exposure factors should be increased (+), decreased (−), or remain the same (0) as compared with the standard exposure factors.

_____  Advanced Paget's disease         _____  Osteoporosis

_____  Joint effusion                   _____  Osteopetrosis

_____  Advanced rheumatoid arthritis    _____  Bursitis

1-15

**REVIEW EXERCISE E:** Positioning of the Forearm, Elbow, and Humerus (see textbook pp. 166-178)

1.  Which basic projections are required for a study of the forearm?  _AP 3 lateral_____

2.  True/False: For a forearm study, the technologist needs to include only the joint closest to the site of the injury.

Both joints + 1.5"

3. To properly position the patient for an AP projection of the elbow, the epicondyles must be _Parallel_
   to the IR.

4. If the patient cannot fully extend the elbow for the AP projection, what alternative projection(s) should be performed?
   _AP partially flexed_

*p 169*

*p 173 ?*

5. Which basic projection of the elbow best demonstrates the radial head, neck, and tuberosity without any
   superimposition? _two AP Proj. one w/ humerus // IR, one w/ forearm // IR_

6. True/False: Gonadal shielding is not required for upper limb radiographs if the patient can sit upright for these exams.
   _Scatter or divergent radiation_

7. Which projection of the elbow best demonstrates the coronoid process? _AP Oblique Medial internal Rotation 45°_

8. The best position to evaluate the posterior fat pads of the elbow joint is _True lateral 90° flexed_

9. Which special projection(s) of the elbow should be performed instead of the basic AP if the patient's elbow is
   tightly flexed and cannot be extended? _Jones method (CR ⊥ forearm & CR ⊥ humerus_

10. The basic positioning routine for a nontraumatic study of the middle or distal humerus is _____
    _? AP, Rotational lateral — lateromedial / mediolateral_

11. How should the epicondyles be aligned for a lateral projection of the humerus? _⊥ to IR_

12. How much and in which direction should the central ray be angled for the Coyle method involving the radial head?
    _lateral Elbow (Flexed 90°) CR directed 45° angle toward shoulder_

13. How much and in which direction should the central ray be angled for the Coyle method involving the coronoid
    process?
    _lateral Elbow (Flexed 80°) CR directed 45° from shoulder_

*pg 175*

14. What is the only difference among the four radial head lateral projections of the elbow?
    _Rotational Position of the hand & wrist_

*s108*

15. Match the nearest skin dose for each of the following:

    _1_   A. PA finger          1.  5 mrad

    _5_   B. AP forearm         2.  10 mrad

    _6_   C. Lateral humerus    3.  15 mrad

    _3_   D. Lateral hand       4.  20 mrad

    _4_   E. Carpal canal wrist 5.  25 mrad

    _2_   F. PA hand            6.  30 mrad

*1-3, 5, 10, 11, 13, 15, 16.*

**REVIEW EXERCISE F:** Problem Solving for Technical and Positioning Errors (see textbook pp. 145-178)

The following radiographic problems involve technical and positioning errors that may lead to substandard images. As you analyze these problems, review your textbook to find solutions to these questions.

Other questions involve situations pertaining to various patient conditions and pathologic findings. If you need more information about a particular pathologic condition, review your textbook or a medical dictionary to learn more about it.

1. A three-projection study of the hand was taken using the following exposure factors: 64 kV, 1000 mA, $\frac{1}{100}$ second, large focal spot, 36-inch (91-cm) SID, and high-speed screens. Which of these factors should be changed on future hand studies to produce more optimal images?

    *MAS ≈ 3, Small focal spot, 40-44 SID, ≤ high speed screen To produce*
                                     *higher quality image*

2. A radiograph of a PA projection of the second digit reveals that the phalanges are not symmetric on both sides of the bony shafts. Which specific positioning error is involved?

    *Rotation*

3. A radiograph of a PA oblique projection of the hand reveals that the midshafts of the fourth and fifth metacarpals are superimposed. Which specific positioning error is involved?

    *Excessive lateral rotation*

4. In a radiographic study of the forearm, the proximal radius crossed over the ulna in the frontal projection. Which specific positioning error led to this radiographic outcome?

    *a PA wase performed not a AP*

5. A PA scaphoid projection of the wrist using a 15° distal central ray angle and ulnar flexion was performed. The resulting radiograph reveals that the scaphoid bone is foreshortened. How must this projection be modified to produce a more diagnostic image of the scaphoid?

    *CR needs To be angled 15° proximal, Toward elbow*

6. A radiograph of an <u>AP</u> elbow projection reveals considerable superimposition between the proximal radius and ulna. Which specific positioning error is involved?

    *The arm was rotated medially*

7. A routine radiograph of an AP oblique elbow with lateral rotation reveals that the radial tuberosity is partially superimposed on the ulna. In what way must this position be modified during the repeat exposure?

    *Increase lateral rotation*

8. A radiograph of a lateral projection of the elbow reveals that the humeral epicondyles are not superimposed and the trochlear notch is not clearly demonstrated. Which specific type of positioning error is involved?

    *The forearm and humerus are not on same plane*

9. **Situation:** A patient with a possible fracture of the radial head enters the emergency room. When the technologist attempts to place the arm in the AP oblique-lateral rotation position, the patient is unable to extend or rotate the <u>elbow laterally</u>. Which other positions can be used to demonstrate the radial head and neck without superimposition on the proximal ulna?

     *Coyle methol w/ CR directed Toward shoulder*

10. **Situation:** A patient with a metallic foreign body in the palm of the hand enters the emergency room. Which specific positions should be used to locate the foreign body?

    *PA 3 Lateral - in Ext/Flexion proj*

*Do* 11. **Situation:** A patient with a trauma injury enters the ER with an evident Colles' fracture. Which positioning routine should be used to determine the extent of the injury?

    AP ; lateral forearm projection To include wrist

*h* 12. **Situation:** A patient with a dislocated elbow enters the ER. The patient has the elbow tightly flexed and is careful not to move it. Which specific positioning routine can be used to determine the extent of the injury?

    Use Jones method ; later proj

*Do* 13. **Situation:** A patient with a possible Bennett's fracture enters the ER. The routine projections do not clearly demonstrate a possible fracture. Which other special projection can be taken?

    Modified Roberts Method

14. **Situation:** A patient with a history of carpal tunnel syndrome comes to the radiology department. The orthopedic physician suspects that bony changes in the carpal sulcus may be causing compression of the median nerve. Which special projection best demonstrates this region of the wrist? _____

_____

*Do* 15. **Situation:** A patient comes to the radiology department for a hand series to evaluate early evidence of rheumatoid arthritis. Which special position can be used in addition to the basic hand projections to evaluate this patient?

     AP Oblique Bilateral Norgaard method / ball catcher's position

*Do* 16. **Situation:** A patient is referred to radiology with a possible injury to the ulnar collateral ligament. The patient complains of pain near the first MCP joint. Initial radiographs of the hand do not indicate any fracture or dislocation. Which special projection can be performed to rule out an injury to the ulnar collateral ligament?

    PA STRESS Skiers Thumb / Folio Method

17. **Situation:** A patient enters the ER with a possible foreign body in the dorsal aspect of the wrist. Initial wrist radiographs are inconclusive in demonstrating the location of the foreign body. What additional projection can be performed to demonstrate this region of the wrist?

    Coyle method for The Coronoid process

*h* 18. **Situation:** A patient has a basic elbow series performed. The AP projection indicates a possible deformity or fracture of the coronoid process. However, the patient is unable to pronate the upper limb for the AP oblique-medial rotation projection because of an arthritic condition. What other projection could be performed to demonstrate the **coronoid process?**

_____

**REVIEW EXERCISE G:** Critique Radiographs of the Upper Limb (see textbook p. 179)

The following questions relate to the radiographs found at the end of Chapter 5 in the textbook. Evaluate these radiographs for the radiographic criteria categories (*A* through *F*) that follow. Describe the corrections needed to improve the overall image. The major, or "repeatable," errors are specific errors that indicate the need for a repeat exposure, regardless of the nature of the other errors.

A.  **PA hand (Fig. C5-174)**
    Description of possible error:

    1.  Structures shown: _____

    2.  Part positioning: _____

3. Collimation and central ray: _____

4. Exposure criteria: _____

5. Markers: _____

Repeatable error(s): _____

B. **Lateral hand (Fig. C5-175)**
Description of possible error:

1. Structures shown: _____

2. Part positioning: _____

3. Collimation and central ray: _____

4. Exposure criteria: _____

5. Markers: _____

Repeatable error(s): _____

C. **AP lateral oblique elbow (Fig. C5-176)**
Description of possible error:

1. Structures shown: _____

2. Part positioning: _____

3. Collimation and central ray: _____

4. Exposure criteria: _____

5. Markers: _____

Repeatable error(s): _____

D. **PA wrist (Fig. C5-177)**
Which special wrist projection is demonstrated on this radiograph?
Description of possible error:

1. Structures shown: _____

2. Part positioning: _____

3. Collimation and central ray: _____

4. Exposure criteria: _____

5. Markers: _____

Repeatable error(s): _____

E.  **PA oblique hand (Fig. C5-178)**
    Description of possible error:

    1.  Structures shown: _____

    2.  Part positioning: _____

    3.  Collimation and central ray: _____

    4.  Exposure criteria: _____

    5.  Markers: _____

    Repeatable error(s): _____

F.  **Lateral elbow (Fig. C5-179)**
    Description of possible error:

    1.  Structures shown: _____

    2.  Part positioning: _____

    3.  Collimation and central ray: _____

    4.  Exposure criteria: _____

    5.  Markers: _____

    Repeatable error(s): _____

## Part III: Laboratory Exercises (see textbook pp. 144-178)

You must gain experience in upper limb positioning before performing the following exams on actual patients. You can get experience in positioning and radiographic evaluation of these projections by performing exercises using radiographic phantoms and practicing on other students (although you will not be taking actual exposures).

   The following suggested activities assume that your teaching institution has an energized lab and radiographic phantoms. If not, perform Laboratory Exercises B and C, the radiographic evaluation and the physical positioning exercises. (Check off each step and projection as you complete it.)

## LABORATORY EXERCISE A: Energized Laboratory

1.  Using the hand radiographic phantom, produce radiographs of the following basic routines:

    _____  Hand (PA, oblique, lateral)        _____  Thumb (AP, oblique, lateral)

    _____  Wrist (PA, oblique, lateral)

2.  Using the elbow radiographic phantom, produce radiographs of the following basic routines:

    _____  AP                    _____  AP oblique, medial rotation

    _____  Lateral elbow          _____  AP oblique, lateral rotation

## LABORATORY EXERCISE B: Radiographic Evaluation

1. Evaluate and critique the radiographs produced above, additional radiographs provided by your instructor, or both. Evaluate each radiograph for the following points:

\_\_\_\_\_ Evaluate the completeness of the study. (Are all of the pertinent anatomic structures included on the radiograph?)

\_\_\_\_\_ Evaluate for positioning or centering errors (e.g., rotation, off centering).

\_\_\_\_\_ Evaluate for correct exposure factors and possible motion. (Are the density and contrast of the images acceptable?)

\_\_\_\_\_ Determine whether markers and an acceptable degree of collimation and/or area shielding are seen on the images.

## LABORATORY EXERCISE C: Physical Positioning

1. On another person, simulate performing all of the following basic and special projections of the upper limb. Include the six steps listed below and described in the textbook. (Check off each step when completed satisfactorily.)

Step 1. Appropriate size and type of IR with correct markers
Step 2. Correct central ray placement and centering of part to central ray and/or IR
Step 3. Accurate collimation
Step 4. Area shielding of patient where advisable
Step 5. Use of proper immobilizing devices when needed
Step 6. Approximate correct exposure factors, breathing instructions where applicable, and "making" exposure

| PROJECTIONS | STEP 1 | STEP 2 | STEP 3 | STEP 4 | STEP 5 | STEP 6 |
|---|---|---|---|---|---|---|
| • Second to fifth digit routines (PA, oblique, lateral) | \_\_\_\_ | \_\_\_\_ | \_\_\_\_ | \_\_\_\_ | \_\_\_\_ | \_\_\_\_ |
| • Thumb routine (AP, oblique, lateral) | \_\_\_\_ | \_\_\_\_ | \_\_\_\_ | \_\_\_\_ | \_\_\_\_ | \_\_\_\_ |
| • Hand (PA, oblique, lateral) | \_\_\_\_ | \_\_\_\_ | \_\_\_\_ | \_\_\_\_ | \_\_\_\_ | \_\_\_\_ |
| • Wrist basic routine (PA, oblique, lateral) | \_\_\_\_ | \_\_\_\_ | \_\_\_\_ | \_\_\_\_ | \_\_\_\_ | \_\_\_\_ |
| • Scaphoid, carpal canal, and carpal bridge projections | \_\_\_\_ | \_\_\_\_ | \_\_\_\_ | \_\_\_\_ | \_\_\_\_ | \_\_\_\_ |
| • Elbow routine (AP, oblique, lateral) | \_\_\_\_ | \_\_\_\_ | \_\_\_\_ | \_\_\_\_ | \_\_\_\_ | \_\_\_\_ |
| • Partial flexion APs | \_\_\_\_ | \_\_\_\_ | \_\_\_\_ | \_\_\_\_ | \_\_\_\_ | \_\_\_\_ |
| • Acute flexion (Jones) | \_\_\_\_ | \_\_\_\_ | \_\_\_\_ | \_\_\_\_ | \_\_\_\_ | \_\_\_\_ |
| • Trauma axial laterals (Coyle) | \_\_\_\_ | \_\_\_\_ | \_\_\_\_ | \_\_\_\_ | \_\_\_\_ | \_\_\_\_ |
| • Radial head projections | \_\_\_\_ | \_\_\_\_ | \_\_\_\_ | \_\_\_\_ | \_\_\_\_ | \_\_\_\_ |
| • Forearm routine (AP, lateral) | \_\_\_\_ | \_\_\_\_ | \_\_\_\_ | \_\_\_\_ | \_\_\_\_ | \_\_\_\_ |
| • AP and rotational lateral projections of midhumerus and distal humerus | \_\_\_\_ | \_\_\_\_ | \_\_\_\_ | \_\_\_\_ | \_\_\_\_ | \_\_\_\_ |

**5**

# *Answers to Review Exercises*

## Review Exercise A: Anatomy of Hand and Wrist

1. A. 14
   B. 5
   C. 8
   D. 27
2. A. Proximal phalanx
   B. Distal phalanx
3. A. Proximal phalanx
   B. Middle phalanx
   C. Distal phalanx
4. A. Head
   B. Body (shaft)
   C. Base
5. A. Base
   B. Body (shaft)
   C. Head
6. Interphalangeal joint
7. Metacarpophalangeal (MCP) joints
8. A. Fifth carpometacarpal (CMC) joint
   B. Body of third metacarpal
   C. Head of fifth metacarpal
   D. Fourth metacarpophalangeal (MCP) joint
   E. Head of proximal phalanx of fifth digit
   F. Base of middle phalanx of fourth digit
   G. Distal interphalangeal (DIP) joint of fourth digit
   H. Body of middle phalanx of second digit
   I. Proximal interphalangeal (PIP) joint of second digit
   J. Body of distal phalanx of first digit
   K. Interphalangeal (IP) joint of first digit
   L. Metacarpophalangeal (MCP) joint of first digit
   M. Head of first metacarpal
   N. Second carpometacarpal (CMC) joint
   O. First carpometacarpal (CMC) joint
9. A. 8
   B. 1
   C. 5
   D. 4
   E. 3
   F. 6
   G. 7
   H. 2
10. Capitate
11. Hamulus or hamular process
12. Scaphoid
13. Either of these two mnemonics is acceptable: (1) **S**end **L**etter **T**o **P**eter **T**o **T**ell'im (to) **C**ome **H**ome or (2) **S**teve **L**eft **T**he **P**arty **T**o **T**ake **C**arol **H**ome
14. A. 3
    B. 9
    C. 2
    D. 5
    E. 1
    F. 8
    G. 6
    H. 7
    I. 4
15. A. Body of first metacarpal (thumb)
    B. Carpometacarpal joint of first digit
    C. Trapezium
    D. Scaphoid
    E. Lunate
    F. Radiocarpal (wrist) joint (between radius and carpals)

## Review Exercise B: Anatomy of the Forearm, Elbow, and Distal Humerus

1. A. Radius
   B. Ulna
2. A. U
   B. U
   C. H
   D. H
   E. U
   F. U
   G. U
   H. H
3. Proximal and distal radioulnar joints
4. A. Trochlea
   B. Capitulum
5. Olecranon fossa
6. A. Trochlear sulcus (groove)
   B. (a) Capitulum
      (b) Trochlea
   C. Trochlear notch
7. A. 1
   B. 5
   C. 1
   D. 2
   E. 2
   F. 4
   G. 1
   H. 3
8. Diarthrodial, 4 (four)
9. True
10. Radial collateral ligament
11. A. Ulnar deviation
    B. Radial deviation
12. Ulnar deviation
13. The proximal radius crosses over the ulna.
14. A. Scaphoid fat stripe
    B. Pronator fat stripe
15. A. Elbow flexed 90°
    B. Optimal exposure techniques used
    C. In a true lateral position
16. False (A nonvisible fat pad suggests a negative exam.)
17. True
18. False
19. Posteroanterior (PA) and oblique wrist
20. Lateral wrist
21. A. Radial tuberosity
    B. Radial neck
    C. Capitulum
    D. Lateral epicondyle
    E. Olecranon fossa
    F. Medial epicondyle
    G. Trochlea
    H. Coronoid tubercle
    I. Olecranon process
    J. Superimposed humeral epicondyles
    K. Radial head
    L. Radial neck
    M. Radial tuberosity
    N. Outer ridges of trochlea and capitulum
    O. Trochlear sulcus (groove)
    P. Trochlear notch
22. A. Radial tubercle
    B. Radial neck
    C. Radial head
    D. Capitulum
    E. Lateral epicondyle
    F. Coronoid process
    G. Trochlea
    H. Olecranon process

## Review Exercise C: Positioning of the Fingers, Thumb, Hand, and Wrist

1. A. Low to medium
   B. Short exposure
   C. Small focal spot
   D. 40 inches (100 cm)
   E. 10 cm
   F. Detail screens
   G. 5 to 7
   H. 8 to 10; 100%
   I. 3 to 4; 25% to 30%
   J. Soft tissue, trabecular
2. Collimation borders should be visible on all four sides if the image receptor (IR) is large enough to allow this without cutting off essential anatomy.
3. B, D, E, F

**5**

4. Child-bearing age or younger
5. True
6. Arthrography
7. PA, PA oblique, and lateral
8. Distal half of metacarpals
9. A. Symmetric appearance of both sides of the shafts of phalanges and distal metacarpals
   B. Equal amounts of tissue on each side of the phalanges
10. A. Perform the medial oblique rather than lateral oblique to decrease OID.
    B. Perform a thumb-down lateral (mediolateral projection) to decrease OID.
11. Proximal interphalangeal (PIP) joint
12. D
13. The AP position produces a decrease in OID and increased resolution.
14. PA oblique
15. 8 × 10 inch (18 × 24 cm)
16. Metacarpophalangeal
17. True
18. C
19. A
20. A. Modified Robert's method
    B. 15° proximal
21. A
22. 1 inch (2.5 cm)
23. True
24. Fan lateral
25. Lateral in extension
26. Norgaard method
27. D
28. 90
29. 45°
30. Anteroposterior (AP) projection (with the hand slightly arched)
31. Excessive lateral rotation from PA
32. B
33. 10 to 15, proximally
34. C
35. 25° to 30°
36. PA projection with radial deviation
37. Carpal canal or Gaynor-Hart projection
38. 45°
39. No difference

### Review Exercise D: Pathologic Features of the Fingers, Thumb, Hand, and Wrist

1. A. Barton's fracture
   B. Multiple myeloma
   C. Osteoporosis
   D. Joint effusion
   E. Achondroplasia
   F. Boxer's fracture
   G. Osteopetrosis
   H. Colles' fracture

2. A. 4
   B. 2
   C. 3
   D. 1
   E. 5
3. Paget's disease (+)
   Joint effusion (0)
   Rheumatoid arthritis (−)
   Osteoporosis (−)
   Osteopetrosis (+)
   Bursitis (0)

### Review Exercise E: Positioning of the Forearm, Elbow, and Humerus

1. AP and lateral
2. False
3. Parallel
4. Two AP projections, one with humerus parallel to IR and one with forearm parallel to IR
5. AP oblique with 45° lateral rotation
6. False (because of scatter, divergent rays, or both reaching gonads)
7. AP oblique with 45° medial rotation
8. Lateral, flexed 90°
9. Two projections—central ray perpendicular to humerus and central ray perpendicular to forearm (Jones method)
10. AP and lateral projections
11. Perpendicular to IR
12. 45° toward shoulder
13. 45° away from shoulder
14. The rotational position of hand and wrist
15. A. 1
    B. 5
    C. 6
    D. 3
    E. 4
    F. 2

### Review Exercise F: Problem Solving for Technical and Positioning Errors

1. Use a small focal spot, minimum 40-inch (102-cm) SID, and detail speed screens to produce a higher-quality study.
2. Rotation
3. Excessive lateral rotation
4. PA forearm projection was performed rather than AP.
5. The central ray needs to be angled 15° proximally, toward the elbow.
6. The elbow is rotated medially.
7. Increase lateral rotation of the elbow to separate the radius from the ulna.
8. The forearm and humerus are not on the same horizontal plane.

9. Coyle method for radial head (lateral elbow, central ray 45° toward shoulder)
10. PA and lateral-in-extension projection
11. AP and lateral forearm projections to include the wrist
12. Two AP projections with acute flexion (Jones method) and a lateral projection
13. Modified Robert's method
14. Carpal canal position
15. Norgaard method—ball catcher's position
16. PA thumb projection—folio method
17. Tangential projection—carpal bridge projection
18. Trauma axial lateral projection—Coyle method for coronoid process

### Review Exercise G: Critique Radiographs of the Upper Limb

A. PA hand (Fig. C5-174)
1. All pertinent anatomic structures included
2. Some lateral rotation evident; asymmetric appearance of distal third, fourth, and fifth metacarpals and slight overlap of distal ulna and radius at distal radioulnar joint
3. No collimation evident on this printed radiograph; centering satisfactory for hand
4. Selected exposure factors acceptable, but streaking artifacts visible on the radiograph (but they may be printing artifacts)
5. Good placement of anatomic markers
Repeatable error(s): 4 (streaking artifacts) and 2

B. Lateral hand (Fig. C5-175)
1. All pertinent anatomic structures included
2. Hand rotated medially; radius and ulna not directly superimposed; metacarpals not all superimposed
3. No collimation evident on this printed radiograph; centering slightly off; central ray centered to the midmetacarpals rather than the second metacarpophalangeal joint; includes too much forearm
4. Acceptable selected exposure factors
5. No anatomic marker evident on this projection

Repeatable error(s): 2 and 5 (unless marker is visible elsewhere on radiograph)

C. AP external (lateral) oblique elbow (Fig. C5-176)
1. All essential anatomic structures included
2. Arm insufficiently rotated; radial tuberosity partially superimposed; capitulum insufficiently elongated and not in total profile
3. No collimation borders evident; central ray centering excellent for elbow
4. Excellent selected exposure factors
5. No anatomic marker evident on this projection

Repeatable error(s): 2 and 5 (unless markers are visible elsewhere on radiograph)

D. PA wrist (Fig. C5-177)
NOTE: This demonstrates a radial deviation for the ulnar side carpals (the opposite of the ulnar deviation for scaphoid).
1. Part of pisiform cut off laterally

2. Excellent part positioning with good radial deviation
3. Central ray centering error—central ray centered over scaphoid and medial carpals; would have excellent collimation if central ray were centered correctly
4. Excellent exposure factors
5. Evidence of satisfactory anatomic marker

Repeatable error(s): 1 and 3

E. PA oblique hand (Fig. C5-178)
1. All pertinent anatomic structures included
2. Excellent part positioning (no overlap of midshafts of third, fourth, and fifth metacarpals)
3. No collimation evident on this printed radiograph; acceptable central ray centering, but centered to middle of third metatarsal rather than to third metacarpophalangeal joint
4. Hand underexposed (soft tissue too evident, trabecular marking of bones not visible)

5. No evident anatomic side marker

Repeatable error(s): 4 and 5 (unless marker is visible elsewhere on radiograph)

F. Lateral elbow (Fig. C5-179)
1. All pertinent anatomic structures demonstrated
2. Elbow overflexed (beyond 90°) and not true lateral; too much distance between parts of concentric circles 1 and 2; trochlear notch space not open
3. Satisfactory collimation (i.e., collimation that is evident); central ray centering slightly off center to the elbow joint
4. Acceptable exposure factors
5. Anatomic side marker partially off radiograph and unacceptable (unless it is demonstrated on the actual radiograph)

Repeatable error(s): 2 and 5 (unless marker is more visible on actual radiograph)

# SELF-TEST

This self-test should be taken only after completing all of the readings, review exercises, and laboratory activities for a particular section. The purpose of this test is not only to provide a good learning exercise but also to serve as a strong indicator of what your final unit evaluation exam will cover. It is strongly suggested that if you do not get at least a 90% to 95% grade on each self-test, you review those areas in which you missed questions before going to your instructor for the final unit evaluation exam. There are 134 questions or blanks—each is worth 0.75 point.

1.   A. How many bones make up the phalanges of the hand?

    A.   14      C.  5

    B.   8       D.  16

    B. How many bones make up the carpal region?

    A.   14      C.  5

    B.   8       D.  7

    C. What is the total number of bones that make up the hand and wrist?

    A.   21      C.  26

    B.   27      D.  32

2.   Match the following joint locations with the correct term:

    _____ A.  Between the two phalanges of the first digit (thumb)                    1.   Radiocarpal

    _____ B.  Between the first metacarpal and the proximal phalanx of the thumb       2.   Fourth DIP

    _____ C.  Between the middle and distal phalanges of the fourth digit              3.   Fourth PIP

    _____ D.  Between the carpals and the first metacarpal                            4.   First MCP

    _____ E.  Between the forearm and the carpals                                     5.   First CMC

    _____ F.  Between the distal radius and ulna                                      6.   Distal radioulnar

                                                                                    7.   IP

3.    Match each of the structures labeled on Fig. 5-12 to its correct term:

_____    A.        1.    Distal phalanx of fourth digit

_____    B.        2.    Head of fifth metacarpal

_____    C.        3.    Base of fourth metacarpal

_____    D.        4.    Scaphoid

_____    E.        5.    Base of first metacarpal

_____    F.        6.    Pisiform

_____    G.        7.    Trapezoid

_____    H.        8.    Body of proximal phalanx of
                          fifth digit

_____    I.        9.    Fifth carpometacarpal joint

_____    J.        10.   Triquetrum

_____    K.        11.   Radius

_____    L.        12.   Proximal phalanx of first digit

_____    M.        13.   Radiocarpal joint

_____    N.        14.   Hamate

_____    O.        15.   Capitate

_____    P.        16.   Distal interphalangeal joint
                          of fifth digit

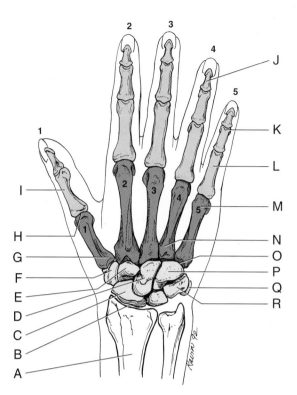

**Fig. 5-12.** Osteology of the hand and wrist.

_____    Q.    17.    Trapezium

_____    R.    18.    First metacarpophalangeal joint

4.    Which carpal contains a "hooklike" process?

A.    Scaphoid          C.    Hamate

B.    Trapezium         D.    Pisiform

5.    Which carpal articulates with the thumb?

A.    Scaphoid          C.    Trapezoid

B.    Lunate            D.    Trapezium

6.    Which carpal is most commonly fractured?

A.    Scaphoid          C.    Trapezium

B.    Capitate          D.    Triquetrum

7.    Which two carpal bones are located most **anteriorly** as seen on a lateral wrist radiograph? (HINT: They are on the
      radial side of the wrist.)

A.    Hamate and pisiform          C.    Capitate and lunate

B.    Trapezium and trapezoid      D.    Scaphoid and trapezium

8. Match each of the structures of the wrist labeled on Figs. 5-13, 5-14, and 5-15 to its correct term:

   _____ A.      1. Pisiform

   _____ B.      2. Trapezoid

   _____ C.      3. Scaphoid

   _____ D.      4. Triquetrum

   _____ E.      5. Base of first metacarpal

   _____ F.      6. Radius

   _____ G.      7. Lunate

   _____ H.      8. Trapezium

   _____ I.      9. Hamate

   _____ J.      10. Ulna

   _____ K.      11. Capitate

9. Which wrist projection does Fig. 5-14 represent?

   A. PA wrist               C. PA—radial deviation

   B. PA—ulnar deviation     D. Carpal canal

10. Which one of the following carpals is *not* well seen in the projection in Fig. 5-14?

    A. Pisiform      C. Scaphoid

    B. Lunate        D. Triquetrum

11. Which projection does Fig. 5-15 represent?

    A. PA—ulnar deviation     C. PA—radial deviation

    B. Carpal canal           D. Modified Stecher method

12. Which one of the following carpal bones is best demonstrated in the projection in Fig. 5-15?

    A. Trapezium     C. Trapezoid

    B. Scaphoid      D. Hamate

13. Which bone of the upper limb contains the coronoid process?

    A. Humerus           C. Radius

    B. First metacarpal  D. Ulna

14. Where are the coronoid and radial fossae located?

    A. Anterior aspect of distal humerus

    B. Posterior aspect of distal humerus

    C. Proximal radius and ulna

    D. Distal end of radius

**Fig. 5-13.** Lateral wrist.

**Fig. 5-14.** Wrist.

**Fig. 5-15.** Wrist.

15. Which two bony landmarks are palpated to assist with positioning of the upper limb?

    A. Coronoid and olecranon processes  C. Lateral and medial epicondyle

    B. Pisiform and hamate  D. Radial and ulnar styloid processes

16. Where is the coronoid tubercle located?

    A. Medial aspect of coronoid process  C. Lateral aspect of proximal radius

    B. Anterior aspect of distal humerus  D. Posterior aspect of distal humerus

17. In an erect anatomic position, which one of the following structures is considered to be most inferior or distal?

    A. Head of ulna  C. Radial tuberosity

    B. Olecranon process  D. Head of radius

18. Match the following articulations to the correct joint movement type (each joint movement type may be used more than once):

    _____ A. Intercarpal joints  1. Sellar

    _____ B. Radiocarpal joint  2. Ginglymus

    _____ C. Elbow joint  3. Ellipsoidal

    _____ D. First carpometacarpal joint  4. Plane

    _____ E. Third carpometacarpal joint

19. The following four radiographs represent the most common routine or basic projections for the elbow. Match each of these projections to the correct figure number:

_____ A.  Fig. 5-16     1.  AP projection

_____ B.  Fig. 5-17     2.  Lateral position

_____ C.  Fig. 5-18     3.  AP oblique—
                               lateral rotation

_____ D.  Fig. 5-19     4.  AP oblique—
                               Medial rotation

Identify the soft tissue and bony structures labeled on Figs. 5-16, 5-17, 5-18, and 5-19 (terms may be used more than once):

**Fig. 5-16.**

_____ E.      1.  Trochlea

_____ F.      2.  Olecranon process

_____ G.      3.  Coronoid process

_____ H.      4.  Medial epicondyle

_____ I.      5.  Supinator fat pad

_____ J.      6.  Capitulum

_____ K.      7.  Anterior fat pad

_____ L.      8.  Radial head and neck

_____ M.      9.  Region of posterior fat pad

_____ N.     10.  Coronoid tubercle

_____ O.

**Fig. 5-17.**          **Fig. 5-18.**          **Fig. 5-19.**

20.  Identify each of the structures labeled on Figs. 5-20 and
     5-21 with its correct term:

     _____  A.        1.   Coronoid fossa

     _____  B.        2.   Medial epicondyle

     _____  C.        3.   Head of radius

     _____  D.        4.   Trochlea

     _____  E.*       5.   Radial tuberosity

     _____  F.*       6.   Coronoid process

     _____  G.        7.   Lateral epicondyle

     _____  H.        8.   Capitulum

     _____  I.        9.   Trochlear sulcus

     _____  J.       10.   Coronoid tubercle

     _____  K.       11.   Radial fossa

*Not visible on radiograph

**Fig. 5-20.** Anterior view of the elbow.

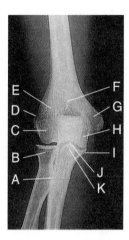

**Fig. 5-21.** Elbow. Anteroposterior (AP) extended.

21.  True/False: To visualize fat pads surrounding the elbow, exposure factors must be adjusted to see both bony and
     soft tissue structures.

22.  True/False: Fat pads of the elbow are normally seen on correctly positioned and correctly exposed anteroposterior
     (AP) elbow projections.

23.  Why should a forearm never be taken as a PA projection?

     A.  Too painful for the patient

     B.  Causes the proximal radius to cross over the ulna

     C.  Causes the distal radius to cross over the ulna

     D.  Increases the object image receptor distance (OID) of the distal radius

24.  In what position should the hand be for an AP elbow projection?

     A.  Supinated        C.  Rotated 20° from supinated position

     B.  Pronated         D.  True lateral position

25.  In what position should the hand be for an AP medial rotation oblique elbow position?

     A.  Supinated        C.  Rotated 20° from supinated position

     B.  Pronated         D.  True lateral position

5

26. Match the projection of the elbow that best demonstrates each of the following structures:

    _____ A. Coronoid process in profile                                    1. Lateral elbow

    _____ B. Radial head and tuberosity without superimposition             2. AP elbow

    _____ C. Olecranon process in profile                                   3. AP, medial rotation oblique

    _____ D. Coronoid tubercle                                              4. AP, lateral rotation oblique

    _____ E. Trochlear notch in profile

    _____ F. Capitulum and lateral epicondyle in profile

    _____ G. Olecranon process seated in olecranon fossa

27. True/False: Lead masking is not required when placing multiple images on the same digital image receptor (IR) plate.

28. The long axis of the anatomic part being imaged should be placed:

    A. Perpendicular to the long axis of the IR

    B. Parallel to the long axis of the IR

    C. 30° angle to the long axis of the IR

    D. Any way that will accommodate multiple images being placed on a single IR

29. *Arthrography* is a radiographic study of:

    A. Fat pads and stripes

    B. Epiphyses of long bones

    C. Medullary aspect of long bones

    D. Soft tissues structures within certain synovial joints

30. Match each of the following pathologic terms to its correct definition:

    _____ 1. Accumulated fluid within the joint cavity                              A. Skier's thumb

    _____ 2. A reduction in the quantity of bone or atrophy of skeletal tissue      B. Bursitis

    _____ 3. Local or generalized infection of bone or bone marrow                  C. Carpal tunnel syndrome

    _____ 4. Reverse of a Colles' fracture                                          D. Bennett's fracture

    _____ 5. Inflammation of the fluid-filled sacs enclosing the joints             E. Smith's fracture

    _____ 6. Fracture of the base of the first metacarpal                           F. Joint effusion

    _____ 7. Sprain or tear of the ulnar collateral ligament                        G. Osteomyelitis

    _____ 8. Painful disorder of hand and wrist from                                H. Osteoporosis
              compression of the median resulting nerve

31. Which one of the following pathologic indications requires a decrease in manual exposure factors?

    A. Achondroplasia       C. Osteoporosis

    B. Osteopetrosis        D. Joint effusion

32. Where is the central ray centered for a PA projection of the second digit?

    A.  Affected PIP joint          C.  Affected MCP joint

    B.  Affected middle phalanx      D.  Affected CMC joint

33. Why is it important to keep the long axis of the digit parallel to the IR?

    A.  To reduce distortion of the phalanges      C.  To demonstrate small fractures

    B.  To properly visualize joints               D.  All of the above

34. Where is the central ray placed for a PA projection of the hand?

    A.  Second MCP joint      C.  Middle phalanx of third digit

    B.  Third MCP joint        D.  Third PIP joint

35. What is the major disadvantage of performing a PA projection of the thumb rather than an AP?

    A.  Increased OID              C.  More painful for patient

    B.  Increase in patient dose    D.  Awkward position for patient

36. What type of fracture is best demonstrated with a modified Robert's method?

    A.  Barton's fracture      C.  Bennett's fracture

    B.  Colles' fracture       D.  Smith's fracture

37. True/False: Both hands are examined with one single exposure when using the Norgaard method.

38. True/False: The hand(s) is(are) placed in a true PA position when using the Norgaard method.

39. Choose the **best** set of exposure factors for upper limb radiography:

    A.  75 kV, 200 mA, $\frac{1}{20}$ second, small focal spot, 40-inch (102-cm) SID, high-speed screens

    B.  75 kV, 600 mA, $\frac{1}{60}$ second, large focal spot, 40-inch (102-cm) SID, detail-speed screens

    C.  64 kV, 100 mA, $\frac{1}{10}$ second, small focal spot, 40-inch (102-cm) SID, high-speed screens

    D.  64 kV, 200 mA, $\frac{1}{20}$ second, small focal spot, 40-inch (102-cm) SID, detail-speed screens

40. True/False: The midline dose for a lateral forearm is greater than the skin dose for a PA finger.

41. A radiograph of a PA oblique of the hand reveals that the midaspect of the third, fourth, and fifth metacarpals is slightly superimposed. What must be done to correct this positioning problem on the repeat exposure?

    A.  Increase obliquity of hand      C.  Decrease obliquity of hand

    B.  Spread fingers out further       D.  Form a tight fist with fingers

42. A radiograph of an AP elbow projection demonstrates total separation between the proximal radius and ulna. What must be done to correct this positioning error on the repeat exposure?

    A.  Rotate upper limb medially      C.  Angle central ray 5° to 10° caudad

    B.  Rotate upper limb laterally     D.  Fully extend elbow

43. A radiograph of the carpal canal (inferosuperior) projection reveals that the pisiform and hamulus are superimposed. What can be done to correct this problem on the repeat exposure?

    A.  Flex wrist slightly          C.  Rotate wrist laterally 5° to 10°

    B.  Extend wrist slightly         D.  Rotate wrist medially 5° to 10°

44. A radiograph of an AP oblique-medial rotation reveals that the coronoid process is not in profile and the radial head is only partially superimposed over the ulna. What specific positioning error was involved?

    A. Insufficient medial rotation    C. Excessive extension of elbow

    B. Excessive medial rotation    D. Excessive flexion of elbow

45. A radiograph of a lateral projection of the elbow reveals that the epicondyles are not superimposed and the trochlear notch is not clearly seen. What must be done to correct this positioning error during the repeat exposure?

    A. Angle central ray 45° toward shoulder    C. Angle central ray 45° away from shoulder

    B. Place humerus/forearm in same horizontal plane    D. Extend elbow to form an 80° horizontal plane angle

46. **Situation:** A patient with a possible Barton's fracture enters the emergency room. Which positioning routine should be performed to confirm the diagnosis?

    A. Elbow    C. Hand

    B. Wrist    D. Thumb

47. **Situation:** A patient with a possible Smith's fracture enters the emergency room. Which positioning routine should be performed to confirm this diagnosis?

    A. Hand    C. Wrist/forearm

    B. Thumb    D. Elbow

48. **Situation:** A patient has a Colles' fracture reduced, and a large plaster cast is placed on the upper limb. The orthopedic surgeon orders a postreduction study. The original technique, used before the cast placement, involved 60 kV and 5 mAs. What new technique measurements should be used with a wet plaster cast?

    A. Same measurements    C. 65 kV and 5 mAs

    B. 75 to 78 kV and 10 mAs    D. 68 to 70 kV or 10 mAs

49. **Situation:** A pediatric patient with a possible radial head fracture is brought into the emergency room. It is too painful for the patient to extend the elbow beyond 90° or rotate the hand. What type of special (i.e., optional) projection could be performed on this patient to confirm the diagnosis without causing further discomfort?

    A. Coyle method    C. Norgaard method

    B. Modified Robert's method    D. Modified Stecher method

50. For the following critique questions, refer to the AP oblique elbow radiograph shown in Fig. C5-176 in your textbook, p. 179.

    A. Which rotation is represented?    (a) Lateral rotation

    (b) Medial rotation

    B. Which positioning error(s) is(are) visible on this radiograph? (More than one answer may be selected.)

    (a) All essential anatomic structures are not demonstrated.

    (b) Central ray is centered incorrectly.

    (c) Collimation is not evident.

    (d) Exposure factors are incorrect.

    (e) No anatomic side marker is visible.

    (f) Excessive rotation in the lateral direction is evident.

    (g) Insufficient rotation in the lateral direction is evident.

    (h) Excessive flexion of the joint is evident.

C. Which criteria error(s) identified above is(are) considered "repeatable"? _____

NOTE: Insufficient lateral rotation itself may only be considered a marginal repeatable error but if no anatomic marker is visible, it is a repeatable error.

D. Which of the following modifications must be made during the repeat exposure? (More than one answer may be selected.)

(a) Increase collimation.

(b) Center central ray correctly.

(c) Decrease exposure factors.

(d) Increase exposure factors.

(e) Place anatomic side marker on IR before exposure.

(f) Rotate elbow slightly more in the medial direction.

(g) Rotate elbow slightly more in the lateral direction.

(h) Extend elbow completely.

51. For the following critique questions, refer to the position of the wrist (shown in Fig. C5-177 in the textbook, p. 179)

A. Which special wrist projection does this represent?     (a) Ulnar deviation

                                                                                 (b) Radial deviation

B. Which positioning error(s) is(are) visible on this radiograph? (More than one answer may be selected.)

(a) All essential anatomic structures are not demonstrated.

(b) Central ray is centered incorrectly

(c) Exposure factors are incorrect.

(d) No anatomic marker is visible.

(e) Excessive rotation in the lateral direction is evident.

(f) Excessive rotation in the medial direction is evident.

(g) Excessive deviation of the joint is evident.

C. Which criteria error(s) identified above is(are) considered "repeatable"? _____

D. Which of the following modifications must be made during the repeat exposure? (More than one answer may be selected.)

(a) Open up collimation to include all soft tissue and bony structures.

(b) Center central ray correctly to midcarpal region.

(c) Decrease exposure factors.

(d) Increase exposure factors.

(e) Place marker on IR before exposure.

(f) Pronate hand toward IR.

(g) Supinate hand away from IR.

(h) Extend wrist.

(i) Increase deviation movement.

(j) Decrease deviation movement.

## CHAPTER 6

# Proximal Humerus and Shoulder Girdle

After you have successfully completed the activities in this chapter, you will be able to:

_____ 1. Identify the bones and specific features of the proximal humerus and shoulder girdle.

_____ 2. On drawings and radiographs, identify specific anatomic structures of the proximal humerus and the shoulder girdle.

_____ 3. Match specific joints of the shoulder girdle to their structural classification and movement type.

_____ 4. Describe anatomic relationships of prominent structures of the proximal humerus and the shoulder girdle.

_____ 5. On radiographic images, identify rotational positions of the proximal humerus.

_____ 6. List the technical and shielding considerations commonly used for proximal humerus and shoulder girdle radiography.

_____ 7. Match specific pathologic indications of the shoulder girdle to the correct definition.

_____ 8. Match specific pathologic indications of the shoulder girdle to the correct radiographic appearance.

_____ 9. For select forms of pathologic conditions of the shoulder girdle, indicate whether manual exposure factors should be increased or decreased or remain the same.

_____ 10. List basic and special projections of the proximal humerus and shoulder, including the type and size of IR holder, the central ray location with correct angles, and the structures best demonstrated.

_____ 11. List the various patient dose ranges for select projections of the proximal humerus and shoulder.

_____ 12. Given various hypothetical situations, identify the correct modification of a position and/or exposure factors to improve the radiographic image.

_____ 13. Given various hypothetical situations, identify the correct position for a specific pathologic feature or condition.

_____ 14. Given radiographs of specific shoulder girdle projections, identify specific positioning and exposure factor errors.

## Positioning and Radiographic Critique

_____ 1. Using a peer, position the patient for basic and special projections of the proximal humerus and shoulder girdle.

_____ 2. Using a shoulder radiographic phantom, produce satisfactory radiographs of the shoulder girdle (if equipment is available).

_____ 3. Critique and evaluate shoulder girdle radiographs based on the four divisions of radiographic criteria: (1) structures shown, (2) position, (3) collimation and central ray, and (4) exposure criteria.

_____ 4. Distinguish between acceptable and unacceptable shoulder girdle radiographs based on exposure factors, motion, collimation, positioning, or other errors.

**6**

## Learning Exercises

Complete the following review exercises after reading the associated pages in the textbook as indicated by each exercise. Answers to each review exercise are given at the end of the review exercises.

## Part I: Radiographic Anatomy

**REVIEW EXERCISE A:** Radiographic Anatomy of the Proximal Humerus and Shoulder Girdle (see textbook pp. 182-186)

1.  The shoulder girdle consists of (A) _proximal humerus_ , (B) _clavical_ , and

    (C) _scapula_ .

2.  Identify the labeled parts on Figs. 6-1 and 6-2. Include secondary terms in parentheses where indicated.

    A. _InterTubercle Groove_ ( _biciptal groove_ )

    B. _Greater Tubercle_ ( _tuberosity_ )

    C. _head of humerus_

    D. _Antomical neck_

    E. _lesser Tubercle_ ( _tuberosity_ )

    F. _Surgical neck_

    _true AP proj G Tubercle lateral ; lesser is anterior_

**Fig. 6-1.** Frontal view, proximal humerus.

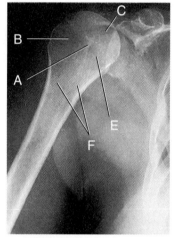

**Fig. 6-2.** Radiograph, proximal humerus.

    G.  Which projection (internal, external, or neutral rotation) of the proximal humerus is represented by this

        drawing and radiograph? _neutral rotation_

3.  The three aspects of the clavicle are the (A) _acromial extremity_ , (B) _body_ , and

    (C) _Sternal extremity_ .

4.  The _male_ (**male** or **female**) clavicle tends to be thicker and more curved in shape.

5.  The three angles of the scapula include the (A) _Superior boarder_ , (B) _Medial boarder_ , and

    (C) _lateral (axillary) boarder_

6.  The anterior surface of the scapula is referred to as the _Costal_ surface.

7.  What is the anatomic name for the armpit? _Axilla_

8.  What are the names of the two fossae located on the posterior scapula?

    A. _Infra spinous fossa_          B. _supraspinous fossa_

9.  All of the joints of the shoulder girdle are classified as being _Synovial (diarthrodial)_

10. List the movement types for the following joints:
   ball ¿ socket
  A. Scapulohumeral: flexion, extension, abduction, adduction, circumduction, medial, lateral    rotation
   plane, gliding
  B. Sternoclavicular: limited gliding motion in nearly every direction
   plane, gliding
  C. Acromioclavicular: gliding (clavical ¿ acromion), rotation (scapula ¿ clavical)

11. Match each of the following anatomic structures with its correct location:

  __C__ 1. Greater tubercle    A. Scapula

  __A__ 2. Coracoid process   B. Clavicle

  __A__ 3. Crest of spine    C. Proximal humerus

  __D__ 4. Coronoid process   D. Not part of the shoulder girdle

  __B__ 5. Acromial extremity

  __C__ 6. Intertubercular groove

  __D__ 7. Condylar process

  __C__ 8. Surgical neck

12. Identify the following structures labeled on Figs. 6-3 and 6-4.
  Include secondary terms in parentheses where indicated.

  A. __Scapula neck__

  B. __scapulohumeral joint__ (__glenohumeral joint__)

  C. __acromion__

  D. __Coronoid process__

  E. __Scapular notch__

  F. __Superior angle__

  G. __medial__ (__vertebra__) border

  H. __lateral__ (__axillary__) border

  I. __Ventral__ (__costal__) surface

  J. __Posterior__ (__dorsal__) surface

  K. __Spine of scapula__

  L. __acromion__

  M. __coronoid process__

  N. __Body__ (__Blade, wing, or ala__)

  O. __Inferior angle__

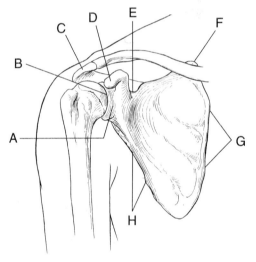

**Fig. 6-3.** Frontal view, scapula.

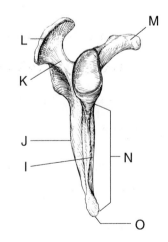

**Fig. 6-4.** Lateral view, scapula.

**6**

13. Identify the structures labeled on Fig. 6-5:

   A. _Coronoid process_

   B. _Scapulohumeral_ joint

   C. _acromion_

   D. _Greater Tubercle_

   E. _lesser Tubercle_

   F. _lateral (axillary) boarder_

   G. Is this an **internal** or **external** rotation AP projection of the proximal humerus and shoulder?

   _internal_

   H. Does Fig. 6-5 represent an **AP** or a **lateral** projection of the proximal humerus? _lateral_

   I. Are the epicondyles of the distal humerus **parallel** or **perpendicular** to the IR on this projection?

   _⊥_

   Identify the structures labeled on Fig. 6-6:

   J. _body of Scapula_

   K. _Spine of scapula & acromion_

   L. _Coronoid process_

   M. _humerus body_

   N. What is the correct term to describe the projection shown in Fig. 6-6? _Scapular Lateral_

14. Identify the structures labeled on Fig. 6-7:

   A. _Coronoid process_

   B. _glenoid process_

   C. _Scapula spine_

   D. _acromion_

   E. What is the name of the projection shown in Fig. 6-7?

   _Inferiorsuperior axial prg_

   F. How much (at what angle) should the affected arm be abducted from the body for this projection?

   _90°_

**Fig. 6-5.** Radiograph.

**Fig. 6-6.** Radiograph.

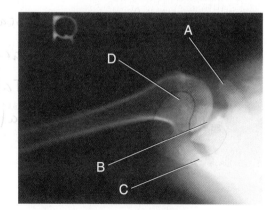

**Fig. 6-7.** Radiograph.

## Part II: Radiographic Positioning

**REVIEW EXERCISE B:** Positioning of the Proximal Humerus and Shoulder Girdle (see textbook pp. 187-207)

1-36
p187

1.  Identify the correct proximal humerus rotation for the each of the following:

    _A_    1.  Greater tubercle profiled laterally                    A.  External rotation

    _C_    2.  Humeral epicondyles angled 45° to image receptor (IR)   B.  Internal rotation

    _B_    3.  Epicondyles perpendicular to IR                         C.  Neutral rotation

    _A_    4.  Supination of hand

 C  _B_    5.  Palm of hand against thigh

    _A_    6.  Epicondyles parallel to IR

 B  _C_    7.  Lesser tubercle profiled medially

 B  _A_    8.  Proximal humerus in a lateral position

    _A_    9.  Proximal humerus in position for an anteroposterior (AP) projection

2.  Identify the proximal humerus rotation represented on the radiographs in Figs. 6-8 to 6-10:

    A.  Fig. 6-8 represents _____Neutral_____ rotation.

    B.  Fig. 6-9 represents _____External_____ rotation.

    C.  Fig. 6-10 represents _____Internal_____ rotation.

Greater
Tubercle
Inter
Tubercle
   groove
Lesser
 tubercle

**Fig. 6-8.** Proximal humerus.
epicondyles 45° to IR

**Fig. 6-9.** Proximal humerus.
epicondyles ||

**Fig. 6-10.** Proximal humerus.
epicondyles ⊥

**6**

3.  Indicate whether each of the following positioning and technical considerations is true or false for the shoulder girdle:

    A.  ~~True~~/False: The use of a grid is not required for shoulders that measure less than 10 cm.  *p 141*

    B.  True/~~False~~: The kilovoltage peak range for adult shoulder projections is between 80 and 90 kV.   *70-80   65-75 kVp*

    C.  True/~~False~~: ~~Low~~ *High* milliamperage with short exposure times should be used for adult shoulder studies.

    D.  True/~~False~~: Large focal spot setting should be selected for most adult shoulder studies.

    E.  ~~True~~/False: A high-speed screen-IR system is recommended for shoulder studies when using a grid.  *P 188*

    F.  True/~~False~~: A 72-inch (180-cm) *40* source-image distance (SID) is recommended for most shoulder girdle studies.

    G.  ~~True~~/False: The gonadal dose for most shoulder projections is 0.1 mrad or less.

    H.  ~~True~~/False: The use of contact shields over the breast, lung, and thyroid regions is recommended for most shoulder projections

4.  Which one of the following kV ranges should be used for a shoulder series on an average adult?

    A.  70 to 80 kV      C.  80 to 90 kV

    B.  55 to 60 kV      (D.)  65 to 75 kV

5.  If physical immobilization is required, which individual should be asked to restrain a child for a shoulder series?

    (A.)  Parent or guardian          C.  Radiography student

    B.  Radiologic technologist       D.  Nurse aide

6.  ~~True~~/False: Arthrography of the shoulder joint requires the use of iodinated contrast media injected into the joint space.  *?*

7.  True/~~False~~: Magnetic resonance imaging (MRI) is an excellent modality for demonstrating nondisplaced fractures of the shoulder girdle.  *P186*   *rotator cuff tears / Soft Tissue*

8.  ~~True~~/False: Nuclear medicine bone scans can demonstrate signs of osteomyelitis and cellulitis.

9.  True/~~False~~: Radiography is *Not* more sensitive than nuclear medicine for demonstrating physiologic aspects of the shoulder girdle.

10. ~~True~~/False: Ultrasound can provide a functional (dynamic) evaluation of joint movement that MRI cannot.

11. Match each of the following pathologic indications to its correct definition:

    __D__  1.  Encroachment of the supraspinous muscle on the anterior acromion

    __B__  2.  Lesion of the anteroinferior glenoid rim

    __G__  3.  Inflammatory condition of the tendon

    __A__  4.  Superior displacement of the distal clavicle

    __C__  5.  Compression fracture of the humeral head

    __F__  6.  Traumatic injury to one or more muscles of the shoulder girdle

    __E__  7.  Atrophy of skeletal tissue

    A.  Acromioclavicular joint dislocation

    B.  Bankart lesion

    C.  Hill-Sachs defect

    D.  Impingement syndrome

    E.  Osteoporosis

    F.  Rotator cuff tear

    G.  Tendonitis

12.  Match the following radiographic appearances to the correct pathologic indication:

_G_  1.  Subacromial spurs                                          A.  Rheumatoid arthritis

_E_  2.  Fluid-filled joint space                                   B.  Bankart lesion

_F_  3.  Thin bony cortex                                           C.  Hill-Sachs defect

_H_  4.  Abnormal widening of acromioclavicular joint space         D.  Osteoarthritis

I  _✗_  5.  Calcified tendons                                       E.  Bursitis

_B_  6.  Lesion on the glenoid rim                                  F.  Osteoporosis

D  ___  7.  Narrowing of joint space                                G.  Impingement syndrome

A  ___  8.  Closed joint space                                      H.  Acromioclavicular joint separation

_C_  9.  Compression fracture of humeral head                       I.  Tendinitis

13.  Which one of the following pathologic indications requires a decrease in manual exposure factors?

   (A.)  Impingement syndrome          C.  Bankart lesion

   B.  Bursitis                        (D.)  Osteoporosis

14.  Which two basic shoulder projections are routinely taken for a shoulder (with no traumatic injury) and proximal humerus?

   A.  _AP External Rotation_                     B.  _AP INTERNAL Rotation_

15.  Specifically, where is the central ray placed for an AP projection of the shoulder?  _3/4" Inferior To AC Joint_
   _To mid scapulohumeral joint 3/4" inferior and lateral to coracoid process_

16.  Which two special projections of the shoulder best demonstrate a possible Hill-Sachs defect (as described in the textbook in the "Pathology Demonstrated" section).

   A.  _Inferosuperior axial_                     B.  _Inferosuperior axial_
       _Lawrence method_                              _west point method_

17.  To best demonstrate a possible Hill-Sachs defect, which additional positioning technique should be used with the projections listed in the previous question?

   A.  Angle central ray 10° to 15° caudad        C.  Angle central ray 3° to 5°caudad

   (B.)  Rotate affected arm externally approximately 45°     D.  Place humeral epicondyles parallel to IR

18.  What type of central ray angulation is required for the inferosuperior axial projection—Lawrence method?  _P 193_

   (A.)  25° to 30° medially     C.  25° anterior and 25° medially

   B.  35° to 45° medially     D.  Central ray perpendicular to IR

19.  The _Posterior Oblique_ projection of the shoulder produces an image of the glenoid process in
   _AP Oblique_

   profile. This projection is also referred to as the  _grashey_  method.

**6**

20. Which one of the following projections produces a tangential projection of the intertubercular groove?

    Ⓐ Fisk method      C. Westpoint method

    B. Grashey method      D. Lawrence method

21. The supine version of the tangential projection for the intertubercular groove requires that the central ray be angled

    _____10° - 15°_____ posteriorly from the horizontal plane.

22. Which one of the following projections would be best for demonstrating a possible dislocation of the proximal humerus?

    A. Grashey method      C. Inferosuperior axiolateral

    B. Fisk method      Ⓓ Scapular Y

23. The ___Tangential___ projection is the special projection of the shoulder that best demonstrates the

    acromiohumeral space for possible subacromial spurs, which create shoulder impingement symptoms.

    This projection is also referred to as the ___Neer. Method___ method.

24. Ⓣrue/False: The transthoracic lateral projection is performed for possible fractures or dislocations of the proximal humerus.

25. Ⓣrue/False: The use of a breathing technique is recommended for the transthoracic lateral projection.

26. True/Ⓕalse: The affected arm must be placed into external rotation for the transthoracic lateral projection.

27. True/Ⓕalse: A central ray angle of 10° to 15° caudad may be used for the transthoracic lateral projections if the patient is unable to elevate the uninjured arm and shoulder sufficiently.

28. Ⓣrue/False: The scapular Y lateral position requires the body to be rotated 45° to 60° anteriorly toward the affected side.

29. Which one of the following shoulder projections delivers the greatest skin dose to the patient?

    A. AP axial clavicle 134      Ⓒ Transthoracic lateral 1005

    B. AP projection, neutral position 45      D. Tangential projection for intertubercular groove 14 or 31

30. Which of the following requires the smallest thyroid dose?

    A. AP neutral rotation shoulder 2      C. AP clavicle 60

    B. Transthoracic lateral 86      Ⓓ Scapular Y lateral 1

31. Which of the following would result in the highest thyroid dose?

    A. AP neutral rotation shoulder      C. AP clavicle

    Ⓑ Transthoracic lateral      D. Scapular Y lateral

32. Which special projection of the shoulder requires that the affected side be rotated 45° toward the cassette and uses

    a 45° caudad central ray angle? _AP Apical Oblique axial proj_

33. A posterior dislocation of the humerus projects the humeral head _____ (Ⓢuperior or

    inferior) to the glenoid cavity with the special projection described in the previous question.

34.   A thin-shouldered patient requires ___10-15°___ (**more** or **less**) CR angle for an AP axial clavicle

projection than a large-shouldered patient.

35.   What must be ruled out before performing the weight-bearing study for acromioclavicular joints?

___fractures___

36.   Match each of the following projections with its corresponding method name. Method names may be used more
than once:

___C___   1.   Inferosuperior axial                           A.   Neer method

___B___   2.   AP oblique for glenoid cavity                  B.   Grashey method

___D___   3.   Tangential for intertubercular (bicipital) groove   C.   Lawrence method

___A___   4.   Supraspinatus outlet tangential                D.   Fisk method

___C___   5.   Transthoracic lateral                          E.   Garth method

___E___   6.   AP apical oblique


**REVIEW EXERCISE C:** Problem Solving for Technical and Positioning Errors

1.   The following factors were used to produce a radiograph of an AP projection of the shoulder: 85 kV, 20 mAs, high-
speed screens, 40-inch (102-cm) SID, grid, and suspended respiration. The resultant radiograph demonstrated poor
radiographic contrast between bony and soft tissue structures. Which of these factors can be altered during the
repeat exposure to improve radiographic quality?

___Change KVp 75KVp ; double mAs To 40mAs___

2.   A radiograph of an AP axial clavicle projection reveals that the clavicle is projected below the superior border of
the scapula. What can the technologist do to correct this problem during the repeat exposure?

___Increase CR cephalad angle by (15-30°)___

3.   A radiograph of an AP scapula reveals that the scapula is within the lung field and difficult to see. Which two
things can the technologist do to improve the visibility of the scapula during the repeat exposure?

___Insure arm is abducted 90° ; using breathing Tech___

4.   A radiograph of an AP projection (with external rotation) of a shoulder (with no traumatic injury) reveals that
neither the greater nor lesser tubercles are profiled. What must be done to correct this during the repeat exposure?

___Insure hand is supinated ; epicondyles are // to IR___

5.   A radiograph of a lateral scapula position reveals that it is not a true lateral projection. (Considerable separation
exists between the axillary and vertebral borders.) The projection was taken using the following factors: erect
position, 40-inch (102-cm) SID, 45° rotation toward cassette from posteroanterior (PA), central ray centered to
midscapula, and no central ray angulation. Based on these factors, how can this position be improved during the
repeat exposure?

___Insure scapular border is True lateral ; increase body oblique to 50°-60°___

6.   A radiograph of the AP oblique (Grashey method) taken as a 35° oblique projection reveals that the borders of the glenoid cavity are not superimposed. The patient had large, rounded shoulders. What must be done to get better superimposition of the cavity during the repeat exposure?

*Increase rotation of affected shoulder toward IR to closer to 45°*

7.   **Situation:** A patient with a possible right shoulder dislocation enters the emergency room. The technologist attempts to perform a erect transthoracic lateral projection, but the patient is unable to raise the left arm and shoulder high enough. The resultant radiograph reveals that the shoulders are superimposed, and the right shoulder and humeral head are not well visualized. What can be done to improve this image during the repeat exposure?

*Angle the CR 10-15° cephalad to separate the shoulders*

8.   **Situation:** A patient with a possible fracture of the right proximal humerus from an automobile accident enters the emergency room. The patient has other injuries and is unable to stand or sit erect. Which positioning routine should

be used to determine the extent of the injury? *AP & Shoulder & humerus w/o rotation & a supine horiz. beam.*

9.   **Situation:** A patient with a clinical history of chronic shoulder dislocation comes to the radiology department. The orthopedic physician suspects that a Hill-Sachs defect may be present. Which specific position(s) may be used to

best demonstrate this pathologic feature? *Lawrence or West Point*

10.  **Situation:** A patient with a possible Bankart lesion comes to the radiology department. Which position of the

shoulder girdle would best demonstrate this? *West Point*

11.  **Situation:** A patient with a possible rotator cuff tear comes to the radiology department. Which one of the following imaging modalities would best demonstrate this injury?

A.   Arthrography       C.   Nuclear medicine

(B.)   MRI                    D.   Radiography

12.  **Situation:** A patient with a clinical history of tendon injury in the shoulder region comes to the radiology department. The orthopedic physician needs a *functional* study of the shoulder joint performed to determine the extent of the tendon injury. Which of the following modalities would best demonstrate this injury?

A.   Arthrography       (C.)   Ultrasound

B.   MRI                    D.   Nuclear medicine

13.  A radiograph of an AP projection with external rotation of the shoulder does not demonstrate either the greater or lesser tubercle in profile. What is the most likely cause for this radiographic outcome?

*Humeral epic. not parallel to IR*

14.  A radiograph of a transthoracic lateral projection demonstrates considerable superimposition of lung markings and ribs over the region of the proximal shoulder. What can the technologist do to minimize this problem during the repeat exposure?

*Breathing technique*

15.  **Situation:** The Garth method is performed on a patient with a shoulder injury. The resultant radiograph demonstrates the proximal humeral head projected below the glenoid cavity. What type of trauma or pathology is indicated with this radiographic appearance?

*Anterior dislocation of prox. humerus*

**REVIEW EXERCISE D:** Critique Radiographs of the Proximal Humerus and Shoulder Girdle
(see textbook p. 208)

The following questions relate to the radiographs found at the end of Chapter 6 of the textbook. Evaluate these radiographs for the radiographic criteria categories (*1* through *5*) that follow. Describe the corrections needed to improve the overall image. The major, or "repeatable," errors are specific errors that indicate the need for a repeat exposure, regardless of the nature of the other errors.

A.  **AP clavicle (Fig. C6-85)**
    Description of possible error:

    1.  Structures shown: _____

    2.  Part positioning: _____

    3.  Collimation and central ray: _____

    4.  Exposure criteria: _____

    5.  Markers: _____

    Repeatable error(s): _____

B.  **AP apical oblique axial shoulder (Fig. C6-86)**
    Description of possible error:

    1.  Structures shown: _____

    2.  Part positioning: _____

    3.  Collimation and central ray: _____

    4.  Exposure criteria: _____

    5.  Markers: _____

    Repeatable error(s): _____

C.  **AP scapula (Fig. C6-87)**
    Description of possible error:

    1.  Structures shown: _____

    2.  Part positioning: _____

    3.  Collimation and central ray: _____

    4.  Exposure criteria: _____

    5.  Markers: _____

    Repeatable error(s): _____

D.  **AP shoulder and proximal humerus (Fig. C6-88)**
    Description of possible error:

    1.  Structures shown: _____

    2.  Part positioning: _____

3.  Collimation and central ray: _____

4.  Exposure criteria: _____

5.  Markers: _____

Repeatable error(s): _____

Which projection (AP, lateral, or oblique) and which rotation of the proximal humerus are evident (internal, external, or

neutral)? _____

## Part III: Laboratory Exercises (see textbook pp. 191-207)

You must gain experience in positioning each part of the proximal humerus and shoulder girdle before performing the following exams on actual patients. You can get experience in positioning and radiographic evaluation of these projections by performing exercises using radiographic phantoms and practicing on other students (although you will not be taking actual exposures).

The following suggested activities assume that your teaching institution has an energized lab and radiographic phantoms. If not, perform Laboratory Exercises B and C, the radiographic evaluation and the physical positioning exercises. (Check off each step and projection as you complete it.)

## LABORATORY EXERCISE A: Energized Laboratory

1.  Using the thorax radiographic phantom, produce radiographs of the following basic routines:

_____ AP shoulder                    _____ AP oblique (Grashey method)

_____ AP and AP axial clavicle       _____ AP and lateral scapula

## LABORATORY EXERCISE B: Radiographic Evaluation

1.  Evaluate and critique the radiographs produced above, additional radiographs provided by your instructor, or both. Evaluate each radiograph for the following points:

_____ Evaluate the completeness of the study. (Are all of the pertinent anatomic structures included on the radiograph?)

_____ Evaluate for positioning or centering errors (e.g., rotation, off centering).

_____ Evaluate for correct exposure factors and possible motion. (Are the density and contrast of the images acceptable?)

_____ Determine whether markers and an acceptable degree of collimation and/or area shielding are seen on the images.

## LABORATORY EXERCISE C: Physical Positioning

On another person, simulate performing all of the following basic and special projections of the proximal humerus and shoulder girdle. Include the six steps listed below and described in the textbook. (Check off each step when completed satisfactorily.)

Step 1.  Appropriate size and type of image receptor with correct markers
Step 2.  Correct central ray placement and centering of part to central ray and/or IR
Step 3.  Accurate collimation
Step 4.  Area shielding of patient where advisable
Step 5.  Use of proper immobilizing devices when needed
Step 6.  Approximate correct exposure factors, breathing instructions where applicable, and "making" exposure

| PROJECTIONS | STEP 1 | STEP 2 | STEP 3 | STEP 4 | STEP 5 | STEP 6 |
|---|---|---|---|---|---|---|
| • Shoulder series (nontrauma) (AP internal and external rotation) | ___ | ___ | ___ | ___ | ___ | ___ |
| • Inferosuperior axiolateral (Lawrence) | ___ | ___ | ___ | ___ | ___ | ___ |
| • AP oblique (Grashey) | ___ | ___ | ___ | ___ | ___ | ___ |
| • Tangential (Fisk) for intertubercular groove | ___ | ___ | ___ | ___ | ___ | ___ |
| • Scapular Y | ___ | ___ | ___ | ___ | ___ | ___ |
| • Transthoracic lateral | ___ | ___ | ___ | ___ | ___ | ___ |
| • AP apical oblique (Garth) | ___ | ___ | ___ | ___ | ___ | ___ |
| • AP and AP axial clavicle | ___ | ___ | ___ | ___ | ___ | ___ |
| • AP and lateral scapula | ___ | ___ | ___ | ___ | ___ | ___ |
| • Acromioclavicular joints (with and without weights) | ___ | ___ | ___ | ___ | ___ | ___ |

6

# *Answers to Review Exercises*

## Review Exercise A: Anatomy of Proximal Humerus and Shoulder Girdle

1. A. Proximal humerus
   B. Scapula
   C. Clavicle
2. A. Intertubercular groove (bicipital groove)
   B. Greater tubercle (tuberosity)
   C. Head of humerus
   D. Anatomic neck
   E. Lesser tubercle (tuberosity)
   F. Surgical neck
   G. Neutral (Neither the greater nor lesser tubercle is in profile.)
3. A. Sternal extremity
   B. Body (shaft)
   C. Acromial extremity
4. Male
5. A. Lateral angle
   B. Superior angle
   C. Inferior angle
6. Costal
7. Axilla
8. A. Infraspinous fossa
   B. Supraspinous fossa
9. Synovial (diarthrodial)
10. A. Spheroidal or ball and socket
    B. Plane or gliding
    C. Plane or gliding
11. 1. C
    2. A
    3. A
    4. D
    5. B
    6. C
    7. D
    8. C
12. A. Neck of scapula
    B. Scapulohumeral joint (gleno-humeral joint)
    C. Acromion
    D. Coracoid process
    E. Scapular notch
    F. Superior angle
    G. Medial (vertebral)
    H. Lateral (axillary)
    I. Ventral (costal)
    J. Dorsal
    K. Spine of scapula
    L. Acromion
    M. Coracoid process
    N. Body (blade, wing, or ala)
    O. Inferior angle
13. A. Coracoid process
    B. Scapulohumeral
    C. Acromion
    D. Greater tubercle
    E. Lesser tubercle
    F. Lateral (axillary) border

G. Internal (Lesser tubercle is in profile medially.)
H. Lateral
I. Perpendicular
J. Body of scapula
K. Spine of scapula and acromion
L. Coracoid process
M. Body (shaft) of humerus
N. Scapular Y lateral
14. A. Coracoid process
    B. Glenoid process
    C. Spine of scapula
    D. Acromion
    E. Inferosuperior axial projection
    F. 90°

## Review Exercise B: Positioning of Proximal Humerus and Shoulder Girdle

1. 1. A
   2. C
   3. B
   4. A
   5. C
   6. A
   7. B
   8. B
   9. A
2. A. Neutral
   B. External
   C. Internal
3. A. True
   B. False
   C. False
   D. False
   E. True
   F. False
   G. True
   H. True
4. D. 65 to 75 kV
5. A. Parent or guardian
6. True
7. False
8. True
9. False
10. True
11. 1. D
    2. B
    3. G
    4. A
    5. C
    6. F
    7. E
12. 1. G
    2. E
    3. F
    4. H
    5. I
    6. B
    7. D

8. A
9. C
13. D. Osteoporosis
14. A. AP, external rotation
    B. AP, internal rotation
15. To midscapulohumeral joint, ¾ inch (2 cm) inferior and lateral to coracoid process
16. A. Inferosuperior axial projection—Lawrence method
    B. Inferosuperior axial projection—Westpoint method
17. B. Rotate affected arm externally approximately 45°
18. A. 25° to 30° medially
19. AP oblique; Grashey
20. A. Fisk method
21. 10° to 15°
22. D. Scapular Y
23. Supraspinatus outlet tangential projection; Neer
24. True
25. True
26. False
27. False
28. True
29. C. Transthoracic lateral
30. D. Scapular Y lateral
31. B. Transthoracic lateral
32. AP apical oblique
33. Superior
34. More
35. Fracture of clavicle
36. 1. C
    2. B
    3. D
    4. A
    5. C
    6. E

## Review Exercise C: Problem Solving for Technical and Positioning Errors

1. Lower kilovoltage peak to 75 kV and double milliamperage seconds (to 40 mAs), which increases radiographic contrast.
2. Increase central ray cephalad angle.
3. Ensure that the affected arm is abducted 90° and use a breathing technique.
4. Supinate the hand and ensure that the epicondyles are parallel to the IR for a true AP.
5. Palpate the scapular borders to ensure true lateral and increase body obliquity if needed to between 50° and 60° from a posteroanterior (PA) position.

6. Increase rotation of affected shoulder toward IR to closer to 45°.
7. Angle the central ray 10° to 15° cephalad to separate the shoulders.
8. The routine includes an anteroposterior (AP) of right shoulder and humerus without rotation (neutral rotation) and a supine, horizontal beam, right transthoracic shoulder. NOTE: In those cases in which the opposite arm cannot be elevated or extended, a supine posterior oblique scapular Y could also be used as a second option for a lateral shoulder position (see Chapter 19).
9. Inferosuperior axial projections—Lawrence or Westpoint method
10. Westpoint method
11. B. MRI
12. C. Ultrasound
13. The humeral epicondyles were not placed parallel to the plane of the IR.
14. Use breathing exposure technique to create blurring of ribs and lung markings.
15. Anterior dislocation of the proximal humerus

## Review Exercise D: Critique Radiographs of the Proximal Humerus and Shoulder Girdle

A. AP clavicle (Fig. C6-85)
1. All of clavicle demonstrated

2. Rotation of body toward the right, superimposing sternal end over the spine and creating overall distortion of the clavicle and associated joints
3. Collimation much too loose and not evident at all; central ray centered too low (inferiorly), which also adds to distorted appearance of clavicle
4. Acceptable but slightly underexposed exposure factors
5. Missing (or not visible) anatomic marker
Repeatable error(s): 2 and 5

B. AP apical oblique axial shoulder (Fig. C6-86)
1. All pertinent anatomic structures demonstrated but severely distorted
2. Correct positioning of shoulder
3. Evidence of acceptable side collimation (no evidence of top and bottom collimation); excessive central ray angulation, leading to distortion of anatomic structures (see p. 201 in textbook for correct appearance of this projection); excessive OID also a possible cause of this distortion
4. Acceptable but slightly underexposed exposure factors
5. Missing (or not visible) anatomic marker
Repeatable error(s): 1, 3, and 5

C. AP scapula (Fig. C6-87)
1. Lower margin of scapula cut off at bottom edge of radiograph
2. Acceptable part positioning
3. Collimation too loose or not evident; need to center central ray and cassette to include the entire scapula
4. Underexposed scapula and blurring of ribs, not evident from breathing technique
5. Missing (or not visible) anatomic marker
Repeatable error(s): 1, 3, 4, and 5

D. AP shoulder and proximal humerus (Fig. C6-88)
1. Majority of the shoulder girdle cut off and not demonstrated
2. Correct part positioning for AP projection, but centering is off
3. Evidence of collimation on one side only, indicating incorrect centering; central ray and IR centering too lateral
4. Acceptable but slightly underexposed exposure factors
5. Acceptable; anatomic marker seen on radiograph
Repeatable error(s): 1 and 3
Position: AP projection, external rotation

# SELF-TEST

My Score = _____ %

This self-test should be taken only after completing all of the readings, review exercises, and laboratory activities for a particular section. The purpose of this test is not only to provide a good learning exercise but also to serve as a strong indicator of what your final unit evaluation exam will cover. It is strongly suggested that if you do not get at least a 90% to 95% grade on each self-test, you review those areas in which you missed questions before going to your instructor for the final unit evaluation exam. There are 50 questions or blanks—each is worth 2 points.

1. Select the term(s) that correctly describes the shoulder joint:

   A. Humeroscapular      C. Glenohumeral

   B. Scapulohumeral      D. B and C

2. Which specific joint is found on the lateral end of the clavicle?

   A. Scapulohumeral      C. Acromioclavicular

   B. Sternoclavicular     D. Glenohumeral

3. Which of the following is *not* an angle found on the scapula?

   A. Inferior angle       C. Lateral angle

   B. Medial angle         D. Superior angle

4. Which one of the following structures of the scapula extends most anteriorly?

   A. Glenoid cavity       C. Scapular spine

   B. Acromion             D. Coracoid process

5. True/False: The male clavicle is shorter and less curved than the female clavicle.

6. Which bony structure separates the supraspinous and infraspinous fossae?

   A. Scapular spine       C. Acromion

   B. Glenoid cavity       D. Superior border of scapula

7. Which one of the following structures is considered to be the most posterior?

   A. Scapular notch       C. Acromion

   B. Coracoid process     D. Glenoid process

8. What is the type of joint movement for the scapulohumeral joint?

   A. Plane                C. Ellipsoidal

   B. Spheroidal           D. Trochoidal

9.  Identify the labeled structures on Fig. 6-11 (terms may be used more than once):

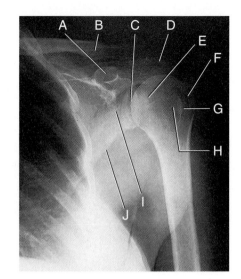

**Fig. 6-11.** Shoulder projection.

_____ A.     1.  Spine of scapula

_____ B.     2.  Lesser tubercle

_____ C.     3.  Coracoid process

_____ D.     4.  Lateral (axillary) border of scapula

_____ E.     5.  Scapulohumeral joint

_____ F.     6.  Clavicle

_____ G.     7.  Intertubercular groove

_____ H.     8.  Acromion of scapula

_____ I.     9.  Neck of scapula

_____ J.    10.  Greater tubercle

K.  Does Fig. 6-11 represent (A) an internal, (B) an external, or

    (C) a neutral rotation of the humerus? _____

Identify the labeled structures on Fig. 6-12 (terms may be used more than once):

**Fig. 6-12.** Shoulder projection.

_____ L.    11.  Lateral extremity of clavicle

_____ M.    12.  Head of humerus

_____ N     13.  Glenoid cavity

_____ O.

_____ P.

_____ Q.

_____ R.

S.  What is the correct term and method for the projection seen on Fig. 6-12?

    A.  Inferosuperior axial projection—Lawrence method

    B.  Transthoracic lateral—Lawrence method

    C.  Posterior oblique—Grashey method

10.  Which one of the following technical considerations does not apply for adult shoulder radiography?

    A.  Center and right automatic exposure control (AEC) chambers activated

    B.  High-speed film-screen system

    C.  40- to 44-in (100- to 110-cm) SID

    D.  70- to 80-kV (with grids)

11. True/False: Even though the amount of radiation exposure is minimal for most shoulder projections, gonadal shielding should be used for children and adults of childbearing age.

12. True/False: The greatest technical concern during a pediatric shoulder study is voluntary motion.

13. Which one of the following imaging modalities/procedures best demonstrates osteomyelitis?

    A. Ultrasound          C. Arthrography

    B. MRI                 D. Nuclear medicine

14. Which one of the following imaging modalities/procedures provides a functional, or dynamic, study of the shoulder joint?

    A. Ultrasound          C. Nuclear medicine

    B. Radiography         D. MRI

15. Match each of the following pathologic indications to its correct definition:

    _____ 1. Disability of the shoulder joint caused by chronic inflammation in and around the joint

    _____ 2. Lesion of the anteroinferior glenoid rim

    _____ 3. Chronic systemic disease with arthritic inflammatory changes throughout the body

    _____ 4. Superior displacement of distal clavicle

    _____ 5. Compression fracture of humeral head

    _____ 6. Traumatic injury to one or more muscles of the shoulder joint

    _____ 7. Reduction in the quantity of bone

    A. Rotator cuff tear

    B. Osteoporosis

    C. Rheumatoid condition

    D. Idiopathic chronic adhesive capsulitis

    E. Bankart lesion

    F. Acromioclavicular joint dislocation

    G. Hill-Sachs defect

16. Which one of the following projections/positions best demonstrates signs of impingement syndrome?

    A. AP and lateral shoulder     C. Transaxillary with exaggerated, external rotation

    B. Transaxillary               D. "Scapular Y" (or Neer method)

17. Which one of the following pathologic conditions produces narrowing of the joint space?

    A. Osteoarthritis      C. Osteoporosis

    B. Bursitis            D. Idiopathic chronic adhesive capsulitis

18. Which one of the following pathologic conditions may require a reduction in manual exposure factors?

    A. Bursitis                    C. Rotator cuff tear

    B. Rheumatoid arthritis        D. Bankart lesion

19. Which basic projection of the shoulder requires that the humeral epicondyles be parallel to the cassette?

    A. External rotation   C. Internal rotation

    B. Neutral rotation    D. Grashey method

20. Where is the central ray centered for an AP projection of the shoulder?

    A. Acromion                                    C. 1 inch (2.5 cm) inferior to coracoid process

    B. 1 inch (2.5 cm) superior to coracoid process    D. 2 inches (5 cm) inferior to acromioclavicular joint

21. Which position of the shoulder and proximal humerus projects the lesser tubercle in profile medially?

    A. External rotation        C. Internal rotation

    B. Neutral rotation         D. Exaggerated rotation

22. What central ray angle should be used for the inferosuperior axial (Lawrence) projection?

    A. 15° medially             C. 25° anteriorly and medially

    B. 25° to 30° medially   D. 35° to 45° medially

23. To best demonstrate the Hill-Sachs defect on the inferosuperior axiolateral projection, which additional positioning maneuver must be used?

    A. Angle central ray 35° medially          C. Use exaggerated internal rotation

    B. Use exaggerated external rotation      D. Abduct arm 120° rotation from midsagittal plane (MSP)

24. The inferosuperior axial projection (Westpoint method) requires a double central ray angulation of:

    A. 25° anterior and medial        C. 15° anterior and medial

    B. 5° medial and 15° anterior    D. 30° medial and 5° anterior

25. Which special projection of the shoulder places the glenoid cavity in profile for an "open" glenohumeral joint?

    A. Garth method                              C. Fisk method

    B. Transthoracic lateral—Lawrence method    D. Grashey method

26. For the erect version of the tangential projection for the intertubercular groove, the patient leans forward

    _____ from vertical.

    A. 5° to 7°          C. 10° to 15°

    B. 20° to 25°       D. 35° to 45°

27. What is the major advantage of the supine, tangential version of the intertubercular groove projection over the erect version?

    A. Less radiation exposure        C. Less risk for motion

    B. Reduced OID                     D. Ability to use automatic exposure control (AEC)

28. Which one of the following projections best demonstrates the supraspinatus outlet region?

    A. Neer method        C. Inferosuperior axial—Lawrence method

    B. Fisk method         D. Inferosuperior axial—Westpoint method

29. With which one of the following projections is a breathing technique preferred?

    A. Grashey method        C. Scapular Y

    B. Transthoracic lateral    D. Garth method

30. What central ray angulation is required for the supraspinatus outlet tangential projection (Neer method)?

    A. 10° to 15° caudad        C. 25° anteriorly and medially

    B. 45° caudad                 D. None; central ray is perpendicular

31. Which pathologic feature is best demonstrated with the Garth method?

    A. Bursitis                         C. Scapulohumeral dislocations

    B. Rheumatoid arthritis       D. Signs of shoulder impingement

32. True/False: A posteroanterior (PA) axial projection of the clavicle requires a 15° to 20° caudal central ray angle.

33. True/False: A 72-inch (180-cm) SID is recommended for acromioclavicular joint studies.

34. Match each of the following dose and projection types (assuming small- to average-size adult with accurate collimation) to its correct patient dose range (dose ranges may be used more than once):

    _____  1.  Thyroid dose for AP acromioclavicular joints            A.  1000 mrad or more

    _____  2.  Breast dose for AP shoulder                             B.  40 to 100 mrad

    _____  3.  Thyroid dose for AP shoulder                            C.  10 mrad or less

    _____  4.  Skin dose for AP shoulder

    _____  5.  Skin dose for transthoracic lateral

    _____  6.  Breast dose for AP acromioclavicular joints (two projections)

    _____  7.  Breast dose for scapular Y lateral

    _____  8.  Breast or thyroid dose for inferosuperior axiolateral shoulder

35. A radiograph of the Grashey method reveals that the anterior and posterior glenoid rims are not superimposed. The following positioning factors were used: erect position, body rotated 35° toward the affected side, central ray perpendicular to scapulohumeral joint space, and affected arm slightly abducted in neutral rotation. Which one of the following modifications will superimpose the glenoid rims during the repeat exposure?

    A.  Angle central ray 10° to 15° caudad       C.  Place affected arm in external rotation position

    B.  Rotate body less toward affected side       D.  Rotate body more toward affected side

36. **Situation:** A patient with a possible shoulder dislocation enters the emergency room. A neutral, AP projection of the shoulder has been taken, confirming a dislocation. Which additional projection should be taken?

    A.  Grashey method                              C.  Garth method

    B.  Inferosuperior axial projection—Lawrence method    D.  AP, external rotation

37. A radiograph of an AP axial clavicle taken on an asthenic type patient reveals that the clavicle is projected in the lung field below the top of the shoulder. The following positioning factors were used: erect position, central ray angled 15° cephalad, 40-inch (100-cm) SID, and respiration suspended at end of expiration. Which one of the following modifications should be made during the repeat exposure?

    A.  Increase central ray angulation             C.  Reverse central ray angulation

    B.  Suspend respiration at end of inspiration    D.  Use 72-inch (180-cm) SID

38. **Situation:** A patient with a possible acromioclavicular separation enters the emergency room. Which one of the following routines should be used?

    A.  Acromioclavicular joint series: non-weight-bearing and weight-bearing projections

    B.  AP neutral projection and Garth method

    C.  AP neutral and transthoracic lateral projections

    D.  AP internal and external projections

**6**

39. **Situation:** A patient comes to the radiology department with a history of tendonitis of the bicep tendon. Which of the following projections will best demonstrate calcification of the tendon within the intertubercular groove?

   A. Garth method

   B. Grashey method

   C. Inferosuperior axial projection—West point method

   D. Tangential projection—Fisk method

40. An AP apical oblique axial (Garth method) radiographic image demonstrates poor visibility of the shoulder joint. The technologist used the following factors: Patient erect, facing the x-ray tube, 45° of rotation of affected shoulder toward the IR, 45° cephalad angle, and the CR centered to the scapulohumeral joint. What of the following factors would have contributed to this poor Garth position?

   A. Wrong direction of CR angle

   B. Incorrect CR centering

   C. Position must be performed recumbent

   D. Shoulder rotated in wrong direction

41. For the following critique questions, see Fig. C6-85, an AP clavicle radiograph, on p. 208 in your textbook.

   A. Which positioning error(s) is(are) visible on this AP left clavicle radiograph? (More than one answer may be selected.)

      (a) All essential anatomic structures are not demonstrated.

      (b) Central ray is centered incorrectly.

      (c) Collimation is not evident.

      (d) Exposure factors are incorrect.

      (e) No anatomic marker is visible on the radiograph.

      (f) Slight rotation toward the right is evident.

      (g) Slight rotation toward the left is evident.

   B. Which error(s) identified above is(are) considered "repeatable"? _____

   C. Which of the following modifications must be made during the repeat exposure? (More than one answer may be selected.)

      (a) Increase collimation.

      (b) Center central ray correctly.

      (c) Decrease exposure factors.

      (d) Increase exposure factors.

      (e) Place anatomic marker on image receptor (IR) before exposure.

      (f) Ensure that no rotation occurs to the right or left.

42.   For the following critique questions, refer to the AP scapula radiograph, Fig. C6-87, on p. 208 in your textbook.

    A.   Which positioning error(s) is(are) visible on this radiograph? (More than one answer may be selected.)

        (a)   All essential anatomic structures are not demonstrated.

        (b)   Central ray is centered incorrectly.

        (c)   Collimation is not evident.

        (d)   Exposure factors are incorrect.

        (e)   No anatomic marker is visible on radiograph.

        (f)   Excessive rotation toward the right is evident.

        (g)   Excessive rotation toward the left is evident.

    B.   Which error(s) identified above is(are) considered "repeatable"? _____

    C.   Which of the following modifications must be made during the repeat exposure? (More than one answer may be selected.)

        (a)   Increase collimation.

        (b)   Center central ray more inferiorly.

        (c)   Decrease exposure factors.

        (d)   Increase exposure factors.

        (e)   Place anatomic marker on IR before exposure.

        (f)   Rotate body slightly toward the left.

        (g)   Rotate elbow slightly toward the right.

# 7

# Lower Limb

After you have successfully completed the activities in this chapter, you will be able to:

_____  1. Identify the bones and specific features of the toes, foot, ankle, lower leg, knee, patella, and distal femur.

_____  2. On drawings and radiographs, identify specific anatomic features of the foot, ankle, leg, knee, patella, and distal femur.

_____  3. Identify specific joints of the foot, ankle, leg, and knee according to the correct classification and movement type.

_____  4. Match specific pathologic indications of the lower limb to the correct definition.

_____  5. Match specific pathologic indications of the lower limb to the correct radiographic appearance.

_____  6. Describe the basic and special projections of the toes, foot, ankle, calcaneus, knee, patella, intercondylar fossa, and femur, including central ray placement and angulation, correct image receptor size and placement, part positioning, technical factors, and evaluation criteria.

_____  7. List the various patient dose ranges for each projection of the lower limb.

_____  8. Given various hypothetical situations, identify the correct modification of a position and/or exposure factors to improve the radiographic image.

_____  9. Given various hypothetical situations, identify the correct position for a specific pathologic form or condition.

_____ 10. Given radiographs of specific lower limb projections, identify specific positioning and exposure factor errors.

## Positioning and Radiographic Critique

_____  1. Using a peer, perform basic and special projections of the lower limb.

_____  2. Using foot and knee phantoms, produce satisfactory radiographs of the lower limb (if equipment is available).

_____  3. Critique and evaluate lower limb radiographs based on the four divisions of radiographic criteria: (1) structures shown, (2) position, (3) collimation and central ray, and (4) exposure criteria.

_____  4. Distinguish between acceptable and unacceptable lower limb radiographs based on exposure factors, motion, collimation, positioning, or other errors.

## Learning Exercises

Complete the following review exercises after reading the associated pages in the textbook as indicated by each exercise. Answers to each review exercise are given at the end of the review exercises.

## Part I: Radiographic Anatomy

**REVIEW EXERCISE A:** Radiographic Anatomy of the Foot and Ankle (see textbook pp. 210-215)

1. Fill in the number of bones for the following:    1— 19

   A.  Phalanges  _14_          C.  Tarsals  _7_

   B.  Metatarsals  _5_         D.  Total  _26_

2. What are two differences in the phalanges of the foot as compared with the phalanges of the hand?

   A.  _feet phalanges are smaller_

   B.  _feet phalanges JOINTS are less moveable_

3. Which tuberosity of the foot is palpable and a common site of foot trauma?

   _At the base of the fifth metatarsal laterally is a tuberosity_
   _Tuberosity of the base of the fifth metatarsal._

4. Where are the sesamoid bones of the foot most commonly located? _1ST metatarsulo phalange joint_
   _The plantar surface of the foot near the 1st metatarophaglx posterior joint_

5. What is the largest and strongest tarsal bone? _Calcaneus_

6. What is the name of the joint found between the talus and calcaneus? _talocalcaneal_

7. List the three specific articular facets found in the joint described in the previous question.

   A.  _anterior_          B.  _middle_          C.  _posterior_

8. The small opening, or space, found between the talus and calcaneus is called the:

   _Sinus Taris_ .

9. Match each of the following characteristics to the correct tarsal bone (answers may be used more than once):

   _B_    1.  Forms an aspect of the ankle joint          A.  Calcaneus

   _F_    2.  The smallest of the cuneiforms             B.  Talus

   _D_    3.  Found on the medial side of the foot       C.  Cuboid
            between the talus
                                                         D.  Navicular
   _G_    4.  The largest of the cuneiforms
                                                         E.  Lateral cuneiform
   _E_    5.  Articulates with the second, third,
            and fourth metatarsal                        F.  Intermediate cuneiform

   _B_    6.  The most superior tarsal bone              G.  Medial cuneiform

   _G_    7.  Articulates with the first metatarsal

   _A_    8.  Contains the sustentaculum tali

   _C_    9.  A tarsal found anterior to the
            calcaneus and lateral to the lateral
            cuneiform

   _B_    10.  The second largest tarsal bone

10.  Identify the labeled structures found in Figs. 7-1 and 7-2:

A.  _Sinus Tarsi_

B.  _Talus_

C.  _Navicular_

D.  _(3rd) lateral cuneiform_

E.  _Base of 1st metatarsal_

F.  _Body of 1st metatarsal_

G.  _Sesamoid_

H.  _1st digit metatarsophalangeal joint_

I.  _Distal phalanx_

J.  _Base of 5th metatarsal_

K.  _Cuboid_

L.  _calcaneal tuberosity_

**Fig. 7-1.** Anatomy of the foot.

M.  Fig. 7-1 represents a radiograph of which projection

of the foot? _AP 45° medial oblique_

N.  _tuberosity of the calcaneus_

O.  _Lateral process of calcaneos_

P.  _Trochlear process_

Q.  _lateral malleolus of fibula_

R.  _sustentaculum Tali_

S.  _Talocalcaneal joint_

T.  Fig. 7-2 represents a radiograph of which projection?

_Plantodorsal (axial) proj_

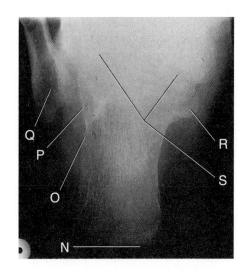

**Fig. 7-2.** Anatomy of the foot.

11.  True/False: The cuboid articulates with the four bones of the foot.

12.  The calcaneus articulates with the talus and the:

A.  Navicular          C.   Medial cuneiform

B.  Cuboid            D.   Lateral cuneiform

13.  List the two arches of the foot:   A.  _Transverse arch_   B.  _longitudinal arch_

14.  Which three bones make up the ankle joint?

A.  _Talus_                    B.  _Tibia_                    C.  _Fibula_

**7**

15. The three bones of the ankle form a deep socket into which the talus fits. This socket is called the _____

_____ Ankle mortise _____ .

16. The distal tibial joint surface forming the roof of the distal ankle joint is called the:

    (A) Tibial plafond         C.   Tibial plateau

    B.   Articular facet        D.   Ankle mortise

17. True/False: The medial malleolus is approximately ½ inch (1 cm) posterior to the lateral malleolus.

18. The ankle joint is classified as a synovial joint with ___ hinge ___ type movement.

19. Identify the structures labeled on Figs. 7-3 and 7-4:

    *Fig. 7-3:*

    A. ___ Tuberosity of the base of the 5th metatarsal ___

    B. ___ lateral malleolus of Fibula ___

    C. ___ Distal tibiofibular joint ___

    D. ___ medial malleolus of Tibia ___

    E. ___ Talus ___

    *Fig. 7-4:*

    F. ___ Calcaneus ___

    G. ___ Sinus tarsi ___

    H. ___ talus ___

    I. ___ tibial plafond ___

    J. ___ Anterior tubercle ___

    K. ___ Navicular ___

    L. ___ Cuboid ___

**Fig. 7-3.** Anatomy of the ankle.     **Fig. 7-4.** Anatomy of the ankle.

    M.  Fig. 7-3 represents a radiograph of which projection of the ankle? ___ AP Mortise proj 10°-15° rotation ___

**REVIEW EXERCISE B:** Radiographic Anatomy of the Lower Leg, Knee, and Distal Femur (see textbook pp. 216-220)

1. The ___ Tibia ___ is the weight-bearing bone of the lower leg.

2. What is the name of the large prominence located on the midanterior surface of the proximal tibia that serves as a distal attachment for the patellar ligament? ___ Tibia tuberosity ___

3. What is the name of the small prominence located on the posterior border of the medial condyle of the femur that is an identifying landmark to determine possible rotation of a lateral knee? ___ Adductor tuberosity ___

4. A small, triangular depression located on the tibia that helps form the distal tibiofibular joint is called the

_Fibular notch_ .

5. The articular facets of the proximal tibia are also referred to as the _Tibia plateau_ .

6. The articular facets slope _10°-15°_ ° posteriorly.

   A. 25      C. 35

   B. 45      D. 10 to 15

7. The most proximal aspect of the fibula is the _Apex or Styloid process_

8. The extreme distal end of the fibula forms the _lateral malleolus_

9. What is the name of the largest sesamoid bone in the body? _Patella_

10. What are two other names for the patellar surface of the femur?

    A. _Intercondylar sulcus_          B. _Trochlear groove_

11. What is the name of the depression located on the posterior aspect of the distal femur?

    _Intercondylar fossa or notch_

12. Why must the central ray be angled 5° to 7° cephalad for a lateral knee position?

    _The medial condyle extends lower than the lateral condyle of the femur 5-7°_

13. The slightly raised area located on the posterolateral aspect of the medial condyle is called the:

    A. Trochlear tubercle      C. Adductor tubercle

    B. Anterior crest          D. Tibial tuberosity

14. What are the two palpable bony landmarks found on the distal femur?

    A. _Medial condyle_          B. _lateral condyle_

15. The general region of the posterior knee is called the _Popliteal region_

16. True/False: Flexion of 20° of the knee forces the patella firmly against the patellar surface of the femur.

17. True/False: The patella acts like a pivot to increase the leverage of a large muscle found in the anterior thigh.

18. True/False: The posterior surface of the patella is normally rough.

19. For which large muscle does the patella serve as a pivot to increase the leverage?

    _quadriceps femoris_ .

20. List the correct terms for the following joints:

    A. Between the patella and distal femur _patellofemoral_

    B. Between the two condyles of the femur and tibia _femorotibial_

21. List the four major ligaments of the knee:

A. _ACl anterior cruciate ligament_    C. _LCL lateral Colateral ligament_

B. _PCl Posterior cruciaTe ligament_    D. _MCL medial Collateral lig._

22. The crescent-shaped fibrocartilage disks that act as shock absorbers in the knee joint are called _lateral & medial meniscus_

23. List the two bursae found in the knee joint.

A. _Infrapatellar_    B. _Suprapatellar_

24. Match each of the following structures to the correct bone (answers may be used more than once):

_A_    1. Tibial plafond          A. Tibia

_A_    2. Medial malleolus        B. Fibula

_C_    3. Lateral epicondyle      C. Distal femur

_C_    4. Patellar surface        D. Patella

_A_    5. Articular facets

_A_    6. Fibular notch

_B_    7. Styloid process

_D_    8. Base

_A_    9. Intercondyloid eminence

_B_   10. Neck

25. Match each of the following articulations to the correct joint classification or movement type (answers may be used more than once):

_B_    1. Ankle joint            A. Synarthrodial (gomphoses type)

_C_    2. Patellofemoral         B. Ginglymus (hinge)

_D_    3. Proximal tibiofibular  C. Sellar (saddle)

_D_    4. Tarsometatarsal        D. Plane (gliding)

_B_    5. Knee joint (femorotibial)   E. Amphiarthrodial (syndesmosis type)

_E_    6. Distal tibiofibular

26.   Identify the labeled structures on Figs. 7-5 through 7-7.

*Fig. 7-5:*

A. fibular notch / distal tibiofibular joint

B. body (shaft) of fibula

C. Articular facets / tibial plateau

D. lateral condyle

E. Intercondylar eminence

F. medial condyle

G. tibia tuberosity

H. Anterior crest of body / shaft

I. medial malleous

*Fig. 7-6:*

J. lateral malleous

K. Fibula body

L. fibula neck

M. fibula head

N. fibula apex

O. 10-120° (degree angle)

P. tibial tuberosity

Q. tibial body

R. medial malleous

*Fig. 7-7:*

S. lateral condyle

T. patellar surface/intercondylar sulcus/ trochlear groove

U. medial condyle

V. patellofemoral joint

W. patella

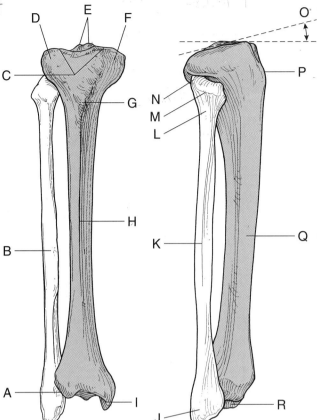

**Fig. 7-5.** Frontal view of tibia and fibula.    **Fig. 7-6.** Lateral view of tibia and fibula.

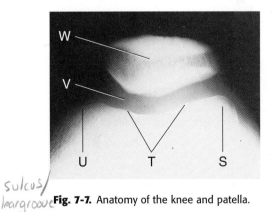

**Fig. 7-7.** Anatomy of the knee and patella.

X.   Which projection does the radiograph in Fig. 7-7 represent?   Tangential projection of patellofemoral joint

27. Identify the bony structures labeled on Figs. 7-8 and 7-9:

*Fig. 7-8:*

A. _Patella Base_

B. _Patella Apex_

C. _Tibial Tuberosity_

D. _Fibula Neck_

E. _Fibula Head_

F. _Fibula Apex of head (styloid process)_

G. _Medial & lateral condyles superimposed_

H. _Patellar surface / intercondylar sulcos / trochlear groove_

**Fig. 7-8.** True lateral radiograph of the knee.

*Fig. 7-9*

I. _Adductor Tubercle_

J. _lateral condyle_

K. _medial condyle_

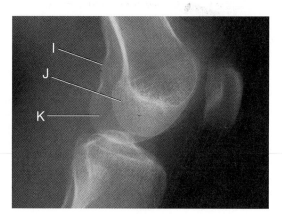

**Fig. 7-9.** Lateral radiograph of the knee.

28. Match the following foot and ankle movements to the correct definition:

   **1**    A. Inward turning or bending of ankle                        1. Inversion (varus)

   **4**    B. Decreasing the angle between the dorsum pedis and anterior lower leg     2. Plantar flexion

   **2**    C. Extending the ankle or pointing the foot and toe downward           3. Eversion (valgus)

   **3**    D. Outward turning or bending of ankle                    4. Dorsiflexion

## Part II: Radiographic Positioning

10·29

**REVIEW EXERCISE C:** Positioning of the Foot and Ankle (see textbook pp. 223-242)

1. True/False: The recommended source image receptor distance (SID) for lower limb radiography is 40 inches (100 cm).

2. True/False: To reduce scatter radiation during table top procedures, the Bucky tray should be positioned over the lower limb being radiographed.

3. True/False: With careful and close collimation, gonadal shielding does not have to be used during lower limb radiography.

4. True/False: During digital radiography, lead masking should be placed on the regions of the imaging plate, not within the collimation field.

5. True/False: A kilovoltage peak range between 50 and 70 should be used for film-screen lower limb radiography.

6. Match the following pathologic indications to the correct definition: p 229

| ___9___ | A. | An inflammatory condition involving the anterior, proximal tibia | 1. | Exostosis |
| ___8___ | B. | Also known as *osteitis deformans* | 2. | Joint effusion |
| ___10___ | C. | Malignant tumor of the cartilage | 3. | Bone cyst |
| ___7___ | D. | Inherited type of arthritis that commonly affects males | 4. | Reiter's syndrome |
| ___1___ | E. | Benign, neoplastic bone lesion caused by overproduction of bone at a joint | 5. | Osteoid osteoma |
| ___5___ | F. | Benign bone lesion usually developing in teens or young adults | 6. | Ewing's sarcoma |
| ___6___ | G. | Most prevalent primary bone malignancy in pediatric patients | 7. | Gout |
| ___3___ | H. | Benign, neoplastic bone lesion filled with clear fluid | 8. | Paget's disease |
| ___2___ | I. | Accumulated fluid in the joint cavity | 9. | Osgood-Schlatter disease |
| ___4___ | J. | Condition affecting the sacroiliac joints and lower limbs of young men, especially the posterosuperior margin of the calcaneus | 10. | Chondrosarcoma |

7. The formal name for "runner's knee" is _Chondromalacia paTellae_ .

8. What is another term for *osteomalacia*? _rickeTs_

9. Match the following radiographic appearances to the correct pathologic indication: p226

| ___7___ | A. | Asymmetric erosion of joint spaces with calcaneal erosion | 1. | Osteoid osteoma |
| ___3___ | B. | Uric acid deposits in joint spaces | 2. | Ewing's sarcoma |
| ___8___ | C. | Well-circumscribed lucency | 3. | Gout |
| ___1___ | D. | Small, round/oval density with lucent center | 4. | Osgood-Schlatter disease |
| ___5___ | E. | Narrowed, irregular joint surfaces with sclerotic articular surfaces | 5. | Osteoarthritis |
| ___4___ | F. | Fragmentation or detachment of the tibial tuberosity | 6. | Osteomalacia |
| ___2___ | G. | Ill-defined area of bone destruction with surrounding "onion peel" | 7. | Reiter's syndrome |
| ___6___ | H. | Decreased bone density and bowing deformities of weight-bearing limbs | 8. | Bone cyst |

10. Why is the central ray angled 10° to 15° toward the calcaneus for an anteroposterior (AP) projection of the toes?

_Open up interphalange joints ʔ mTp joinTs_

11. Where is the central ray centered for an AP oblique projection of the foot? _base of Third metatarsal_

12. Which projection is best for demonstrating the sesamoid bones of the foot? _Tangential proj_

13. The foot should be dorsiflexed so that the plantar surface of the foot is __15-20__ ° from vertical for the sesamoid projection.

14. Why should the central ray be angled 10° posterior for an AP projection of the foot?
_Opens up metatarsophalangeal & interophalangeal joints_   (MTP)   (I P)

15. If a foreign body is lodged in the plantar surface of the foot, which type of central ray angle should be used for the AP projection?

    A.   10° posterior          C.   10° anterior

    B.   15° posterior          (D.)  None; use a perpendicular central ray

16. Rotation can be determined on a radiograph of an AP foot projection by the near-equal distance between the
    _2nd to 5th_ _____ metatarsals.

17. Which oblique projection of the foot best demonstrates the majority of the tarsal bones?
    _AP Oblique w/ medial rotation_

18. Which oblique projection of the foot best demonstrates the navicular and the first and second cuneiforms with
    minimal superimposition? _AP Oblique w/ lateral rotation_

19. Which projection tends to place the foot into a truer lateral position—mediolateral or lateromedial?
    _lateromedial proj_

20. Which type of study should be performed to best evaluate the condition of the longitudinal arches of the foot?
    _AP & lateral weight Bearing proj_

21. How should the central ray be angled from the long axis of the foot for the plantodorsal axial projection of the
    calcaneus? _40° Cephalad_

22. Which calcaneal structure should appear medially on a well-positioned plantodorsal projection?
    _Sustentaculum Tali_

23. Where is the central ray placed for a lateral projection of the calcaneus? _____
    _1/4" inferior To the medial malleolus_

24. Which joint surface is *not* visualized with a correctly positioned AP projection of the ankle?

    A.   Medial aspect of joint        (C.)  Lateral aspect of joint

    B.   Superior aspect of joint      D.   All of the above aspects of the joint *are* visualized.

25. Why should AP, 45° oblique, and lateral ankle radiographs include the proximal metatarsals?
    _To demonstrate a fracture on The 5th metatarsal tuberosity._

26.   How much (if any) should the foot and ankle be rotated for a mortise projection of the ankle?

_____ 15°-20° medial _____

27.   Which projection of the ankle best demonstrates a possible fracture of the lateral malleolus?

_____ AP Oblique w/ medial rotation _____

28.   With a true lateral projection of the ankle, the lateral malleolus is:

A.   Projected over the anterior aspect of the distal tibia

(B.)   Projected over the posterior aspect of the distal tibia

C.   Directly superimposed over the distal tibia

D.   Directly superimposed over the medial malleolus

29.   Which projections of the ankle require forced inversion and eversion movements?

_____ AP STress proj _____

15-25

**REVIEW EXERCISE D:** Positioning of the Tibia, Fibula, Knee, and Distal Femur (see textbook pp. 243-258)

1.   What is the basic positioning routine for a study of the tibia and fibula?   AP ; lateral proj

2.   Why is it important to include the knee joint for an initial study of tibia trauma, even if the patient's symptoms involve the middle and distal aspect?

_____ because a fracture may exist proximal tibia in addition to distally _____

3.   To include both joints for a lateral projection of the tibia and fibula for an adult, the technologist may place the

cassette _____ in relation to the part.

A.   Parallel          (C.) Diagonally

B.   Perpendicular     D.   Transverse

4.   What is the recommended central ray angulation for an AP projection of the knee for a patient with thick thighs and buttocks (i.e., measuring greater than 24 cm)?

A.   3° to 5° caudad        C.   Central ray perpendicular to IR

(B.)   3° to 5° cephalad      D.   Central ray perpendicular to patellar plane

5.   Where is the central ray centered for an AP projection of the knee?

(A.)   ½ inch (1.25 cm) distal to apex of patella          C.   Midpatella

B.   1 inch (2½ cm) proximal to apex of patella          D.   Level of tibial tuberosity

6.   Which basic projection of a knee best demonstrates the proximal fibula free of superimposition?

A.   True AP          (C.) AP oblique, 45° medial rotation

B.   True lateral     D.   AP oblique, 45° lateral rotation

7.   For the AP oblique projection of the knee, the _____ rotation (**medial [internal]** or

**lateral [external]**) best visualizes the lateral condyle of the tibia and the head and neck of the fibula.

7

8. What is the recommended central ray placement for a lateral knee position on a tall, slender male patient with a narrow pelvis?

   A. 3° to 5° caudad    C. Central ray perpendicular to IR

   B. 3° to 5° cephalad    D. Central ray perpendicular to patellar plane

9. How much flexion is recommended for a lateral projection of the knee?

   A. No flexion    C. 30° to 35°

   B. 20° to 30°    D. 45°

10. Which positioning error is present if the distal borders of the femoral condyles are not superimposed on a

    radiograph of a lateral knee? _Improper cephalic angle of The CR_

11. Which positioning error is present if the posterior portions of the femoral condyles are not superimposed on a

    lateral knee radiograph? _Over or under roTation of The knee_

12. Which anatomic structure of the femur can be used to determine which rotation error (overrotation or underrotation) is present on a slightly rotated lateral knee radiograph?

    _adductor tubercle on posTerolateral aspect of medial femoral condyle_

13. Which special projection of the knee best evaluates the knee joint for cartilage degeneration or deformities?

    _AP wt-bearing Bilateral knee proj_

14. AP knee stress projections are performed to demonstrate:

    A. Patellar dislocation    C. Medial or collateral ligament damage

    B. Osgood-Schlatter disease    D. Osteoarthritis

15. Which one of the following special projections of the knee best demonstrates the intercondylar fossa?

    A. Holmblad    C. AP weight-bearing, bilateral projections

    B. Merchant    D. Settegast

16. How much flexion of the lower leg is required for the Camp-Coventry projection when the central ray is angled 40°

    caudad? _40° flexion_

17. Why is the posteroanterior (PA) axial projection for the intercondylar fossa recommended instead of an AP axial

    projection? _DisTorTion caused by The CR angle ¿ increased OID for The AP_

18. True/False: To place the interepicondylar line parallel to the image receptor for a PA projection of the patella, the lower limb must be rotated approximately 5° internally.    _p252_

19. How much part flexion is recommended for a lateral projection of the patella?

    _p253_    _5° - 10°_

20. The skin dose range for an AP knee projection is:

    A. 5 to 10 mrad    C. 50 to 60 mrad

    B. 20 to 30 mrad    D. More than 100 mrad

21. How much central ray angle from the long axis of the femora is required for a Merchant bilateral projection?

    _30° from horizontal_

22.   How much part flexion is required for the following methods?

    A.   Hughston method _____45°_____

    B.   Settegast method _____90°_____

23.   Which of these methods (Hughston or Settegast) is preferred, and why?

*Stop*   Because acute knee flexion draws patella into intercondylar sulcus reducing the diagonostic value of this projection

24.   Match each of the following descriptions of positioning for projections of the knee and/or patella to its correct name (using each answer only once):

    __F__   1.   Patient on "all fours" on table

    __E__   2.   Patient prone; requires 90° knee flexion

    __D__   3.   Patient prone with 40° to 50° knee flexion and with equal 40° to 50° caudad CR angle

    ? __G__   4.   Curved cassette preferred

    __C__   5.   Patient prone with 45° knee flexion and 10° to 20° cephalad CR angle from long axis of lower leg.

    __A__   6.   Patient supine with cassette resting on midthighs

    __B__   7.   Patient supine with 40° knee flexion and with 30° caudad CR angle from horizontal

    A.   Inferosuperior axial for patellofemoral joint

    B.   Merchant method

    C.   Hughston method

    D.   Camp-Coventry method

    E.   Settegast method

    F.   Holmblad method

    G.   Béclere method ?

25.   To best utilize the anode-heel effect on a mediolateral hip projection, the hip should be placed under the

    _____ (**cathode** or **anode**) end?

11/4/2

*All*   **REVIEW EXERCISE E:** Problem Solving for Technical and Positioning Errors

1.   **Situation:** A radiograph of an AP projection of the foot reveals that the metatarsophalangeal joints are not open and the metatarsals are somewhat foreshortened. What was the positioning error involved, and what modification should be made to improve this image on the repeat exposure?

    CR angle is not correct it should be; CR↓ metatarsal ophalanges

2.   **Situation:** A radiograph of an AP oblique-medial rotation projection of the foot reveals that the proximal first and second metatarsals are completely superimposed. What type of positioning error led to this radiographic outcome?

    Over medial rotation of foot toward medial Direction

3.   **Situation:** A radiograph of a plantodorsal axial projection of the calcaneus reveals considerable foreshortening of the calcaneus. What type of positioning modification is needed on the repeat exposure?

    Increase cephalic angle of the central ray to correctly elongate calcaneus

4.   **Situation:** A radiograph of an AP projection of the ankle reveals that the lateral surface of the ankle joint is totally open. (It should not be open on a true AP projection.) The technologist is positive that the ankle was in the correct, true AP position with the long axis of the foot perpendicular to the IR. What else could have led to this joint space being open?

    A possible spread of the ankle mortise cause by rupture ligaments

5. **Situation:** A radiograph of an intended AP oblique-mortise projection reveals that the lateral malleolus is superimposed over the talus, and the distal tibiofibular joint is not well demonstrated. What is the most likely reason for this radiographic outcome?

Under rotation of the ankle toward the medial direction
The describe is an AP

6. **Situation:** A radiograph of an AP knee projection demonstrates that the femorotibial joint space is not open at all. The patient is young and has no history of degenerative disease. What type of positioning modification may improve the outcome of this projection?

Angle the CR to keep the jt parralld w/the tibial plateau

7. **Situation:** A radiograph of an intended AP oblique with **medial** rotation of the knee to demonstrate the proximal fibula reveals that there is total superimposition of the proximal tibia and the fibula. What must be modified to correct this projection?

This is the description of the lateral oblique proj (external rotation)

8. **Situation:** A radiograph of a lateral recumbent knee reveals that the posterior border of the medial femoral condyle (identified by the adductor tubercle) is not superimposed but is slightly posterior to the lateral condyle. The fibular head is also completely superimposed by the tibia. What type of positioning error led to this radiographic outcome?

Slightly rotated knee, Underrotated

9. **Situation:** A patient with trauma to the medial aspect of the foot comes to the emergency room. A heavy object was dropped on the foot near the base of the first metatarsal. Basic foot projections do not clearly demonstrate this region. What other projection of the foot could be used to better delineate this area?

Use AP lateral oblique proj w/ 30° external rotation of foot

10. **Situation:** A radiograph of an AP and lateral tibia and fibula reveals that the ankle is not included on the AP projection, but both the knee and the ankle are included on the lateral projection. What should the technologist do in this situation?

Repeat AP proj of tibia & fibula

11. **Situation:** A radiograph obtained by using the Camp-Coventry method reveals that the distal femoral condyles and intercondylar fossa are asymmetric. Which specific positioning error is present?

Rotattaion of affected leg

12. **Situation:** A radiograph of a lateral patella reveals that the patella is drawn tightly against the intercondylar sulcus. Which positioning modification should be performed to improve the quality of the image during the repeat exposure?

Decrease knee flexion to 5° - 10°

13. **Situation:** A patient with a history of degenerative disease of the left knee joint comes to the radiology department. The orthopedic surgeon orders a radiographic study to determine the extent of damage to the joint space. Which projection(s) should be performed?

AP or PA Bilateral wt bearing knee proj

14. **Situation:** A patient with a history of pain in the feet comes to the radiology department. The referring physician orders a study to examine the sesamoid bones. Which projection(s) would demonstrate these structures?

Tangental proj; Toes Sesamoids

15. **Situation:** A patient with a history of pain in the feet comes to the radiology department. The referring physician orders a study to evaluate the longitudinal arches of the feet. Which positioning routine should be used?

   _AP p lateral wT-Bearing proj; feet_

16. **Situation:** A patient with bony, loose bodies (or "joint mice") within the knee joint comes to radiology for a knee series. The AP and lateral knee projections fail to demonstrate any loose bodies. What additional knee projection can be taken to better demonstrate them?

   _Do PA Axial proj-Tunnel view; Knee   Intercondylar Fossa_

17. **Situation:** A young male patient comes to the radiology department with a clinical history of Osgood-Schlatter disease. Which single projection of the basic knee series will best demonstrate this condition?

   _Do a lateral knee proj._

18. **Situation:** A radiograph of a mediolateral knee projection demonstrates that the medial femoral condyle is projected inferior to the lateral condyle. What can the technologist do to correct this problem during the repeat exposure?

   _Use a CR 5-7° cephalic or more if angle wase used already_

**REVIEW EXERCISE F:** Critique Radiographs of the Lower Limbs (see textbook p. 259)

The following questions relate to the radiographs found at the end of Chapter 7 of the textbook. Evaluate these radiographs for the radiographic criteria categories (1 through 5) that follow. Describe the corrections needed to improve the overall image. The major, or "repeatable," errors are specific errors that indicate the need for a repeat exposure, regardless of the nature of the other errors.

   Comparing these radiographs with the correctly positioned and exposed radiographs in this chapter of the textbook will help you evaluate each of them for errors.

A. **Bilateral tangential patella (Fig. C7-146)**
   Description of possible error:

   1. Structures shown: _____

   2. Part positioning: _____

   3. Collimation and central ray: _____

   4. Exposure criteria: _____

   5. Markers: _____

   Repeatable error(s): _____

B. **AP foot (Fig. C7-147)**
   Description of possible error:

   1. Structures shown: _____

   2. Part positioning: _____

   3. Collimation and central ray: _____

   4. Exposure criteria: _____

   5. Markers: _____

   Repeatable error(s): _____

C. **Lateral ankle (Fig. C7-148)**
   Description of possible error:

   1. Structures shown: _____

   2. Part positioning: _____

   3. Collimation and central ray: _____

   4. Exposure criteria: _____

   5. Markers: _____

   Repeatable error(s): _____

D. **AP knee (Fig. C7-149)**
   Description of possible error:

   1. Structures shown: _____

   2. Part positioning: _____

   3. Collimation and central ray: _____

   4. Exposure criteria: _____

   5. Markers: _____

   Repeatable error(s): _____

E. **Lateral knee (Fig. C7-150)**
   Description of possible error:

   1. Structures shown: _____

   2. Part positioning: _____

   3. Collimation and central ray: _____

   4. Exposure criteria: _____

   5. Markers: _____

   Repeatable error(s): _____

F. **Lateral knee (Fig. C7-151)**
   Description of possible error:

   1. Structures shown: _____

   2. Part positioning: _____

   3. Collimation and central ray: _____

   4. Exposure criteria: _____

   5. Markers: _____

   Repeatable error(s): _____

## Part III: Laboratory Activities (see textbook pp. 228-258)

You must gain experience in positioning each part of the lower limb before performing the following exams on actual patients. You can get experience in positioning and radiographic evaluation of these projections by performing exercises using radiographic phantoms and practicing on other students (although you will not be taking actual exposures).

The following suggested activities assume that your teaching institution has an energized lab and radiographic phantoms. If not, perform Laboratory Exercises B and C, the radiographic evaluation and the physical positioning exercises. (Check off each step and projection as you complete it.)

### LABORATORY EXERCISE A: Energized Laboratory

1.   Using the foot/ankle radiographic phantom, produce radiographs of the basic routines for the following:

_____   Foot

_____   Ankle

_____   Calcaneus

2.   Using the knee radiographic phantom, produce radiographs of the following basic routines:

_____   AP

_____   AP oblique, medial rotation

_____   Lateral (horizontal beam lateral if flexed knee is not available)

### LABORATORY EXERCISE B: Radiographic Evaluation

1.   Evaluate and critique the radiographs produced above, additional radiographs provided by your instructor, or both. Evaluate each radiograph for the following points:

_____   Evaluate the completeness of the study. (Are all of the pertinent anatomic structures included on the radiograph?)

_____   Evaluate for positioning or centering errors (e.g., rotation, off centering).

_____   Evaluate for correct exposure factors and possible motion. (Are the density and contrast of the images acceptable?)

_____   Determine whether markers and an acceptable degree of collimation and/or area shielding are seen on the images.

### LABORATORY EXERCISE C: Physical Positioning

1.   On another person, simulate performing all basic and special projections of the lower limb as follows. Include the six steps listed below and described in the textbook. (Check off each step when completed satisfactorily.)

Step 1.  Appropriate size and type of image receptor with correct markers
Step 2.  Correct central ray placement and centering of part to central ray and/or image receptor
Step 3.  Accurate collimation
Step 4.  Area shielding of patient where advisable
Step 5.  Use of proper immobilizing devices when needed
Step 6.  Approximate correct exposure factors, breathing instructions where applicable, and "making" exposure

| *PROJECTIONS* | *STEP 1* | *STEP 2* | *STEP 3* | *STEP 4* | *STEP 5* | *STEP 6* |
|---|---|---|---|---|---|---|
| • Positioning routine for a specific toe | ____ | ____ | ____ | ____ | ____ | ____ |
| • Basic foot routine | ____ | ____ | ____ | ____ | ____ | ____ |
| • Special projection for sesamoid bones | ____ | ____ | ____ | ____ | ____ | ____ |
| • Basic projections of the calcaneus | ____ | ____ | ____ | ____ | ____ | ____ |
| • Weight-bearing foot projections | ____ | ____ | ____ | ____ | ____ | ____ |
| • Basic ankle routine, including mortise and 45° oblique projections | ____ | ____ | ____ | ____ | ____ | ____ |
| • AP and lateral tibia and fibula | ____ | ____ | ____ | ____ | ____ | ____ |
| • Basic knee routine | ____ | ____ | ____ | ____ | ____ | ____ |
| • Special projections for intercondylar fossa | ____ | ____ | ____ | ____ | ____ | ____ |
| • Weight-bearing AP knee projections | ____ | ____ | ____ | ____ | ____ | ____ |
| • Special projections for patellofemoral joint space | ____ | ____ | ____ | ____ | ____ | ____ |
| • AP and lateral midfemur projections | ____ | ____ | ____ | ____ | ____ | ____ |

7

# Answers to Review Exercises

## Review Exercise A: Radiographic Anatomy of the Foot and Ankle

1. A. 14
   B. 5
   C. 7
   D. 26
2. A. Phalanges of the foot are smaller.
   B. The joint movements of the foot are more limited than those of the hand.
3. Tuberosity of base of the fifth metatarsal
4. The plantar surface of the foot near the first metatarsophalangeal joint
5. Calcaneus
6. Subtalar or talocalcaneal
7. A. Posterior facet
   B. Anterior facet
   C. Middle facet
8. Sinus tarsi or tarsal sinus
9. 1. B
   2. F
   3. D
   4. G
   5. E
   6. B
   7. G
   8. A
   9. C
   10. B
10. A. Sinus tarsi (tarsal sinus)
    B. Talus
    C. Navicular
    D. Lateral cuneiform
    E. Base of first metatarsal
    F. Body (shaft) of first metatarsal
    G. Sesamoid bone
    H. Metatarsophalangeal (MTP) joint of first digit
    I. Distal phalanx of first digit
    J. Tuberosity at base of fifth metatarsal
    K. Cuboid
    L. Calcaneal tuberosity
    M. Anteroposterior (AP) 45° medial oblique
    N. Tuberosity of calcaneus
    O. Lateral process of calcaneus
    P. Peroneal trochlea (trochlear process)
    Q. Lateral malleolus of fibula
    R. Sustentaculum tali
    S. Talocalcaneal joint
    T. Plantodorsal (axial) projection of calcaneus
11. True
12. B. Cuboid
13. A. Longitudinal arch
    B. Transverse arch
14. A. Talus
    B. Tibia
    C. Fibula
15. Ankle mortise
16. A. Tibial plafond
17. False
18. Ginglymus or hinge
19. A. Tuberosity at base of fifth metatarsal (see fracture on radiograph in Fig. 7-3)
    B. Lateral malleolus of fibula
    C. Distal tibiofibular joint
    D. Medial malleolus
    E. Talus
    F. Calcaneus
    G. Sinus tarsi (tarsal sinus)
    H. Talus
    I. Tibial plafond
    J. Anterior tubercle
    K. Navicular
    L. Cuboid
    M. AP mortise, 15° to 20° medial rotation

## Review Exercise B: Radiographic Anatomy of the Lower Leg, Knee, and Distal Femur

1. Tibia
2. Tibial tuberosity
3. Adductor tubercle
4. Fibular notch
5. Tibial plateau
6. D. 10 to 15
7. Apex or styloid process
8. Lateral malleolus
9. Patella
10. A. Intercondylar sulcus
    B. Trochlear groove
11. Intercondylar fossa or notch
12. Because the medial condyle extends lower than the lateral condyle of the femur
13. C. Adductor tubercle
14. A. Medial epicondyle
    B. Lateral epicondyle
15. Popliteal region
16. False
17. True
18. False
19. Quadriceps femoris muscle
20. A. Patellofemoral
    B. Femorotibial
21. A. Fibular (lateral) collateral
    B. Tibial (medial) collateral
    C. Anterior cruciate
    D. Posterior cruciate
22. Medial and lateral menisci
23. A. Suprapatellar bursa
    B. Infrapatellar bursa
24. 1. A
    2. A
    3. C
    4. C
    5. A
    6. A
    7. B
    8. D
    9. A
    10. B
25. 1. B
    2. C
    3. D
    4. D
    5. B
    6. E
26. A. Fibular notch of tibia (also may be identified as distal tibiofibular joint)
    B. Body (shaft) of fibula
    C. Articular facets (or tibial plateau)
    D. Lateral condyle of tibia
    E. Intercondyloid eminence (tibial spine)
    F. Medial condyle of tibia
    G. Tibial tuberosity
    H. Anterior crest of body (shaft of tibia)
    I. Medial malleolus
    J. Lateral malleolus
    K. Body (shaft) of fibula
    L. Neck of fibula
    M. Head of fibula
    N. Apex or styloid process of fibula
    O. 10° to 20°
    P. Tibial tuberosity
    Q. Body (shaft) of tibia
    R. Medial malleolus
    S. Lateral condyle of femur
    T. Patellar surface of femur
    U. Medial condyle of femur
    V. Patellofemoral joint space
    W. Patella
    X. Tangential (patellofemoral joint)
27. A. Base of patella
    B. Apex of patella
    C. Tibial tuberosity
    D. Neck of fibula
    E. Head of fibula
    F. Apex or styloid process of fibula
    G. Superimposed medial and lateral condyles
    H. Patellar surface/intercondylar sulcus or trochlear groove
    I. Adductor tubercle
    J. Lateral femoral condyle
    K. Medial femoral condyle
28. A. 1
    B. 4
    C. 2
    D. 3

**7**

## Review Exercise C: Positioning of the Foot and Ankle

1. True
2. False
3. False
4. True
5. True
6. A. 9
   B. 8
   C. 10
   D. 7
   E. 1
   F. 5
   G. 6
   H. 3
   I. 2
   J. 4
7. Chondromalacia patellae
8. Rickets
9. A. 7
   B. 3
   C. 8
   D. 1
   E. 5
   F. 4
   G. 2
   H. 6
10. Opens up the interphalangeal and metatarsophalangeal joints
11. Base of third metatarsal
12. Tangential projection
13. 15° to 20°
14. Opens up metatarsophalangeal and certain intertarsal joints
15. D. None; use perpendicular central ray
16. Second to fifth
17. AP oblique with medial rotation
18. AP oblique with lateral rotation
19. Lateromedial
20. AP and lateral weight-bearing projections
21. 40° cephalad
22. Sustentaculum tali
23. 1½ inches (4 cm) inferior to the medial malleolus
24. C. Lateral aspect of joint
25. To demonstrate a possible fracture of the fifth metatarsal tuberosity (a common fracture site)
26. 15° to 20° (medially)
27. 45° AP oblique with medial rotation
28. B. Projected over the posterior aspect of the distal tibia
29. AP stress projections

## Review Exercise D: Positioning of the Tibia, Fibula, Knee, and Distal Femur

1. AP and lateral projections
2. A fracture may also be present at the proximal fibula in addition to the distal portion.
3. C. Diagonally
4. B. 3° to 5° cephalad
5. A. ½ inch (1.25 cm) distal to apex of patella
6. C. AP oblique, 45° medial rotation
7. Medial (internal)
8. B. 3° to 5° cephalad
9. B. 20° to 30°
10. Improper cephalad angle of the central ray
11. Overrotation or underrotation of the knee
12. Adductor tubercle on posterolateral aspect of the medial femoral condyle
13. AP or PA weight-bearing knee
14. C. Medial or collateral ligament damage
15. A. Holmblad
16. 40° flexion
17. Distortion caused by central ray angle and increased OID for AP
18. True
19. 5° to 10°
20. B. 20 to 30 mrad
21. 30° from horizontal
22. A. 45° to 55°
    B. 90°
23. Hughston method. Acute knee flexion of 90° tends to draw the patella into the intercondylar sulcus, reducing the diagnostic value of this projection.
24. 1. F
    2. E
    3. D
    4. G
    5. C
    6. A
    7. B
25. Cathode

## Review Exercise E: Problem Solving for Technical and Positioning Errors

1. Central ray is not angled correctly; adjust central ray angle to keep it perpendicular to metatarsals.
2. Overrotation of foot (toward the medial direction)
3. Increase cephalad angle of the central ray to correctly elongate the calcaneus.
4. Possibly a spread of the ankle mortise caused by ruptured ligaments
5. Underrotation of the ankle (toward the medial direction). The described appearance is that of a true AP ankle with little or no obliquity.
6. Angling the central ray correctly to keep it parallel to the articular facets (tibial plateau)
7. The wrong oblique position of the knee was obtained. This description is that of a laterally or externally oblique position of the knee.
8. Underrotation of knee (excessive rotation of patella away from table top)
9. An AP lateral oblique projection with 30° of external rotation will separate the bases of the first and second metatarsals.
10. Repeat the AP projection to ensure the ankle joint is demonstrated.
11. Rotation of the affected limb
12. Decrease the amount of flexion of the knee to only 5° to 10°.
13. An AP or PA weight-bearing bilateral knee projection will best evaluate the joint spaces.
14. Tangential projection for the sesamoid bones
15. AP and lateral weight-bearing projections
16. Intercondylar fossa projections, including the Holmblad and/or Camp-Coventry methods, demonstrate the entire knee joint and intercondylar fossa region, which may be hiding "joint mice."
17. The lateral knee projection will best demonstrate any separation of the tibial tuberosity from the shaft of the tibia.
18. By angling the central ray 5° to 7° cephalad, the medial femoral condyle will be superimposed with the lateral condyle. If CR angulation was used on the initial projection, increase the amount of angle with the repeat exposure.

## Review Exercise F: Critique Radiographs of the Lower Limb

A. Bilateral tangential patella (Fig. C7-146)
   1. Portion of each patella superimposed over intercondylar sulcus of femur
   2. Excessive flexion of knee most likely cause of superimposition of patella over femur
   3. Evidence of collimation; correct central ray centering and IR placement; may be an error in central ray angle, which would have contributed to the superimposition
   4. Underexposed
   5. Anatomic side marker present
   Repeatable error(s): 1, 2, and 3 (possibly 4)

B. AP foot (Fig. C7-147)
  1. Proximal metatarsals and all tarsals totally obscured; metatarsopha-langeal joints not open; fourth and fifth metatarsals partially superimposed (can compare with textbook Fig. 7-57, p. 232)
  2. Acceptable but superimposed part centering; obscured anatomic structures, indicating foot was not extended (plantar flexion) sufficiently and was rotated slightly externally
  3. Evidence of collimation; insufficient central ray angle, which could also have contributed to some of the distortion and closure of joint spaces and to obscuring of proximal metatarsals and tarsals
  4. Acceptable exposure factors, but lack of contrast
  5. Anatomic side marker only partially visible
  Repeatable error(s): 1, 2, and possibly 3

C. Lateral ankle (Fig. C7-148)
  1. Joint space between tibia and talus not open; obscured anterior tubercle
  2. Excessive rotation of anterior foot toward cassette (overrotation)

  3. No evidence of collimation; correct central ray centering and IR placement
  4. Acceptable exposure factors
  5. Anatomic side marker present
  Repeatable error(s): 1 and 2

D. AP knee (Fig. C7-149)
  1. Joint space not totally open
  2. Leg rotated slightly laterally (and note slight medial location of patella; can compare with textbook Fig. 7-101, p. 245)
  3. No evidence of collimation; incorrect central ray angle, which led to narrowing and closing of joint space; correct IR placement
  4. Acceptable exposure factors
  5. Anatomic side marker not present; patient ID marker should be on top, away from fibular area
  Repeatable error(s): 3 (not a repeatable error in most situations)

E. Lateral knee (Fig. C7-150)
  1. All pertinent anatomic structures included but patellofemoral joint not open* (presence of superimposition of patella over lateral condyle because of rotation)
  2. Rotation of anterior knee away from cassette (underrotation); almost total superimposition of

proximal fibula; visibility of adductor tubercle identifies medial condyle as being posterior; overflexed knee (should be flexed only 15° to 20° rather than the almost 45° used in this radiograph)
  3. No evidence of collimation; correct central ray centering and IR placement
  4. Acceptable exposure factors
  5. Anatomic side marker present
  Repeatable error(s): 1 and 2

F. Lateral knee (Fig. C7-151)
  1. Closure of patellofemoral joint space caused by positioning error
  2. Excessive rotation of anterior knee toward cassette (overrotation); separation of proximal fibula from tibia; outline of adductor tubercle on medial condyle also anterior to lateral condyle; knee slightly underflexed
  3. No evidence of collimation; correct central ray centering and IR placement
  4. Acceptable exposure factors
  5. Anatomic side marker present
  Repeatable error(s): 1 and 2

7

# SELF-TEST

This self-test should be taken only after completing all of the readings, review exercises, and laboratory activities for a particular section. The purpose of this test is not only to provide a good learning exercise but also to serve as a strong indicator of what your final evaluation exam will be. It is strongly suggested that if you do not get at least a 90% to 95% grade on this self-test, you review those areas in which you missed questions before going to your instructor for the final evaluation exam for this chapter. There are 92 questions or blanks—each is worth 1.1 points.

1. Which of the following is not an aspect of the metatarsal?

   A. Head     C. Body

   B. Tail     D. Base

2. True/False: The distal portion of the fifth metatarsal is a common fracture site.

3. Where are the sesamoid bones of the foot most commonly located?

   A. Plantar surface near head of first metatarsal

   B. Plantar surface at first tarsometatarsal joint

   C. Dorsum aspect near base of first metatarsal

   D. Plantar surface near cuboid bone

4. What is the name of the tarsal bone found on the medial side of the foot between the talus and three cuneiforms?

   A. Calcaneus     C. Cuboid

   B. Lateral malleolus     D. Navicular

5. Which tarsal bone is considered to be the smallest?

   A. Medial cuneiform     C. Intermediate cuneiform

   B. Navicular     D. Lateral cuneiform

6. What is another term for the talocalcaneal joint?

   A. Tarsometatarsal joint     C. Mortise joint

   B. Subtalar joint     D. Tibiocalcaneal joint

7. The distal tibial joint surface is called the:

   A. Medial malleolus     C. Lateral malleolus

   B. Tibial plafond     D. Anterior tubercle

8. True/False: The mortise of the ankle should be totally open and visible on a correctly positioned anteroposterior (AP) projection of the ankle.

9.   Match each of the following structures or characteristics to the correct bone of the foot or ankle (using each choice only once):

　　　 _____   1.   Trochlear process                                                            A.   Metatarsal

　　　 _____   2.   Lateral malleolus                                                            B.   Talus

　　　 _____   3.   The second largest tarsal bone                                        C.   Tibia

　　　 _____   4.   Found between the navicular and base of first metatarsal     D.   Calcaneus

　　　 _____   5.   Base                                                                            E.   Sinus tarsi

　　　 _____   6.   Found between the calcaneus and talus                              F.   Medial cuneiform

　　　 _____   7.   Anterior tubercle                                                            G.   Fibula

10.  Match the structures labeled on Fig. 7-10 (using each choice only once):

　　　 _____   A.   1.   Talus

　　　 _____   B.   2.   First metatarsal

　　　 _____   C.   3.   Lateral malleolus

　　　 _____   D.   4.   Distal tibiofibular joint

　　　 _____   E.   5.   Medial malleolus

**Fig. 7-10.** Anatomy of the ankle.

　　 F.   What projection does this radiograph represent?

　　　 A.  AP mortise ankle              C.  AP ankle

　　　 B.  AP stress ankle—inversion      D.  AP stress ankle—eversion

11.  Match the structures labeled on the radiographs in Figs. 7-11 through 7-13 (answers may be used more than once):

　　　 _____   A.   1.   Distal phalanx, second digit

　　　 _____   B.   2.   Proximal phalanx, first digit

　　　 _____   C.   3.   Interphalangeal joint

　　　 _____   D.   4.   Head of second metatarsal

　　　 _____   E.   5.   Metatarsophalangeal joint
                              of first digit

　　　 _____   F.   6.   Base of first metatarsal

　　　 _____   G.   7.   Proximal phalanx,
                              second digit

　　　 _____   H.   8.   Head of first metatarsal

　　　 _____   I.   9.   Distal phalanx, first digit

　　　 _____   J.

　　　 _____   K.

**Fig. 7-11.** Anatomy of the metatarsal bones and digits.

**Fig. 7-12.** Anatomy of the metatarsal bones and digits.

**Fig. 7-13.** Anatomy of the metatarsal bones and digits.

12. Which of the radiographs in the previous question represents an AP oblique projection of the toes?

    A. Fig. 7-11        C. Fig. 7-12

    B. Fig. 7-13        D. None of the above

13. What is the correct central ray centering placement for an AP projection of the toes?

    A. Affected MTP joint        C. Affected PIP joint

    B. Affected DIP joint        D. Head of affected metatarsal

14. Which type of central ray angle is required for an AP projection of the toes?

    A. None (central ray is perpendicular)        C. 5° posterior

    B. 10° to 15° posterior                       D. 20° to 25° posterior

15. Which of the following projections is used for the sesamoid bones of the foot?

    A. AP and lateral weight-bearing        C. Tangential

    B. Camp-Coventry                        D. AP mortise

16. How much foot rotation is required for the AP oblique, medial rotation projection of the foot?

    A. 3° to 5°        C. 15° to 20°

    B. 45°             D. 30° to 40°

17. What is another name for the AP projection of the foot?

    A. Mortise projection        C. Weight-bearing study

    B. Plantodorsal projection        D. Dorsoplantar projection

18. Which central ray angle and direction are generally required for the AP projection of the foot?

    A. 10° posterior        C. 15° posterior

    B. 10° anterior         D. None (central ray is perpendicular)

19. Which projection of the foot best demonstrates the cuboid?

    A. AP                              C. AP oblique—medial rotation

    B. AP oblique—lateral rotation        D. Lateromedial

20. What is another term for the intercondyloid eminence?

    A. Tibial plateaus        C. Tibial tuberosity

    B. Intercondylar fossa        D. Intercondylar tubercles

21. What is the name of the deep depression found on the posterior aspect of the distal femur?

    A. Intercondylar fossa        C. Patellar surface

    B. Intercondylar sulcus        D. Articular facets

22. A line drawn across the most distal aspect of the medial and lateral femoral condyles would be _____ from being at a right angle (90°) to the long axis of the femur.

    A. 5° to 7°        C. 0°

    B. 3° to 5°        D. 10° to 20°

23. True/False: The angle referred to in question 22 would be less on a tall, slender person.

24.   The upper, or superior, portion of the patella is called the:

    A.   Apex      C.   Styloid process

    B.   Base      D.   Patellar head

25.   Which two ligaments of the knee joint help stabilize the knee from the anterior and posterior perspective?

    A.   Collaterals      C.   Cruciate

    B.   Patellar      D.   Quadriceps femoris

26.   Which structures serve as shock absorbers within the knee joint?

    A.   Articular facets      C.   Menisci

    B.   Infrapatellar and suprapatellar bursae      D.   Infrapatellar fat pads

27.   Match the structures labeled on Figs. 7-14 and 7-15 (using each choice only once):

    _____ A.    1.   Medial condyle of tibia

    _____ B.    2.   Neck of fibula

    _____ C.    3.   Head of fibula

    _____ D.    4.   Articular facets

    _____ E.    5.   Patella

    _____ F.    6.   Lateral condyle of femur

    _____ G.    7.   Proximal tibiofibular joint

    _____ H.    8.   Intercondyloid eminence

    _____ I.    9.   Femorotibial joint space

    _____ J.    10.   Lateral condyle of tibia

**Fig. 7-14.** AP radiograph of the knee.    **Fig. 7-15.** Radiograph of the knee.

28. Which knee projection does Fig. 7-15 represent?

   A. AP

   B. AP oblique—medial rotation

   C. AP oblique—lateral rotation

   D. AP weight-bearing

29. Match the parts labeled on Figs. 7-16 and 7-17 (answers may be used more than once):

   _____ A.    1. Adductor tubercle

   _____ B.    2. Head of fibula

   _____ C.    3. Medial femoral condyle

   _____ D.    4. Anterior aspect of medial condyle

   _____ E.    5. Lateral femoral condyle

   _____ F.    6. Anterior aspect of lateral condyle

   _____ G.    7. Tibial tuberosity

   _____ H.

   _____ I.

   _____ J.

**Fig. 7-16.** Anatomy of the knee.

**Fig. 7-17.** Anatomy of the knee.

30. What is the *primary* positioning error present on Fig. 7-16?*

   A. Overangulation of central ray

   B. Underrotation toward image receptor

   C. Overrotation of knee toward image receptor

   D. Underangulation of central ray

31. True/False: The lateral knee position in Fig. 7-16 is excessively flexed.

32. What is the *primary* positioning error in Fig. 7-17?*

   A. Overangulation of central ray

   B. Underrotation toward image receptor

   C. Overrotation of knee toward image receptor

   D. Underangulation of central ray

*HINT: Two methods can be used to detect rotational errors on a lateral knee radiograph. Note the relative differences of the proximal fibula and superimposition by the tibia. In addition to identifying the medial or lateral femoral condyle by the appearance of the adductor, the amount of superimposition of the fibular head also allows you to determine overrotation or underrotation of the knee if the radiograph is not a true lateral.

33.  Which one of the following conditions may cause the tibial tuberosity to be pulled away from the tibial shaft?

A.  Gout

B.  Reiter's syndrome

C.  Osteomalacia

D.  Osgood-Schlatter disease

34.  A condition that literally means "bone softening" is:

A.  Exostosis

B.  Paget's disease

C.  Osteoclastoma

D.  Osteomalacia

35.  Which one of the following conditions may produce the radiographic appearance of a destructive lesion with irregular periosteal reaction?

A.  Osteogenic sarcoma

B.  Gout

C.  Bone cyst

D.  Osteoid osteoma

36.  What is the common term for *chondromalacia patellae?*

A.  Brittle bone disease

B.  Runner's knee

C.  Degenerative joint disease

D.  Giant cell tumor

37.  Where is the central ray placed for a plantodorsal axial projection of the calcaneus?

A.  Calcaneal tuberosity

B.  Sustentaculum tali

C.  Base of third metatarsal

D.  1 inch (2½ cm) inferior to medial malleolus

38.  Which ankle projection is best for demonstrating the mortise of the ankle?

A.  AP

B.  AP oblique (15° to 20° medial rotation)

C.  AP oblique (15° to 20° lateral rotation)

D.  Mediolateral

39.  Which imaginary plane should be placed parallel to the IR for an AP projection of the knee?

A.  Intermalleolar

B.  Midcoronal

C.  Midsagittal

D.  Interepicondylar

40.  Which joint space should be open or almost open for a well-positioned AP oblique knee projection with medial rotation?

A.  Both sides of knee joint

B.  Proximal tibiofibular

C.  Distal tibiofibular

D.  Patellofemoral

41.  True/False: A 5° to 7° cephalad angle of the central ray for a lateral projection of the knee helps superimpose the distal borders of the medial and lateral condyles of the femur.

42.  Why is a PA projection of the patella preferred to an AP projection?

A.  Less object image receptor distance (OID)

B.  Less distortion of patella

C.  Less magnification of patella

D.  All of the above

43.  **Situation:** A projection is performed for the patellofemoral joint with the patient supine and the knee flexed 40°. The central ray is angled 30° caudad from horizontal. The cassette is resting on the lower legs supported by a special cassette-holding device. Which one of the following methods has been described?

A.  Camp-Coventry

B.  Settegast

C.  Hughston

D.  Merchant

44. What is the major *disadvantage* of the Settegast method?

    A. Requires use of specialized equipment
    C. Requires overflexion of knee

    B. Requires AP positioning
    D. Requires the use of a long OID

45. **Situation:** A radiograph of an AP knee reveals that the joint spaces are not equally open and the proximal fibula is superimposed over the tibia. Which specific positioning error lead to this radiographic outcome?

    A. Underangulation of central ray
    C. Overangulation of central ray

    B. Lateral rotation of lower limb
    D. Medial rotation of lower limb

46. **Situation:** A radiograph of the Camp-Coventry method was produced, but the intercondylar fossa is not open and is foreshortened. The following positioning factors were used: prone position, lower leg flexed 45°, and central ray angled 30° caudad and centered to the popliteal crease. Which of the following should be done during the repeat exposure to produce a more diagnostic image?

    A. Decrease lower leg flexion to 30°
    C. Increase CR angle to 45°

    B. Rotate lower limb 5° internally
    D. Increase flexion of lower limb to 50° to 60°

47. **Situation:** A radiograph of a plantodorsal axial projection of the calcaneus reveals that the calcaneus is foreshortened. The following positioning factors were used: supine position, foot dorsiflexed perpendicular to image receptor, and central ray angled 30° cephalad and centered to base of third metatarsal. Which of the following should be done during the repeat exposure to produce a more diagnostic image?

    A. Increase central ray angulation to 40°
    C. Reduce dorsiflexion of foot

    B. Reverse direction of central ray angulation
    D. Center central ray to sustentaculum tali

48. **Situation:** A patient with a possible fracture of the middle and distal femur enters the emergency room. The patient cannot be turned from the supine position. The physician orders a portable study because the patient is in a splint and in great pain. What specific positioning routine would be used with this patient?

    A. AP and lateral recumbent femur
    C. AP projection only

    B. Lateral position only
    D. AP and horizontal beam lateral position

49. For the following critique questions, refer to the bilateral patella radiograph in Fig. C7-146 on p. 259 in your textbook.

    A. Which positioning error(s) is(are) visible on this radiograph? (More than one answer may be selected.)

      (a) All essential anatomic structures are not demonstrated.

      (b) Central ray is centered incorrectly.

      (c) Collimation is not evident.

      (d) Exposure factors are incorrect.

      (e) Central ray is angled incorrectly.

      (f) No anatomic marker is visible on the radiograph.

      (g) Excessive flexion of knees is evident.

      (h) Insufficient flexion of knees is evident.

    B. Which error(s) identified above is(are) considered "repeatable"? _____

    C.  Which of the following modifications must be made during the repeat exposure? (More than one answer may be selected.)

      (a)  Increase collimation.

      (b)  Center central ray correctly.

      (c)  Decrease exposure factors.

      (d)  Increase exposure factors.

      (e)  Alter central ray angulation.

      (f)  Place anatomic marker on image receptor before exposure.

      (g)  Decrease flexion of knees.

      (h)  Increase flexion of knees.

50.  For the following critique questions, refer to the lateral ankle radiograph in Fig. C7-148 on p. 259 in your textbook.

    A.  Which positioning error(s) is(are) visible on this radiograph? (More than one answer may be selected.)

      (a)  All essential anatomic structures are not demonstrated.

      (b)  Central ray is centered incorrectly.

      (c)  Collimation is not evident.

      (d)  Exposure factors are incorrect.

      (e)  No anatomic marker is visible on the radiograph.

      (f)  Excessive rotation of anterior foot toward cassette is evident.

      (g)  Excessive rotation of anterior foot away from cassette is evident.

    B.  Which error(s) identified above is(are) considered "repeatable"? _____

    C.  Which of the following modifications must be made during the repeat exposure? (More than one answer may be selected.)

      (a)  Increase collimation.

      (b)  Center central ray correctly.

      (c)  Decrease exposure factors.

      (d)  Increase exposure factors.

      (e)  Place anatomic marker on image receptor before exposure.

      (f)  Rotate anterior foot away from image receptor.

      (g)  Rotate anterior foot toward image receptor.

## CHAPTER 8

# Proximal Femur and Pelvic Girdle

After you have successfully completed the activities in this chapter, you will be able to:

_____ 1. Identify the bones and specific features of the proximal femur and pelvic girdle on drawings and radiographs.

_____ 2. Identify the location of the major landmarks of the pelvis and hip and describe two methods of locating the femoral head and neck on an anteroposterior (AP) hip and pelvis radiograph.

_____ 3. List the structural and functional differences of the greater and lesser pelvis and the structural difference between the male and female pelvis.

_____ 4. List the correct classification and movement type for the pelvic joints.

_____ 5. Identify the specific pediatric and geriatric applications for pelvis and hip radiographic examinations as described in the textbook.

_____ 6. Match specific pathologic indications of the pelvic girdle to the correct definition.

_____ 7. Match specific pathologic indications of the pelvic girdle to the correct radiographic appearance.

_____ 8. Determine whether a pelvis or hip is in a true AP position based on the established radiographic criteria.

_____ 9. List the patient dose ranges for each projection of the hip and pelvis and know the approximate difference among patient doses when using a higher kilovoltage, lower milliamperage seconds technique.

_____ 10. List the basic projections, type, and size of image receptor (IR), automatic exposure control (AEC) chamber selection, central ray location, and anatomic structures best demonstrated for radiographic examinations of the hips, pelvis, and sacroiliac (SI) joints.

_____ 11. Given various hypothetical clinical situations, identify the correct modification of a position and/or exposure factors to improve the radiographic image.

_____ 12. Given radiographs of specific shoulder girdle projections, identify positioning and exposure factor errors.

## Positioning and Radiographic Critique

_____ 1. Using a peer, position for the basic and special projections of the proximal femur and pelvic girdle.

_____ 2. Using a pelvic radiographic phantom, produce satisfactory radiographs of specific positions (if equipment is available).

_____ 3. Critique and evaluate pelvic girdle radiographs based on the four divisions of radiographic criteria: (1) structures shown, (2) position, (3) collimation and central ray, and (4) exposure criteria.

_____ 4. Distinguish between acceptable and unacceptable pelvic girdle radiographs based on exposure factors, motion, collimation, positioning, or other errors.

## Learning Exercises

Complete the following review exercises after reading the associated pages in the textbook as indicated by each exercise. Answers to each review exercise are given at the end of the review exercises.

## Part I: Radiographic Anatomy

**REVIEW EXERCISE A:** Radiographic Anatomy of the Hips and Pelvis (see textbook pp. 262-268)

1. The largest and strongest bone of the body is the ___Femur___ .

2. A small depression located in the center of the femoral head is the ___Fovea Capitis___.

3. The lesser trochanter is located on the _____ (**medial** or **lateral**) aspect of the proximal femur.

   It projects _____ (**anteriorly** or **posteriorly**) from the junction between the neck and shaft.

4. Because of the alignment between the femoral head and pelvis, the lower limb must be rotated

   ___15°-20°___ ° internally to place the femoral neck parallel to the plane of the image receptor to

   achieve a true anteroposterior (AP) projection.

5. True/False: According to *Gray's Anatomy* reference textbook, the terms *pelvis* and *pelvic girdle* are **not** synonymous.

   A. List the **four** bones comprising the **pelvis:** ___Two hip bones, one sacrum, one Coccyx___

   B. List the **two** bones comprising the **pelvic girdle:** ___Two hip bones___

   C. List two additional terms used for the bones identified in *B:*

       1. ___Innominate bones___        2. ___Ossa coxae___

6. List the three divisions of the hip bone:

   A. ___ilium___       B. ___Ischium___       C. ___pubis___

7. All three divisions of the hip bone eventually fuse at the ___aceTabulum___ at the age of ___mid Teens___

8. What are the two important radiographic landmarks found on the ilium?

   A. ___AnTerior superior ilium spine___       B. ___ilium cresS___

9. Which bony landmark is found on the most **inferior** aspect of the posterior pelvis? ___Ischuial Tuberosity___

10. What is the name of the joint found between the superior rami of the pubic bones? ___Symphysis pubis___

11. The ___ObTurator foramina___ of the pelvis is the largest foramen in the skeletal system.

12. The upper margin of the greater trochanter is approximately (A) ___1"___ above the level of

    the superior border of the symphysis pubis, and the ischial tuberosity is about (B) ___1½"-2"___ below.

13. An imaginary plane that divides the pelvic region into the greater and lesser pelvis is called the

    ___pelvic brium___

14. List the alternate terms for the greater and lesser pelvis:

    A. Greater pelvis ___false pelvis___       B. Lesser pelvis ___True peluis___

15. List the major function of the greater pelvis and the lesser pelvis:

    A. Greater pelvis ___SuporTs The lower abdominal organs and feTus___       B. Lesser pelvis ___Forms actual birTh Canal___

16. List the three aspects of the lesser pelvis, which also describe the birth route during the delivery process.

    A. _Inlet_                          B. _Outlet_                          C. _Cavity_

17. Match the following structures or characteristics to the correct hip bone (answers may be used more than once):

    _B_ 1. Possesses a large tuberosity found at the most inferior aspect of the pelvis          A. Ilium

    _B_ 2. Lesser sciatic notch                                                                 B. Ischium

    _A_ 3. Ala                                                                                  C. Pubis

    _A_ 4. Posterior superior iliac spine (PSIS)

    _C_ 5. Possesses a slightly movable joint

    _A_ 6. Anterior superior iliac spine (ASIS)

    _C_ 7. Forms the anterior, inferior aspect of the lower pelvic girdle

    _A_ 8. Articulates with the sacrum to form the SI joints

18. In the past, which radiographic examination was performed to measure the fetal head in comparison with the maternal pelvis to predict possible birthing problems? _Cephalopelvimetry_

19. What imaging modality has replaced the procedure identified in the previous question?

    _Sonography (ultrasound_

20. Indicate whether the following radiographic characteristics apply to a male (M) or female (F) in relation to an AP projection of the pelvis:

    _F_ 1. Wide, more flared ilia                      M. Male

    _F_ 2. Pubic arch angle of 110°                    F. Female

    _M_ 3. A heart-shaped inlet

    _M_ 4. Narrow ilia that are less flared

    _M_ 5. Pubic arch angle of 75°

    _F_ 6. Larger and more round-shaped inlet

21. List the joint classification, mobility type, and movement type for the joints of the pelvis. Write *N/A* (not applicable) if the mobility or movement type does not apply.

| | CLASSIFICATION | MOBILITY TYPE | MOVEMENT TYPE |
|---|---|---|---|
| A. Hip | Synovial | diarthrodial | spheroidal |
| B. Sacroiliac | Synovial | ampharthrodial | N/A |
| C. Symphysis pubis | Cartilaginous | ampharthrodial | N/A |
| D. Acetabulum (union) | Cartilaginous | ampharthrodial | N/A |

8

22. Identify the structures labeled on Figs. 8-1 and 8-2. Where indicated, use the following abbreviations to identify with which bone of the pelvis each labeled part is associated: *IL,* ilium; *IS,* ischium; *P,* pubis.

| | STRUCTURE | BONE |
|---|---|---|
| A. | iliac crest | ilium |
| B. | Anterior Superior iliac Spine | ilium |
| C. | Greater Trochanter | Femur |
| D. | body | IS |
| E. | superior ramus | P |
| F. | ischial Tuberosity | IS |
| G. | Inferior ramus | P |
| H. | obturator foamen | |
| I. | body | P |
| J. | body | IS |
| K. | ala | ilium |
| L. | sacroiliac joint | |
| M. | Ischial spine | IS |
| N. | sacrum | |
| O. | Body | ilium |
| P. | Posterior Superior iliac Spine | ilium |
| Q. | Posterior Inferior iliac Spine | ilium |
| R. | Greater sciatic notch | ilium |
| S. | ischial Spine | IS |
| T. | lesser siatioc knotch | IS |
| U. | ischival Tuberosity | IS |
| V. | ramus | IS |
| W. | Inferior ramus | P |
| X. | acetabulum | IL, IS, P |
| Y. | Anterior Inferior iliac Spine | |
| Z. | ASIS | |

**Fig. 8-1.** Frontal view, pelvis.

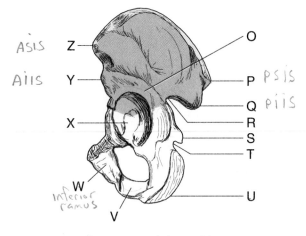

ASIS

AIIS

PSIS

PIIS

Inferior ramus

**Fig. 8-2.** Lateral view, pelvis.

## Part II: Radiographic Positioning

**REVIEW EXERCISE B:** Positioning of the Hips, Pelvis, and Sacroiliac Joints (see textbook pp. 269-285)

1. Which two bony landmarks need to be palpated for hip localization?

   A. _ASIS_                                                          B. _Symphysis pubis_

2. From the midpoint of the imaginary line created by the two landmarks identified in the previous question, where

   would the femoral neck be located? _2.5" below the midpoint of the line_

3. A second method for locating the femoral head is to palpate the _ASIS_ and go _1-2_ inches

   (_3-5_ cm) medial at the level of the _symphysis pubis ?_, which is _3-4_ inches (_8-10_ cm) distal to
   _greater trochanter_

   the original palpation point.

4. To achieve a true AP position of the proximal femur, the lower limb must be rotated _15-20°_ internally.

5. Which structures on an AP pelvis or hip radiograph indicate whether the proximal head and neck are in position for
   a true AP projection?

   _lesser trochanter should not be visible or slightly visible_

6. Which physical sign may indicate that a patient has a hip fracture? _pt foot is rotated externally_

7. Which projection should be taken first and reviewed by a radiologist before attempting to rotate the hip into a
   lateral position (if trauma is suspected)?

   _AP Pelvis_

8. Gonadal shielding should be used for all patients of reproductive age, unless _it cover antomical_
   _area of interest_

9. Should a gonadal shield be used for a hip study on a young female? _yes_ If *yes*, describe how it should be
   placed on the patient.

   _use ovarian shaped shield, top at ASIS ; bottom at symphysis pubis_

10. Should a gonadal shield be used for a hip study on a young male? _yes_ If *yes*, describe how it should be placed
    on the patient.

    _The top willbe placed at interior margin of the symphysis pubis_

11. What is the advantage of using 90 kV rather than 80 kV range for hip and pelvis studies on younger patients?

    _reduce pt dosage by 30%_

12. What is the disadvantage of using 90 kV for hip and pelvis studies, especially on older patients with some bone
    mass loss?

    _It reduces radiograph contrast._

8

13.  Which one of the following conditions is a common clinical indication for performing pelvic and hip examinations on a pediatric (newborn) patient?

A.  Osteoporosis                             C.  Ankylosing spondylitis

B.  Developmental dysplasia of hip (DDH)     D.  Osteoarthritis

14.  True/False: Geriatric patients are more prone to hip fractures because of their increased incidence of osteoporosis.

15.  Which one of the following imaging modalities can be used on a newborn to assess hip joint stability during movement of the lower limbs?

A.  Sonography                    C.  Magnetic resonance imaging

B.  Computed tomography           D.  Nuclear medicine

16.  Which one of the following imaging modalities is most sensitive in diagnosing early signs of metastatic carcinoma of the pelvis?

A.  Sonography                    C.  Magnetic resonance imaging

B.  Computed tomography           D.  Nuclear medicine

*STOP*

17.  Match each of the following pathologic indications to the correct definition (using each choice only once):

___7___  A.  A degenerative joint disease

___5___  B.  Most common fracture in older patients because of high incidence of osteoporosis or avascular necrosis

___4___  C.  A malignant tumor of the cartilage of hip

___2___  D.  A disease producing extensive calcification of the longitudinal ligament of the spinal column

___6___  E.  A fracture resulting from a severe blow to one side of the pelvis

___1___  F.  Malignancy spread to bone via the circulatory and lymphatic systems or direct invasion

___3___  G.  Now referred to as *developmental dysplasia of the hip*

1.  Metastatic carcinoma

2.  Ankylosing spondylitis

3.  Congenital dislocation

4.  Chondrosarcoma

5.  Proximal hip fracture

6.  Pelvic ring fracture

7.  Osteoarthritis

*START* 18.  Where is the central ray placed for an AP pelvis projection?  *Midway between symphysis pubis & ASIS*

19.  Which ionization chamber(s) should be activated when using automatic exposure control (AEC) for an AP pelvis projection?

A.  Center chamber only             C.  Center and upper left or right chambers

B.  Upper right and left chambers   D.  Upper left chamber only

20.  Which specific positioning error is present when the left iliac wing is elongated on an AP pelvis radiograph?

_____ *LT ROTATION (toward left side)* _____

21.  Which specific positioning error is present when the left obturator foramen is more open than the right side?

_____ *RT ROTATION* _____

22. Indicate whether each of the following projections is used for patients with traumatic (T) injuries or nontraumatic (NT) injuries:

    _I_     A.  Danelius-Miller projection                T.    Traumatic

    _NT_    B.  Unilateral frog-leg                        NT.   Not traumatic

    _NT_    C.  Modified Cleaves (bilateral frog-leg)

    _T_     D.  Clements-Nakayama

    _T_     E.  Anterior pelvic bones

23. When gonadal shielding is *not* used, __3X_____ (**males** or **females**) receive a greater gonadal

    dose with an AP pelvis projection.

24. How many degrees are the femurs abducted (from the vertical plane) for the bilateral frog-leg projection?

    _____40°-45°_____

25. Where is the central ray placed for a unilateral frog-leg projection? _Mid femoral neck_

26. Which cassette size should be used for an adult bilateral frog-leg projection? ___14"×17"_____

27. Where is the central ray placed for an AP bilateral frog-leg projection? _1" Superior To symphysis pubis_

28. Which central ray angle is required for the "outlet" projection (Taylor method) for a female patient?

    A.  15° to 25° caudad       C.  20° to 35° cephalad  MALE

    B.  30° to 45° cephalad      D.  None (central ray is perpendicular)

29. Which type of pathologic feature is best demonstrated with the Judet method?

    A.  Acetabular fractures      C.  Proximal femur fractures
        Dislocations
    B.  Anterior pelvic bone fractures   D.  Femoral neck fractures

30. How much obliquity of the body is required for the Judet method?

    A.  None (central ray is perpendicular)   C.  30°

    B.  20°                                    D.  45°

31. True/False: Any orthopedic device or appliance of the hip should be seen in its entirety on an AP hip radiograph.

32. The axiolateral inferosuperior projection is designed for _____ (**traumatic**) or
        Danelius-Miller

    **nontraumatic**) situations.

                                                  Danelius-Miller
33. How is the unaffected leg positioned for the axiolateral hip projection? _Flex & elvaTe To prevent_

    _____Superinposition_____

34. Which one of the following factors does **not** apply to an axiolateral projection of the hip on a male patient?

    A.  Cassette parallel to femoral neck     C.  Use of gonadal shielding

    B.  80 to 90 kV                           D.  Use of a stationary grid

35. True/False: An AP pelvis projection using 90 kV and 8 mAs results in a patient dose of approximately 30% less than a projection using 80 kV and 12 mAs (for both males and females).

36. True/False: During an axiolateral (inferosuperior) projection of the hip, a male patient receives more than 20 times the gonadal dose than a female.

37. The Clements-Nakayama method requires the CR to be angled _____ 15°-20° ° posteriorly from horizontal.

38. Which special projection of the hip demonstrates the **anterior** and posterior rims of the acetabulum and the ilioischial and iliopubic columns? (Include the projection name and the method name.)

    A. _____ Judet - Posterior Obl. Acetabulum _____

    B. Which central ray angle (if any) is used for this projection? _____ ⊥ IR _____

39. What is the name of a special AP axial projection of the pelvis used to assess trauma to pubic and ischial

    structures? (Include the projection name and the method name.) _____ Taylor method     AP Axial Outlet _____

40. The _____ (**right** or **left**) SI joint is best demonstrated with the left posterior oblique (LPO) position.

41. Does an anterior oblique projection demonstrate the downside or upside SI joint? _____ Downside _____

   *279*

42. Which type of central ray angle is required for an AP axial projection of the SI joints? _____ 30°-35° cephalic _____
    *Female*

43. Match each of the following projections with its corresponding proper name (using each choice only once):

    D   1. Axiolateral (inferosuperior)              A.   Judet

    C   2. Modified axiolateral                      B.   Taylor

    F   3. Bilateral or unilateral frog-leg          C.   Clements-Nakayama

    E   4. Modified frog-leg with affected side in   D.   Danelius-Miller
           contact with table top
                                                     E.   Modified Lauenstein and Hickey
    B   5. AP axial for pelvic "outlet" bones
                                                     F.   Modified Cleaves
    A   6. Posterior oblique for acetabulum

*STOP* 44. True/False: The gonadal dose for female patients for posterior oblique projections of the SI joints is similar (±5 mrad) to the dose for anterior oblique projections of the SI joints.

                        *All          1-5, 9, 10*

**REVIEW EXERCISE C: Problem Solving for Technical and Positioning Errors (see textbook pp. 275-285)**

1. **Situation:** A radiograph of an AP pelvis projection reveals that the lesser trochanters are readily demonstrated on the medial side of the proximal femurs. The patient is ambulatory but has a history of early osteoarthritis in both hips. Which positioning modification needs to be made to prevent this positioning error?

   Rotate legs 15-20° internally To place proximal femurs in True AP position

2. **Situation:** A radiograph of an AP pelvis reveals that the right iliac wing is foreshortened as compared with the left side. Which specific positioning error has been made?

   _Pt is rotated left as in a LPO_

3. **Situation:** A radiograph of a lateral frog-leg projection reveals that the greater trochanter is superimposed over the femoral neck. Based on the AP hip projection, the radiologist suspects a nondisplaced fracture of the femoral neck. What can the technologist do to better define this region?

   _Repeat exposure using a 20°-25° Cephalad CR to seperate greater trochanter from the femoral neck_

4. **Situation:** A radiograph of an axiolateral (inferosuperior) projection reveals that the posterior aspect of the _Danelius- miller_ acetabulum and femoral head were cut off of the bottom of the image. The emergency room physician requests that the position be repeated. What can be done to avoid this problem on the repeat exposure?

   _Elevate pt by 2" using blanckets or sheets beneth the pelvis_

5. **Situation:** A radiograph of an AP axial projection for anterior pelvic bones reveals that the pubic and ischial bones _Taylor_ are not elongated sufficiently. The following factors were used for this study: 86 kV, 7 mAs, Bucky, 20° to 30° central ray cephalad angle, and 40-inch (102-cm) source image receptor distance (SID). The female patient was p 277 placed in a supine position on the table. What must be changed to improve the quality of the image during the repeat exposure?

   _Greater CR angle is required for females change CR to 30°-45° cephalad_

6. **Situation:** Bilateral posterior oblique radiographs of the SI joints demonstrate that the right joint is open but the p 284 left one is not. The left iliac wing slightly overlaps the region of the left SI joint. The right posterior oblique (RPO) p 285 and LPO positions were performed. Which positioning error led to this radiographic outcome?

   _The RPO was positioned w/ too much obliquity, No More Than 30°_

7. **Situation:** A radiograph of an AP pelvis reveals that overall the image is underexposed (underpenetrated). The following factors were used: 80 kV, 40-inch (102-cm) SID, Bucky, and AEC with the center chamber activated. Which one of these factors should be changed to produce a darker and more diagnostic image?

   _When using AEC use both the ctr & rt or lt ionogitation cells_

8. **Situation:** A radiograph from a modified axiolateral projection reveals excessive grid lines on the image, which _Clements- Nakayama_ p 28 also appears underexposed. What can be done to avoid this problem during the repeat exposure?

   _Insure that the CR is ctr near midline of the grid & that the face of the cassettes is ⊥ to the CR_

9. **Situation:** A portable AP and lateral hip study is ordered for a patient who is in recovery following hip replacement surgery. The radiograph of the AP hip reveals that the upper portion of the acetabular prosthesis is slightly cut off but is included on the lateral projection. Should the technologist repeat the AP projection? Why or why not?

   Yes, any orthopedic appliance must be seen in it entirety in both projections

10. **Situation:** A patient with hip pain from a fall enters the emergency room. The physician orders a left hip study. When moved to the radiographic table, the patient complained loudly about the pain in the left hip. Which positioning routine should be used for this patient?

   AP pelvis ; ok'ed by Doc before pt is moved

11. **Situation:** A patient has just been moved to his hospital room after a bilateral hip replacement surgery. The surgeon has ordered a postoperative hip routine for both hips. Which specific positioning routine should be used? (The patient can be brought to the radiology department.)

   AP pelvis ; modified axiolateral (Clements + Nakayama)

12. **Situation:** A patient with a possible pelvic ring fracture from a trauma enters the emergency room. The AP pelvis projection, which was taken to determine whether the right acetabulum is fractured, is inconclusive. Which other projection can be taken to better visualize the acetabulum?

   Posterior Oblique Judet Method

13. **Situation:** A young patient comes to the radiology department with a chronic pain near the ASIS. She is an active athlete who injured her pelvis while running hurdles. Her physician suspects an avulsion fracture. Which position(s) may best diagnose this condition? Must the technologist increase or decrease kV for this projection to demonstrate the fracture?

   AP pelvis. Decrease kV to 65-70 from 80-90 kV

14. **Situation:** A technologist notices that his AP pelvis projections often demonstrate a moderate degree of rotation. What positioning technique can the technologist perform to eliminate (or at least minimize) rotation on his AP pelvis projections?

   Palpate both ASIS ; ensure they are equal distance from Table Top

15. **Situation:** A very young child comes to the radiology department with a clinical history of DDH. What is the most common positioning routine for this condition?

   AP pelvis ; bilateral frogleg (Modified Cleaves)

**REVIEW EXERCISE D:** Critique Radiographs of the Proximal Femur and Pelvis (see textbook p. 286)

The following questions relate to the radiographs found at the end of Chapter 8 of the textbook. Evaluate these radiographs for the radiographic criteria categories *(1* through *5)* that follow. Describe the corrections needed to improve the overall image. The major, or "repeatable," errors are specific errors that indicate the need for a repeat exposure, regardless of the nature of the other errors.

A.  **AP pelvis (83-year-old) (Fig. C8-76)**
    Description of possible error:

    1.  Structures shown: _____

    2.  Part positioning: _____

    3.  Collimation and central ray: _____

    4.  Exposure criteria: _____

    5.  Markers: _____

    Repeatable error(s): _____

B.  **Unilateral frog-leg (84-year-old) (Fig. C8-77)**
    Description of possible error:

    1.  Structures shown: _____

    2.  Part positioning: _____

    3.  Collimation and central ray: _____

    4.  Exposure criteria: _____

    5.  Markers: _____

    Repeatable error(s): _____

C.  **AP pelvis (57-year-old) (Fig. C8-78)**
    Description of possible error:

    1.  Structures shown: _____

    2.  Part positioning: _____

    3.  Collimation and central ray: _____

    4.  Exposure criteria: _____

    5.  Markers: _____

    Repeatable error(s): _____

D.  **Bilateral frog-leg (2-year-old) (Fig. C8-79)**
    Description of possible error:

    1.  Structures shown: _____

    2.  Part positioning: _____

3.  Collimation and central ray: _____

4.  Exposure criteria: _____

5.  Markers: _____

Repeatable error(s): _____

## Part III: Laboratory Exercises (see textbook pp. 275-285)

You must gain experience in positioning each part of the proximal femur and pelvis before performing the following exams on actual patients. You can get experience in positioning and radiographic evaluation of these projections by performing exercises using radiographic phantoms and practicing positioning on other students (although you will not be taking actual exposures).

The following suggested activities assume that your teaching institution has an energized lab and radiographic phantoms. If not, perform Laboratory Exercises B and C, the radiographic evaluation and the physical positioning exercises. (Check off each step and projection as you complete it.)

## LABORATORY EXERCISE A: Energized Laboratory

1.  Using the pelvic radiographic phantom, produce radiographs of the following basic routines:

_____  AP pelvis projection

_____  AP axial projection for SI joints

_____  Posterior or anterior oblique positions for SI joints

_____  Posterior oblique positions for acetabulum, Judet method

_____  AP axial projection, Taylor method

## LABORATORY EXERCISE B: Radiographic Evaluation

1.  Evaluate and critique the radiographs produced above, additional radiographs provided by your instructor, or both. Evaluate each radiograph for the following points:

_____  Evaluate the completeness of the study. (Are all of the pertinent anatomic structures included on the radiograph?)

_____  Evaluate for positioning or centering errors (e.g., rotation, off centering).

_____  Evaluate for correct exposure factors and possible motion. (Are the density and contrast of the images acceptable?)

_____  Determine whether markers and an acceptable degree of collimation and/or area shielding are visible on the images.

## LABORATORY EXERCISE C: Physical Positioning

On another person, simulate performing all basic and special projections of the proximal femur and pelvic girdle as follows. Include the six steps listed below and described in the textbook. (Check off each step when completed satisfactorily.)

Step 1. Appropriate size and type of image receptor with correct markers
Step 2. Correct central ray placement and centering of part to central ray and/or image receptor
Step 3. Accurate collimation

Step 4. Area shielding of patient where advisable
Step 5. Use of proper immobilizing devices when needed
Step 6. Approximate correct exposure factors, breathing instructions when applicable, and "making" exposure

| PROJECTIONS | STEP 1 | STEP 2 | STEP 3 | STEP 4 | STEP 5 | STEP 6 |
|---|---|---|---|---|---|---|
| • AP pelvis | ___ | ___ | ___ | ___ | ___ | ___ |
| • AP hip, unilateral | ___ | ___ | ___ | ___ | ___ | ___ |
| • Unilateral frog-leg | ___ | ___ | ___ | ___ | ___ | ___ |
| • Bilateral frog-leg | ___ | ___ | ___ | ___ | ___ | ___ |
| • Axiolateral (inferosuperior) | ___ | ___ | ___ | ___ | ___ | ___ |
| • Modified axiolateral | ___ | ___ | ___ | ___ | ___ | ___ |
| • Anterior oblique for acetabulum | ___ | ___ | ___ | ___ | ___ | ___ |
| • AP axial for anterior pelvic bones | ___ | ___ | ___ | ___ | ___ | ___ |
| • AP axial for SI joints | ___ | ___ | ___ | ___ | ___ | ___ |
| • Posterior obliques, SI joints | ___ | ___ | ___ | ___ | ___ | ___ |
| • Anterior obliques, SI joints | ___ | ___ | ___ | ___ | ___ | ___ |

8

# *Answers to Review Exercises*

## Review Exercise A: Anatomy of Hips and Pelvic Girdle

1. Femur
2. Fovea capitis
3. Medial; posteriorly
4. 15 to 20
5. True
   A. Right and left hip bones, sacrum and coccyx
   B. Right and left hip bones
   C. Ossa coxae and/or innominate bones
6. A. Ilium
   B. Ischium
   C. Pubis
7. Acetabulum, mid teens
8. A. Crest of ilium (iliac crest)
   B. Anterior superior iliac spine (ASIS)
9. Ischial tuberosity
10. Symphysis pubis
11. Obturator foramen
12. A. 1 inch (2½ cm)
    B. 1½ to 2 inches (4 to 5 cm)
13. Pelvic brim
14. A. False pelvis
    B. True pelvis
15. A. Supports the lower abdominal organs and fetus
    B. Forms the actual birth canal
16. A. Inlet
    B. Cavity
    C. Outlet
17. 1. B
    2. B
    3. A
    4. A
    5. C
    6. A
    7. C
    8. A
18. Cephalopelvimetry
19. Sonography (ultrasound)
20. 1. F
    2. F
    3. M
    4. M
    5. M
    6. F
21. A. Synovial, diarthrodial, spheroidal
    B. Synovial, amphiarthrodial, N/A
    C. Cartilaginous, amphiarthrodial, N/A
    D. Cartilaginous, amphiarthrodial, N/A
22. A. Crest, IL
    B. ASIS, IL
    C. Greater trochanter
    D. Body, IS

E. Superior ramus, P
F. Ischial tuberosity, IS
G. Inferior ramus, P
H. Obturator foramen
I. Body, P
J. Body, IL
K. Wing (ala), IL
L. Right sacroiliac (SI) joint
M. Ischial spine, IS
N. Sacrum
O. Body, IL
P. Posterior superior iliac spine (PSIS), IL
Q. Posterior inferior iliac spine, IL
R. Greater sciatic notch, IL
S. Ischial spine, IS
T. Lesser sciatic notch, IS
U. Ischial tuberosity, IS
V. Ramus, IS
W. Inferior ramus, P
X. Acetabulum, IS, IL, P
Y. Anterior inferior iliac spine, IL
Z. ASIS, IL

## Review Exercise B: Positioning of Hips, Pelvis, and Sacroiliac Joints

1. A. ASIS
   B. Symphysis pubis
2. Approximately 2½ inches (6 to 7 cm) below the midpoint of the line
3. ASIS; 1 to 2 inches (3 to 5 cm); symphysis pubis and greater trochanter; 3 to 4 inches (8 to 10 cm)
4. 15 to 20
5. Lesser trochanter should not be visible, or should only be slightly visible, on the radiograph.
6. The patient's foot is rotated externally.
7. AP pelvis
8. It covers anatomic structures of primary interest.
9. Yes. Use a shaped ovarian shield with top of shield at level of ASIS and bottom at symphysis pubis.
10. Yes. The top of the shield should be placed at the inferior margin of the symphysis pubis.
11. It reduces patient dose by about 30%.
12. It reduces radiographic contrast.
13. B. DDH (development dysplasia of hip)
14. True
15. A. Sonography
16. D. Nuclear medicine
17. A. 7

B. 5
C. 4
D. 2
E. 6
F. 1
G. 3
18. Midway between ASIS and symphysis pubis
19. B. Upper right and left chambers
20. Rotation toward left side
21. Right rotation
22. A. T
    B. NT
    C. NT
    D. T
    E. T
23. Females (nearly 3 times more)
24. 40° to 45°
25. Midfemoral neck
26. 35 × 43 cm (14 × 17 inches) crosswise
27. 1 inches (2½ cm) superior to the symphysis pubis
28. B. 30° to 45° cephalad
29. A. Acetabular fractures
30. D. 45°
31. True
32. Traumatic
33. It is flexed and elevated to prevent it from being superimposed over the affected hip.
34. C. Use of gonadal shielding
35. True
36. True
37. 15 to 20
38. A. Posterior oblique projections of acetabulum (Judet method)
    B. 0° (perpendicular)
39. AP axial outlet projection (Taylor method)
40. Right
41. Downside
42. 30° to 35° cephalad
43. 1. D
    2. C
    3. F
    4. E
    5. B
    6. A
44. True

## Review Exercise C: Problem Solving for Technical and Positioning Errors

1. Rotate the lower limbs 15° to 20° internally to place the proximal femurs in a true AP position. (With general chronic pain, the lower limbs can usually be rotated safely.)

2. The patient is rotated toward the left—left posterior oblique (LPO).
3. Repeat the exposure using a 20° to 25° cephalad central ray angle. (It will separate the greater trochanter from the femoral neck.)
4. If possible, elevate the patient at least 2 inches (or 5 cm) by placing sheets or blankets beneath the pelvis.
5. A greater central ray angle is required. Female patients require a central ray angle of 30° to 45°.
6. The right posterior oblique (RPO) position was performed with too much obliquity. The obliques must be no more than 30° of rotation.
7. When using automatic exposure control (AEC) for an AP pelvis projection, both the center and left or right ionization chambers must be activated. The center chamber is over the less dense pelvic cavity, which may lead to an underexposed image.
8. Ensure that the central ray is centered to near the midline of the grid cassette and that the face of the cassette is perpendicular to the central ray.
9. Yes. Any orthopedic appliance or prosthesis must be seen in its entirety in both projections.
10. AP pelvis and axiolateral left hip. The AP pelvis radiograph should be taken initially without leg rotation; the radiograph must be reviewed by the physician and checked for fractures or dislocations before attempting an internal rotation of the left leg for the axiolateral (inferosuperior) projection.
11. AP pelvis and modified axiolateral—Clements-Nakayama method
12. Posterior oblique—Judet method
13. AP pelvis projection. Decrease kV to 65 to 70 (from standard 80 to 90 kV).
14. Palpate both ASIS and ensure they are equal distance from tabletop.
15. AP pelvis and bilateral "frog-leg" projections

## Review Exercise D: Critique Radiographs of the Proximal Femur and Pelvis

A. AP pelvis (83-year-old) (Fig. C8-76)
1. Both hands of patient superimposed over hips, obscuring hip detail; watch on left wrist
2. Slight rotation **toward the right** with left side of pelvis elevated; no internal rotation of legs (acceptable in this case because of evidence of right hip fracture)
3. No evidence of collimation (but only slight collimation should be visible for this projection); pelvis slightly off center to the left and centered a little high
4. Acceptable exposure factors
5. Anatomic side marker present (but a better placement would be to the midlateral margin away from the hip region)
   Repeatable error(s): 1
B. Unilateral frog-leg (84-year-old) (Fig. C8-77)
1. Distal part of orthopedic prosthesis cut off—needs to be seen in its entirety
2. Correct part positioning
3. Excellent collimation; correct centering but a larger cassette required
4. Acceptable exposure factors
5. Anatomic side marker cut off
   Repeatable error(s): 1
C. AP pelvis (57-year-old) (Fig. C8-78)
1. Superior iliac wings cut off (may be acceptable if patient history indicates hip region is area of interest)
2. Rotation of pelvis toward the right (and note the elongation of the right ilium); to viewer's right, film incorrectly placed for viewing; lesser trochanters visible and femoral necks severely foreshortened, indicating the legs were not rotated internally for a true AP projection
3. Acceptable collimation; central ray centering/film placement too high (which cut off upper iliac wings)
4. Acceptable exposure factors
5. Anatomic side marker present (but better placement would have been higher up under patient ID blocker, away from hip region)
   NOTE: Radiograph is incorrectly placed for viewing and should be flipped right to left.
   Repeatable error(s): 1 and 2
D. Bilateral frog-leg (2-year-old) (Fig. C8-79)
1. Left hip (assuming that this is the left side because the side marker is not visible) obscured by artifact (superimposition of patient's hand)
2. Tilted pelvis (and note that the gonadal shield placement is useless for either males *or* females—a serious error for a small child)
3. No visible collimation, which should be visible for this pediatric patient; central ray centering/film placement too high for pelvis centering but acceptable for bilateral hip projection
4. Very low contrast (may have been caused by not using a grid)
5. No visible anatomic side marker
   Repeatable error(s): 1

# SELF-TEST

My Score = _____ %

This self-test should be taken only after completing all of the readings, review exercises, and laboratory activities for a particular section. The purpose of this test is not only to provide a good learning exercise but also to serve as a strong indicator of what your final evaluation exam for this chapter will cover. It is strongly suggested that if you do not get at least a 90% to 95% grade on each self-test, you review those areas in which you missed questions before going to your instructor for the final evaluation exam. There are 90 questions and/or blanks—each is worth 1.1 point.

1. List the four bones of the pelvis:

     A. _____      C. _____

     B. _____      D. _____

2. List the three divisions of the hip bone:

     A. _____      B. _____      C. _____

3. *Innominate bone* is another name for:

     A. One half of pelvic girdle      C. Ossa coxae

     B. Hip bone      D. All of the above

4. What is the largest foramen in the body? _____

5. Which one of the following landmarks is **not** a palpable bony landmark?

     A. Greater trochanter      C. Ischial tuberosity

     B. Lesser trochanter      D. Anterior superior iliac spine (ASIS)

6. What are the two aspects of the ischium?

     A. _____      B. _____

7. What is the name of the imaginary plane that separates the greater from the lesser pelvis?

     _____

8. Match the following structures or characteristics to the correct division of the pelvis:

     _____ 1. True pelvis               A. Greater pelvis

     _____ 2. Supports the lower abdominal organs      B. Lesser pelvis

     _____ 3. Formed primarily by the ala of the ilium

     _____ 4. Cavity

     _____ 5. False pelvis

     _____ 6. Forms the actual birth canal

     _____ 7. Found below the pelvic brim

9. The pubic arch angle on an average male pelvis is an _____ (**acute** or **obtuse**) angle that is

     _____ (**greater than** or **less than**) 90 degrees.

10. Identify the labeled structures found on the
    following radiographs.

    *Fig. 8-3:*

    A. _____

    B. _____

    C. _____

    D. _____

    E. _____

    F. _____

    G. _____

    H. _____

    I. _____

    J. Is this a male or female pelvis? _____

    *Fig. 8-4:*

    K. _____

    L. _____

    M. _____

    N. _____

    O. Which projection of the hip is represented on
       this radiograph? _____

    *Fig. 8-5*

    P. _____

    Q. _____

    R. _____

    S. _____

    T. _____

    U. _____

    V. _____

    W. Which projection of the hips is represented

       on this radiograph? _____

**Fig. 8-3.** AP pelvis radiograph.

**Fig. 8-4.** Lateral hip radiograph.

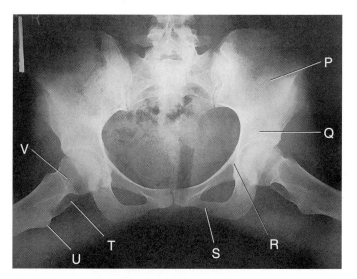

**Fig. 8-5.** Bilateral hip radiograph.

11. Indicate whether the following characteristics are those of a male (M) or female (F) pelvis:

    _____  1. Heart-shaped inlet                          F.  Female

    _____  2. Acute pubic arch (less than 90°)            M.  Male

    _____  3. Iliac wings that are more flared

    _____  4. Obtuse pubic arch (greater than 90°)

    _____  5. Larger and more rounded inlet

    _____  6. Iliac wings that are less flared

12. Which one of the following structures is considered to be the most posterior?

    A. Ischial spines        C. Symphysis pubis

    B. ASIS                  D. Acetabulum

13. The small depression near the center of the femoral head where a ligament is attached is called the

    _____ .

14. A geriatric patient with an externally rotated lower limb may have:

    A. A normal hip joint        C. Fractured proximal femur

    B. Osteoarthritis            D. Slipped capital femoral epiphyses (SCFE)

15. Which one of the following pathologic indications may result in the early fusion of the sacroiliac (SI) joints?

    A. Chondrosarcoma            C. Developmental dysplasia of the hip

    B. Metastatic carcinoma      D. Ankylosing spondylitis

16. Match each of the following radiographic appearances with the correct pathologic indications (using each choice only once):

    _____  1. Usually consists of numerous small lytic lesions              A.  Pelvic ring fracture

    _____  2. Increased hip joint space and misalignment                    B.  DDH

    _____  3. Bilateral radiolucent lines across                            C.  Osteoarthritis
                  bones and misalignment of SI joints
                                                                              D.  SCFE
    _____  4. Early fusion of SI joints and "bamboo spine"
                                                                              E.  Ankylosing spondylitis
    _____  5. Epiphyses appear shorter and epiphyseal plate wider
                                                                              F.  Metastatic carcinoma
    _____  6. Hallmark sign of spurring and narrowing of joint space

17. Which one of the following radiographic signs indicates that the proximal femurs are in position for a true AP projection?

    A. Appearance of the greater trochanter in profile

    B. Limited view of fovea capitis

    C. Limited view of the lesser trochanter in profile

    D. Symmetric appearance of iliac wings

18. The gonadal dose for an average-size male with a routine axiolateral (inferosuperior) lateral trauma hip projection is in the _____ mrad range.

    A. 50 to 100        C. 10 to 50

    B. 200 to 500       D. 600 to 800

19. True/False: The female gonadal dose for an AP pelvis is in the 50 to 100 mrad range, which is about 3 times greater than the dose for a male when no gonadal shields are used.

20. Which one of the following projections/methods is often performed to evaluate a pediatric patient for congenital hip dislocation?

    A. Bilateral frog-leg          C. Taylor method

    B. Clements-Nakayama       D. Judet

21. What type of central ray angle is required when using the Taylor method for a female patient?

    A. None (central ray is perpendicular)      C. 20° to 25° cephalad

    B. 10° to 15° caudad                        D. 30° to 45° cephalad

22. True/False: The modified Cleaves method is designed for nontraumatic hip projections.

23. True/False: Centering for the AP pelvis projection is 1 inch, or 2½ cm, superior to the symphysis pubis.

24. True/False: The Clements-Nakayama method is considered a nontraumatic lateral hip projection.

25. Which position of the pelvic girdle is designed to demonstrate the acetabulum? _____

26. Which one of the following projections/methods is used to evaluate the pelvic inlet for possible fracture?

    A. Danelius-Miller     C. Taylor

    B. AP axial            D. Clements-Nakayama

27. Where is the central ray centered for posterior oblique projections of the SI joints?

    _____

28. Does the AP axial projection for SI joints of a male generally require more or less central ray angle than the same

    projection for a female? _____

29. Does a right anterior oblique (RAO) position for SI joints demonstrate the right or left SI joints?

    _____

30. **Situation:** An initial AP pelvis radiograph reveals possible fractures involving the lower anterior pelvis. The emergency room physician asks for another projection to better demonstrate this area of the pelvis. The patient is traumatized and must remain in a supine position. Which projection should be taken?

    _____

31. **Situation:** A radiograph of an axiolateral (inferosuperior) projection of a hip demonstrates a soft tissue density that is visible across the affected hip and acetabulum. This artifact is obscuring the image of the proximal femur. What is the most likely cause of the artifact, and how can it be prevented from showing up on the repeat exposure?

    _____

    _____

32. **Situation:** A radiograph of an LPO projection for sacroiliac joints reveals that the ilium is superimposed over the involved joint. What type of positioning error is present on this radiograph?

_____

_____

33. **Situation:** A radiograph of an AP hip reveals that the lesser trochanter is not visible. Should the technologist repeat

the projection? _____ If yes, what should be modified to improve the image during the repeat exposure?

_____

_____

34. **Situation:** A young patient with a clinical history of SCFE comes to the radiology department. Which projection(s) are most often taken for this condition?

_____

_____

35. **Situation:** A radiograph produced using the Taylor method demonstrates that the anterior pelvic bones of a female patient are foreshortened. The following positioning factors were used: supine position, 40-inch (100-cm) SID, and central ray angled 30° caudad and centered 1 to 2 inches (3 to 5 cm) distal to symphysis pubis. Which one of the following modifications should be made during the repeat exposure?

    A.  Increase central ray angle          C.  Center central ray at level of ASIS

    B.  Reverse central ray angle            D.  Place patient prone on table

36. **Situation:** A radiograph of an AP projection of the pelvis demonstrates that the left obturator foramen is narrowed and the right one is open. What is the specific positioning error present on this radiograph?

_____

_____

37. **Situation:** A patient enters the emergency room with a possible pelvic ring fracture. The AP pelvis projection is inclusive on the extent and location of the fracture(s). What additional pelvis projection(s) can be taken on this patient to demonstrate possible pelvic fractures? (More than one correct answer is possible)

_____

_____

38. What type of CR angle is required for the AP axial, "inlet" projection?

    A.  20° to 35° cephalad      C.  40° caudad

    B.  10° to 15° cephalad      D.  None (CR is perpendicular to IR)

39. **Situation:** A radiograph of posterior oblique projections of the SI joints reveals that the lower aspects of the joints are not well defined. The radiologist asks the technologist to repeat both projections and open up the lower SI joints. What can the technologist do to open up the inferior aspect of the joints?

_____

_____

8

40. For the following critique questions, refer to the unilateral frog-leg radiograph in Fig. C8-77 on p. 286 in the textbook:

   A. Which positioning error(s) is(are) visible on this radiograph? (More than one answer may be selected.)

      (a) All essential anatomic structures are not demonstrated.

      (b) Central ray is centered incorrectly.

      (c) Collimation is not evident.

      (d) Exposure factors are incorrect.

      (e) No anatomic marker is visible on the radiograph.

   B. Which error(s) identified above is(are) considered "repeatable"? _____

   C. Which of the following modifications must be made during the repeat exposure? (More than one answer may be selected.)

      (a) Increase collimation.

      (b) Center central ray to femoral neck.

      (c) Decrease exposure factors.

      (d) Increase exposure factors.

      (e) Reposition anatomic marker on image receptor (IR) before exposure.

      (f) Use larger IR.

41. For the following critique questions, refer to the AP pelvis radiograph in Fig. C8-78 on p. 286 in the textbook.

   A. Which positioning error(s) is(are) visible on this radiograph? (More than one answer may be selected.

      (a) All essential anatomic structures are not demonstrated.

      (b) Central ray is centered incorrectly.

      (c) Collimation is not evident.

      (d) Exposure factors are incorrect.

      (e) No anatomic marker is visible on the radiograph.

      (f) Slight rotation toward the right is evident.

      (g) Slight rotation is evident.

      (h) Proximal femurs are not placed in a true AP position.

   B. Which error(s) identified above is(are) considered "repeatable"? _____

   C. Which of the following modifications must be made during the repeat exposure? (More than one answer may be selected.)

      (a) Increase collimation.

      (b) Center central ray correctly.

      (c) Decrease exposure factors.

      (d) Increase exposure factors.

      (e) Place anatomic marker on IR before exposure.

      (f) Rotate body slightly toward the left.

      (g) Rotate body slightly toward the right.

      (h) Rotate proximal femurs 15° to 20° internally.

# Cervical and Thoracic Spine

## CHAPTER OBJECTIVES

After you have successfully completed the activities in this chapter, you will be able to:

_____ 1. Using drawings and radiographs, identify specific anatomic structures of the cervical and thoracic spine.

_____ 2. Identify specific features of the cervical and thoracic vertebrae that distinguish them from other aspects of the vertebral column.

_____ 3. Identify the location, angulation, classification, and type of movement for specific joints of the cervical and thoracic spine.

_____ 4. List additional terms for the first, second, and seventh cervical vertebrae.

_____ 5. Identify topographic landmarks that can be palpated to locate specific thoracic and cervical vertebrae.

_____ 6. Match specific pathologic indications of the cervical and thoracic spine to the correct definition.

_____ 7. Identify which radiographic projection and/or procedure best demonstrates specific pathologic indications.

_____ 8. Identify structures that are best demonstrated with each position of the cervical and thoracic spine.

_____ 9. List the patient dose ranges, including thyroid and female breast doses, for specific projections of the cervical and thoracic spine.

_____ 10. Identify basic and special projections of the cervical and thoracic spine and list the correct size and type of image receptor (IR) and the central ray location, direction, and angulation for each position.

_____ 11. Given various hypothetical situations, identify the correct modification of a position and/or exposure factors to improve the radiographic image.

_____ 12. Given radiographs of specific cervical and thoracic spine projections, identify positioning and exposure factor errors.

### Positioning and Radiographic Critique

_____ 1. Using a peer, position for basic and special projections of the cervical and thoracic spine.

_____ 2. Using appropriate radiographic phantoms, produce satisfactory radiographs of specific positions (if equipment is available).

_____ 3. Critique and evaluate cervical and thoracic spine radiographs based on the four divisions of radiographic criteria: (1) structures shown, (2) position, (3) collimation and central ray, and (4) exposure criteria.

_____ 4. Distinguish between acceptable and unacceptable spine radiographs based on exposure factors, motion, collimation, positioning, or other errors.

## Learning Exercises

Complete the following review exercises after reading the associated pages in the textbook as indicated by each exercise. Answers to each review exercise are given at the end of the review exercises.

## Part I: Radiographic Anatomy

1-26, 29, 30

**REVIEW EXERCISE A:** Radiographic Anatomy of the Cervical and Thoracic Spine (see textbook pp. 288-290)

1. List the number of bones found in each division in the **adult** vertebral column:

   A. Cervical ___7___        D. Sacrum ___1___

   B. Thoracic ___12___       E. Coccyx ___1___

   C. Lumbar ___5___          F. Total ___26___

   Refer to Fig. 9-1 to answer questions 2 through 4.

2. List the two **primary** or **posterior convex** curves seen in the vertebral column:

   A. ___Thoracic___

   B. ___Sacral___

3. Indicate which two portions of the vertebral column are classified as **secondary** or **compensatory** curves:

   A. ___Cervical___

   B. ___Lumbar___

4. Match the correct aspect(s) of the vertebral column with the following characteristics (may be more than one answer):

   _B, D_  1. Convex curve (with respect to posterior)        A. Cervical spine

   _A, C_  2. Concave curve (with respect to posterior)        B. Thoracic spine

   _A, C_  3. Secondary curve                                  C. Lumbar spine

   _B, D_  4. Primary curve                                    D. Sacrum

   _A_     5. Develops as child learns to hold head erect

**Posterior    Anterior**

Centerline of gravity

**Fig. 9-1.** Lateral view, spinal column.

5. An abnormal, or exaggerated, "sway back" lumbar curvature is called ___Lordosis___ .

6. An abnormal lateral curvature seen in the thoracolumbar spine is called ___Scoliosis___ .

7. The two main parts of a typical vertebra are the ___body___ and the ___Vertebral arch___ .

8. The ___laminae___ are two bony aspects of the vertebral arch that extend posteriorly from each pedicle to join at the midline.

9. The ___Intervertebral___ foramina are created by two small notches on the superior and inferior aspects of the pedicles.

10.  The opening, or passageway, for the spinal cord is the _Vertebral (spinal) canal_.

11.  The spinal cord begins with the (A) _medulla oblongata_ of the brain and extends down to the

(B) _first lumbar L1_ vertebra, where it tapers and ends. This tapered ending is called the

(C) _Conus medullaris_ .

12.  Which structures pass through the intervertebral foramina? _nerves and blood vessels_

13.  Identify the following structures labeled on these drawings of typical thoracic vertebrae (Fig. 9-2):

*Superior view*

A.  _Spinous process_

B.  _Laminae_

C.  _Transverse process_

D.  _Facet of superior articular process_

E.  _Pedicle_

F.  _Vertebral foramen_

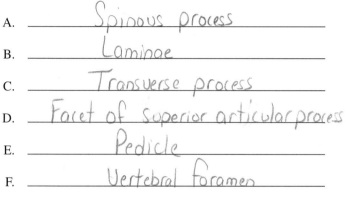

Superior view

*Lateral view*

G.  _Spinous process_

H.  _Superior articular process facet_

I.  _Pedicle_

J.  _Body_

K.  _Inferior articular process_

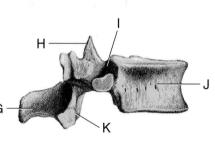

Lateral view

*Lateral oblique view*

L.  _Superior articular process_

M.  _Zygapophyseal_ joint

N.  _Facet for head of rib articulation_

O.  _Intervertebral foramen_

P.  _Facet for rib articulation_

Lateral oblique view

Q.  The joints between the ribs and vertebrae at *N* are called:

_Costovertebral_

R.  The joints between the ribs and vertebrae at *P* are called:

_Costotransverse_

**Fig. 9-2.** Typical thoracic vertebra.

9

14. Which of the following is found between the superior and inferior articular processes?

    A. Intervertebral joints      C. Zygapophyseal joints

    B. Articular joints           D. Intervertebral facets

15. True/False: Only T1, T11, and T12 have **full** facets for articulation with ribs.

16. True/False: The zygapophyseal joints of all cervical vertebrae are visualized only in a true lateral position.    *between C1, C2 AP*

17. List the outer and inner aspects of the intervertebral disk:

    A. Outer aspect *annulus fibrosus*      B. Inner aspect *nucleus pulposus*

18. The condition involving a "slipped disk" is correctly referred to as *herniated nucleus pulposus (HNP)*

_____ .

19. List the alternative names for the following cervical vertebrae:

    A. C1: *the atlas*

    B. C2: *the axis*

    C. C7: *vertebra prominens*

20. List three features that make the cervical vertebrae unique:

    A. *Transverse foramina*          C. *Overlapping vertebral bodies*

    B. *bifid spinous process tips*

21. A short column of bone found between the superior and articular processes in a typical cervical vertebra is called

    *articular pillar* _____ .

22. What is the term for the same structure, identified in the previous question, for the C1 vertebra?

    _____ *lateral mass* _____

23. The zygapophyseal joints for the second through seventh cervical vertebrae are at a *90* ° angle to the midsagittal plane; the thoracic vertebrae are at a *20-25*° angle to the midsagittal plane.

24. What is the name of the joint found between the superior articular processes of C1 and the occipital condyles of the

    skull? *atlantooccipital articulations*

25. The modified body of C2 is called the *dens* or *odontoid process* .

26. A lack of symmetry of the zygapophyseal joints between C1 and C2 may be caused by injury or may be associated

    with *rotation of the skull* _____ .

27. What is the unique feature of all thoracic vertebrae that distinguishes them from other vertebrae?

    *their facets for articulation with ribs*

28. Which specific thoracic vertebrae are classified as typical thoracic vertebrae (i.e., they least resemble cervical or

    lumbar vertebrae)? *T5-T8*

29.  Identify the labeled structures on the radiographs of the cervical spine in Figs. 9-3 and 9-4. (Indicate the specific structure and the vertebra of which it is a part.)

|   | STRUCTURE | VERTEBRA |
|---|-----------|----------|
| A. | Body | C4 |
| B. | Dens (odontoid) | C1 |
| C. | Posterior arch and tubercle | C1 |
| D. | Zygapophyseal joint | C5-6 |
| E. | Spinous process (verteba prominens) | C7 |
| F. | Posterior arch and tubercle | C1 |
| G. | Pedicle | C4 |
| H. | Intervertebral foramen | C4-5 |

**Fig. 9-3.** Lateral view, cervical spine.

**Fig. 9-4.** 45-degree oblique view, cervical spine.

30.  For the central ray to pass through and "open" the intervertebral spaces on a 45° posterior oblique projection of the cervical vertebrae, what central ray angle (if any) would be required? __15° cephalad__

## Part II: Radiographic Positioning

1-3, 10, 17-37, 39-41

**REVIEW EXERCISE B:** Positioning of the Cervical and Thoracic Spine (see textbook pp. 300-319)

1.  Name the following parts of the sternum or associated topographic landmarks.

     A.  Upper portion of sternum: __manubrium__

     B.  Superior margin of this upper section (landmark): __jugular notch__

     C.  Main center portion of sternum: __body__

     D.  Joint between top and center portions (landmark): __Sternal angle__

     E.  Most inferior aspect of sternum (landmark): __Xiphoid process (tip)__

2.  Match the following topographic landmarks to the correct vertebral level (using each choice only once):

| | | | |
|---|---|---|---|
| H | 1. Gonion | A. | T1 |
| E | 2. Xiphoid process (tip) | B. | T2-3 |
| F | 3. Thyroid cartilage | C. | C1 |
| B | 4. Jugular notch | D. | T4-5 |
| D | 5. Sternal angle | E. | T10 |
| C | 6. Mastoid tip | F. | C4-6 |
| A | 7. Vertebra prominens | G. | T7 |
| G | 8. 3 to 4 inches (8 to 10 cm) below jugular notch | H. | C3 |

9

3.  In addition to the gonads, which other radiosensitive organs are of greatest concern during cervical and thoracic spine radiography?

    thyroid, parathyroid, breasts

4.  List the two advantages of using higher kilovoltage exposure factors for spine radiography, especially on an anteroposterior (AP) thoracic spine radiograph:

    A.  _____    B.  _____

5.  True/False: When using digital imaging for spine radiography, it is important to use close collimation, grids, and lead masking.

6.  True/False: If close collimation is used during conventional radiography of the spine, the use of lead masking is generally not required.

7.  True/False: To a certain degree, magnetic resonance imaging (MRI) and computed tomography (CT) are replacing myelography as the imaging modalities of choice for the diagnosis of a ruptured intervertebral disk.

8.  True/False: Nuclear medicine is often performed to diagnose bone tumors of the spine.

9.  To ensure that the intervertebral joint spaces are open for lateral thoracic spine projections, it is important to:

    A.  Keep the vertebral column parallel to the image receptor (IR)

    B.  Use a small focal spot

    C.  Use a breathing technique

    D.  Angle the central ray cephalad

10. For lateral and oblique projections of the cervical spine, it is important to minimize magnification and maximize detail by (more than one answer may be used):

    A.  Keeping vertebral column parallel to image receptor

    (B) Using a small focal spot

    (C) Increasing source image receptor distance (SID)

    D.  Using a breathing technique

11. Match each of the following pathologic indications of the spine to the correct definition (using each choice only once):

    _____  A.  Fracture through the pedicles and anterior arch of C2 with forward displacement upon C3

    _____  B.  Inflammation of the vertebrae

    _____  C.  Abnormal or exaggerated convex curvature of the thoracic spine

    _____  D.  Comminuted fracture of the vertebral body with posterior fragments displaced into the spinal canal

    _____  E.  Avulsion fracture of the spinous process of C7

    _____  F.  Abnormal lateral curvature of the spine

    _____  G.  A form of rheumatoid arthritis

    _____  H.  Impact fracture from axial loading of the anterior and posterior arch of C1

    _____  I.  Mild form of scoliosis and kyphosis developing during adolescence

    _____  J.  Produces the "bow tie" sign

    1.  Ankylosing spondylitis

    2.  Clay shoveler's fracture

    3.  Unilateral subluxation

    4.  Kyphosis

    5.  Scheuermann's disease

    6.  Scoliosis

    7.  Jefferson fracture

    8.  Teardrop burst fracture

    9.  Hangman's fracture

    10. Spondylitis

12. List the conventional radiographic examination/projections performed for the following pathologic indications:

   A. Scoliosis: _____

   B. Teardrop burst fracture: _____

   C. Jefferson fracture: _____

   D. Scheuermann's disease: _____

   E. Unilateral subluxation of cervical spine: _____

   F. HNP: _____

13. What are the major differences between spondylosis and spondylitis? _____

14. True or False: Many geriatric patients have a fear of falling off the radiographic table.

15. What is the name of the radiographic procedure that requires the injection of contrast media into the subarachnoid

   space? _____

16. Which imaging modality is ideal for detecting early signs of osteomyelitis?

   _____

17. Which two landmarks must be aligned for an AP "open mouth" projection? *lower margin of upper incisors and base of the skull*

18. What is the purpose of the 15° to 20° angle for the AP axial projection of the cervical spine?

   *because of overlapping, to better demonstrate the intervertebral disk spaces*

19. For an AP axial of the cervical spine, a plane through the tip of the mandible and _____ should be parallel to the angled central ray.

   A. Mastoid process      C. Base of skull

   B. Gonion               D. External auditory meatus (EAM)

20. What are two important benefits of an SID longer than 40 to 44 inches (102 to 112 cm) for the lateral cervical spine projection?

   A. *Comp. for OID; reduce magnification*  B. *less divergence of beam to reduce shoulder superimposition of C7*

21. What central ray angulation must be used with a posterior oblique projection of the cervical spine?

   *15° Cephalad*

22. Which foramina are demonstrated with a left posterior oblique (LPO) position of the cervical spine?

   *Right intervertebral foramina (Upside)*

23. Which foramina are demonstrated with a left anterior oblique (LAO) position of the cervical spine?

   *Left intervertebral foramina (downside)*

24. In addition to extending the chin, which additional positioning technique can be performed to ensure that the mandible is not superimposed over the upper cervical vertebrae for the oblique projections?

   *rotate skull into a near lateral position*

9

25.  What is the recommended SID for a lateral projection of the cervical spine?

_____60-72 inches_____

26.  The lateral projection of the cervical spine should be taken during __expiration__ (inspiration, expiration, or suspended respiration). Why?

_for maximum Shoulder depression_____

27.  Which specific projection must be taken first if trauma to the cervical spine is suspected and the patient is in a

supine position on a backboard?  ____lateral position, horizontal beam_____

28.  The proper name of the method for performing the cervicothoracic (swimmer's lateral) projection is the

_____Twining Method_____ .

29.  Where should the central ray be placed for a cervicothoracic (swimmer's lateral) projection?

_____T1; 1 inch above jugular notch or at vertebra prominens____

30.  Which region of the spine must be demonstrated with a cervicothoracic (swimmer's lateral) projection?

_____C4 -T3_____

31.  Which one of the following projections is considered a "functional study" of the cervical spine?

A.  AP "wagging jaw" projection          C.  Fuchs or Judd method

B.  AP "open mouth" position             (D.)  Hyperextension and flexion lateral positions

32.  When should the Judd or Fuchs method be performed?

_When dens is not well visualized on AP Open Mouth_____

33.  Which AP projection of the cervical spine demonstrates the entire **upper** cervical spine with one single projection?

_AP Wagging Jaw "Ottonello Method"_____

34.  Which two things can be done to produce equal density along the entire thoracic spine for the AP projection

(especially for a patient with a thick chest)?  _Anode Heel Effect; use of_

_Compensating (wedge) filter_____

35.  What is the purpose of using a breathing technique for a lateral projection of the thoracic spine?

_blurs out unwanted rib and lung markings overlying vertebrae_

36.  Which zygapophyseal joints are demonstrated in a right anterior oblique (RAO) projection of the thoracic spine?

_____right (downside)_____

37.  Which one of the following projections delivers the greatest skin dose to the patient?

A.  AP thoracic spine projection          (C.)  Swimmer's lateral projection

B.  Lateral cervical spine projection       D.  Fuchs or Judd method

9

38. Which of the following results in the lowest midline and skin doses for the patient? (Note dose relationship to milliampere seconds.)

    A.  AP thoracic spine at 90 kV, 7 mAs       C.  Lateral thoracic spine at 80 kV, 50 mAs

    B.  AP thoracic spine at 80 kV, 12 mAs      D.  Oblique thoracic spine at 80 kV, 20 mAs

39. True/False: The thyroid dose used during a posterior oblique cervical spine projection is more than 10 times greater than the dose used for an anterior oblique projection of the cervical spine.

40. Which one of the following structures is best demonstrated with an AP axial vertebral arch projection?

    A.  Spinous processes of lumbar spine                 C.  Zygapophyseal joints of thoracic spine

    B.  Articular pillar (lateral masses) of cervical spine       D.  Cervicothoracic spine region

41. What central ray angle must be used with the AP axial—vertebral arch projection?

    A.  15° to 20° cephalad       C.  20° to 30° caudad

    B.  5° to 10° cephalad        D.  None (central ray is perpendicular to IR)

42. What ancillary device should be placed behind the patient on the table top for a recumbent lateral projection of the thoracic spine when using computed radiography?

_____

*1-5, 7-12*

**REVIEW EXERCISE C:** Problem Solving for Technical and Positioning Errors (see textbook pp. 306-319)

1. A radiograph of an AP "open mouth" projection of the cervical spine reveals that the base of the skull is superimposed over the upper dens. Which **specific** positioning error is present on this radiograph?

    _____ *excessive rotation of the skull* _____

2. A radiograph of an AP axial projection of the cervical spine reveals that the intervertebral disk spaces are not open. The following positioning factors were used: extension of the skull, central ray angled 10° cephalad, central ray centered to the thyroid cartilage, and no rotation or tilt of the spine. Which of these factors need(s) to be modified to produce a more diagnostic image?

    _____ *CR 15-20°* _____

3. A radiograph of a right posterior oblique (RPO) cervical spine projection reveals that the lower intervertebral foramina are *not* open. The upper intervertebral foramina are well visualized. What positioning error most likely led to this radiographic outcome?

    *Shoulders incorrectly rotated , Should be rotated 45°*

4. A radiograph on a lateral projection of the cervical spine reveals that C7 is not clearly visible. The following factors were used: erect position, 44-inch (112-cm) SID, arms down by the patient's side, and exposure made during inspiration. Which two of these factors should be changed to produce a more diagnostic image during the repeat exposure?

    *Increase SID to 72" and Suspend resp. on expiration*

5. A radiograph of an AP "chewing" or "wagging jaw" projection taken at 75 kV, 20 mAs, and ½ second demonstrates that part of the image of the mandible is still visible and obscuring the upper cervical spine. Which modification needs to be made to produce a more diagnostic image during the repeat exposure?

    *reduce mA and increase exposure time to produce more blurring*

9

6. A radiograph of a lateral thoracic spine reveals that lung markings and ribs make it difficult to visualize the vertebral bodies. The following factors were used: recumbent position, 40-inch (102-cm) SID, short exposure time, and exposure made during full expiration. Which one of these factors needs to be modified to produce a more diagnostic image during the repeat exposure?

_____

7. A radiograph of an AP projection of the thoracic spine reveals that the upper thoracic spine is greatly overexposed but the lower vertebrae are well visualized. The head of the patient was placed at the anode end of the table. What can be modified during the repeat exposure to produce a more diagnostic image?

_Use a wedge filter with thicker part placed over upper t-spine_
_to equalize density_

8. A radiograph of a cervicothoracic lateral projection demonstrates superimposition of the humeral heads over the upper thoracic spine. Because of an arthritic condition, the patient is unable to rotate the shoulders any further apart. What can the technologist do to further separate the shoulders during the repeat exposure?

_Angle CR 3-5° Caudad_

9. **Situation:** A patient with a possible cervical spine injury enters the emergency room. The patient is on a backboard. Which projection of the cervical spine should be taken first?

_lateral position horizontal beam_

10. **Situation:** A patient who has been in a motor vehicle accident (MVA) enters the emergency room. The basic projections of the cervical spine reveal no subluxation (partial dislocation) or fracture. The physician wants the spine evaluated for whiplash injury. Which additional projections would best demonstrate this type of injury?

_hyperextension and flexion lateral positions_

11. **Situation:** A patient comes to the radiology department for a cervical spine series. An AP "open mouth" radiograph indicates that the base of the skull and lower edge of the front incisors are superimposed, but the top of the dens is not clearly demonstrated. What should the technologist do to demonstrate the upper portion of the dens? (A horizontal beam lateral has ruled out a C-spine fracture or subluxation.

_either Fuchs or Judd Method_

12. **Situation:** A patient comes to the radiology department for a routine cervical spine series. The lateral projection only demonstrates the C1 to C6 region. The radiologist wants to see C7-T1. What additional projection can be taken to demonstrate this region of the spine?

_Cervicothoracic "Swimmers" lateral_

13. **Situation:** A patient enters the ER with a possible cervical spine fracture, but the initial projections do not demonstrate any gross fracture or subluxation. After reviewing the initial radiographs, the ER physician suspects either a congenital defect or fracture of the lateral mass on C4. He wants an additional projection taken to better see this aspect of the vertebrae. What additional projection can be taken to demonstrate the lateral masses of C4?

_____

14. **Situation:** A patient comes to the ER with a possible Jefferson fracture. Other than a lateral projection or a CT scan, what specific radiographic projection will best demonstrate this type of fracture?

_____

15. **Situation:** A patient comes to the radiology department with a clinical history of Scheuermann's disease. Which radiographic procedure is often performed for this condition?

_____

**REVIEW EXERCISE D:** Critique Radiographs of the Cervical and Thoracic Spine (see textbook p. 320)

The following questions relate to the radiographs found at the end of Chapter 9 of the textbook. Evaluate these radiographs for the radiographic criteria categories *(1 through 5)* that follow. Describe the corrections needed to improve the overall image. The major, or "repeatable," errors are specific errors that indicate the need for a repeat exposure, regardless of the nature of the other errors.

A. **AP open mouth (Fig. C9-91)**
   Description of possible error:

   1. Structures shown: _____

   2. Part positioning: _____

   3. Collimation and central ray: _____

   4. Exposure criteria: _____

   5. Markers: _____

   Repeatable error(s): _____

B. **AP open mouth (Fig. C9-92)**
   Description of possible error:

   1. Structures shown: _____

   2. Part positioning: _____

   3. Collimation and central ray: _____

   4. Exposure criteria: _____

   5. Markers: _____

   Repeatable error(s): _____

C. **AP axial projection (Fig. C9-93)**
   Description of possible error:

   1. Structures shown: _____

   2. Part positioning: _____

   3. Collimation and central ray: _____

   4. Exposure criteria: _____

   5. Markers: _____

   Repeatable error(s): _____

**9**

D. **Oblique (RPO) (Fig. C9-94)**
   Description of possible error:

   1. Structures shown: _____

   2. Part positioning: _____

   3. Collimation and central ray: _____

   4. Exposure criteria: _____

   5. Markers: _____

   Repeatable error(s): _____

E. **Lateral (trauma) (Fig. C9-95)**
   Description of possible error:

   1. Structures shown: _____

   2. Part positioning: _____

   3. Collimation and central ray: _____

   4. Exposure criteria: _____

   5. Markers: _____

   Repeatable error(s): _____

F. **Lateral (nontrauma) (Fig. C9-96)**
   Description of possible error:

   1. Structures shown: _____

   2. Part positioning: _____

   3. Collimation and central ray: _____

   4. Exposure criteria: _____

   5. Markers: _____

   Repeatable error(s): _____

## Part III: Laboratory Exercises (see textbook pp. 306-319)

You must gain experience in positioning each part of the cervical and thoracic spine before performing the following exams on actual patients. You can get experience in positioning and radiographic evaluation of these projections by performing exercises using radiographic phantoms and practicing positioning on other students (although you will not be taking actual exposures).

The following suggested activities assume that your teaching institution has an energized lab and radiographic phantoms. If not, perform Laboratory Exercises B and C, the radiographic evaluation and the physical positioning exercises. (Check off each step and projection as you complete it.)

## LABORATORY EXERCISE A: Energized Laboratory

1.  Using the radiographic phantom, produce radiographs of the following basic routines:

    A.  AP, lateral, and oblique cervical spine

    B.  AP, lateral, and oblique thoracic spine

## LABORATORY EXERCISE B: Radiographic Evaluation

1.  Evaluate and critique the radiographs produced above, additional radiographs provided by your instructor, or both. Evaluate each radiograph for the following points:

    _____ Evaluate the completeness of the study. (Are all of the pertinent anatomic structures included on the radiograph?)

    _____ Evaluate for positioning or centering errors (e.g., rotation, off centering).

    _____ Evaluate for correct exposure factors and possible motion. (Are the density and contrast of the images acceptable?)

    _____ Determine whether anatomic side markers and an acceptable degree of collimation and/or area shielding are visible on the images.

## LABORATORY EXERCISE C: Physical Positioning

On another person, simulate performing all basic and special projections of the cervical and thoracic spine as follows. Include the six steps listed below and described in the textbook. (Check off each step when completed satisfactorily.)

Step 1. Appropriate size and type of image receptor with correct markers
Step 2. Correct central ray placement and centering of part to central ray and/or image receptor
Step 3. Accurate collimation
Step 4. Area shielding of patient where advisable
Step 5. Use of proper immobilizing devices when needed
Step 6. Approximate correct exposure factors, breathing instructions where applicable, and "making" exposure

| PROJECTIONS | STEP 1 | STEP 2 | STEP 3 | STEP 4 | STEP 5 | STEP 6 |
|---|---|---|---|---|---|---|
| • Cervical spine series (AP axial, AP C1-2, obliques, lateral) | _____ | _____ | _____ | _____ | _____ | _____ |
| • Thoracic spine series (AP and lateral) | _____ | _____ | _____ | _____ | _____ | _____ |
| • Swimmer's lateral | _____ | _____ | _____ | _____ | _____ | _____ |
| • Hyperextension and flexion laterals | _____ | _____ | _____ | _____ | _____ | _____ |
| • AP "chewing" or "wagging jaw" | _____ | _____ | _____ | _____ | _____ | _____ |
| • AP (Fuchs) for dens | _____ | _____ | _____ | _____ | _____ | _____ |
| • PA (Judd) for dens | _____ | _____ | _____ | _____ | _____ | _____ |
| • Thoracic spine obliques | _____ | _____ | _____ | _____ | _____ | _____ |

**9**

# *Answers to Review Exercises*

## Review Exercise A: Radiographic Anatomy of the Cervical and Thoracic Spine

1. A. 7
   B. 12
   C. 5
   D. 1
   E. 1
   F. 26
2. A. Thoracic
   B. Sacral
3. A. Cervical
   B. Lumbar
4. 1. B and D
   2. A and C
   3. A and C
   4. B and D
   5. A
5. Lordosis
6. Scoliosis
7. Body; vertebral arch
8. Lamina
9. Intervertebral
10. Vertebral (spinal) canal
11. A. Medulla oblongata
    B. Lower border of L1
    C. Conus medullaris
12. Spinal nerves and blood vessels
13. A. Spinous process
    B. Lamina
    C. Transverse process
    D. Facet of superior articular process
    E. Pedicle
    F. Vertebral foramen
    G. Spinous process
    H. Facet of superior articular process
    I. Pedicle
    J. Body
    K. Inferior articular process
    L. Superior articular process
    M. Zygapophyseal joint
    N. Facet for head of rib articulation
    O. Intervertebral foramen
    P. Facet for rib articulation
    Q. Costovertebral joints
    R. Costotransverse joints
14. C. Zygapophyseal joints
15. True
16. False (between C1 and C2 visualized on a frontal or AP projection)
17. A. Annulus fibrosus
    B. Nucleus pulposus
18. Herniated nucleus pulposus (HNP)
19. A. C1: Atlas
    B. C2: Axis
    C. C7: Vertebra prominens
20. A. Transverse foramina
    B. Bifid spinous process
    C. Overlapping vertebral bodies
21. Articular pillar

22. Lateral mass
23. 90; 70 to 75
24. Atlanto-occipital articulation
25. Dens or odontoid process
26. Rotation of the skull
27. Presence of facets for articulation with ribs
28. T5 to T8
29. A. Body, C4
    B. Dens (odontoid), C2
    C. Posterior arch and tubercle, C1
    D. Zygapophyseal joint, C5-6
    E. Spinous process (vertebra prominens), C7
    F. Posterior arch and tubercle, C1
    G. Pedicle, C4
    H. Intervertebral foramen, C4-5
30. 15° cephalad

## Review Exercise B: Positioning of the Cervical and Thoracic Spine

1. A. Manubrium
   B. Jugular (suprasternal) notch
   C. Body
   D. Sternal angle
   E. Xiphoid process
2. 1. H
   2. E
   3. F
   4. B
   5. D
   6. C
   7. A
   8. G
3. Thyroid gland, parathyroid glands, and female breasts
4. A. Increase in exposure latitude
   B. Decrease in patient dose
5. True
6. False (Lead masking should be used even if close collimation is used.)
7. True
8. True
9. A. Keep vertebral column parallel to image receptor (IR)
10. B. Using a small focal spot
    C. Increasing SID
11. A. 9
    B. 10
    C. 4
    D. 8
    E. 2
    F. 6
    G. 1
    H. 7
    I. 5
    J. 3
12. A. Erect (AP/PA) and lateral spine including bending laterals

B. Lateral cervical
   C. AP open mouth C1-2, tomography—following lateral projection
   D. Scoliosis series
   E. Lateral cervical spine
   F. Lateral of affected spine
13. Spondylitis is an inflammatory process of the vertebrae. Spondylosis is a condition of the spine characterized by rigidity of a vertebral joint.
14. True
15. Myelography
16. Nuclear medicine
17. Lower margin of upper incisors and base of skull
18. To open up the intervertebral disk spaces
19. C. Base of skull
20. A. Compensates for increased object image receptor distance (OID); reduces magnification
    B. Less divergence of x-ray beam to reduce shoulder superimposition of C7
21. 15° cephalad
22. Right intervertebral foramina (upside)
23. Left intervertebral foramina (downside)
24. Rotate the skull into a near lateral position
25. 60 to 72 inches (150 to 180 cm)
26. Expiration; for maximum shoulder depression
27. Lateral, horizontal beam projection
28. Twining method
29. To T1; 1 inch (2.5 cm) above the jugular notch, or at vertebra prominens
30. C4 to T3
31. D. Hyperextension and flexion lateral positions
32. If unable to demonstrate the upper portion of the dens with the AP "open mouth" projection
33. AP "wagging jaw" projection (Ottonello method)
34. Correct use of anode-heel effect; use of compensating (wedge) filter
35. To blur out rib and lung markings that obscure detail of thoracic vertebrae
36. Right (downside)
37. C. Swimmer's lateral projection
38. A. 90 kV, 7 mAs
39. True (anterior oblique < 5 mrad; posterior oblique < 69 mrad)
40. B. Articular pillar (lateral masses)
41. C. 20° to 30° caudad
42. Lead mat or masking

**9**

## Review Exercise C: Problem Solving for Technical and Positioning Errors

1. Excessive extension of the skull
2. Increase central ray angulation to 15°.
3. The shoulders are incorrectly rotated. They need to be rotated 45°.
4. Initiate exposure during suspended expiration and increase SID to 72 inches (183 cm).
5. Reduce milliamperage and increase exposure time to produce more blurring of the mandible
6. Use of a breathing technique to blur lung markings and ribs more effectively
7. Utilize a compensating (wedge) filter with thicker part of filter placed over the upper thoracic spine to equalize the density along the thoracic spine.
8. Angle CR 3° to 5° caudad
9. Lateral, horizontal beam projection
10. Hyperextension and flexion lateral positions
11. Perform either the Fuchs or Judd method.
12. Cervicothoracic (swimmer's) lateral projection
13. AP axial—vertebral arch (pillar) projection
14. AP open mouth projection
15. Scoliosis series

## Review Exercise D: Critique Radiographs of the Cervical and Thoracic Spine

A. AP open mouth (Fig. C9-91)
   1. Upper aspect of dens obscured by base of skull
   2. Overextension of skull, causing superimposition of base of skull over dens
   3. Collimation too loose, resulting in excessive exposure to face, eyes, and neck region; correct central ray and IR placement
   4. Acceptable exposure factors
   5. No evidence of anatomic side marker

   Repeatable error(s): 1 and 2

B. AP open mouth (Fig. C9-92)
   1. Upper aspect of dens and joint space obscured by front incisors
   2. Overflexion of skull causing superimposition of front incisors over top of dens
   3. Collimation too loose, resulting in excessive exposure to face, eyes, and neck region; slightly low central ray and IR
   4. Acceptable exposure factors
   5. No evidence of anatomic side marker

   Repeatable error(s): 1 and 2

C. AP axial projection (Fig. C9-93)
   1. Distorted vertebral bodies and intervertebral joint spaces; base of skull superimposed over upper cervical spine
   2. Overextension of skull and/or excessive central ray cephalic angle, which probably led to poor definition of vertebral bodies and joint spaces
   3. Evidence of collimation; slightly low central ray centering but correct IR placement
   4. Acceptable exposure factors
   5. Evidence of anatomic side marker

   Repeatable error(s): 1 and 2

   Note: Unsure of the origin of the artifact seen on lower, left cervical spine region

D. Oblique (RPO) (Fig. C9-94)
   1. Intervertebral joint spaces and foramina not clearly demonstrated; superimposition of mandible over upper cervical spine
   2. Appears that body is underrotated from AP position (with appearance of upper rib cage suggesting underrotation rather than overrotation), an error that led to narrowing and obscuring of the intervertebral foramina; can place the skull into lateral position to remove mandible from the upper C spine (department option)
   3. No evidence of collimation; insufficient or incorrect central ray angulation (and foreshortened cervical spine)—may have led to closure of disk spaces
   4. Acceptable exposure factors
   5. No evidence of anatomic side marker

   Repeatable error(s): 1, 2, and 3

E. Lateral (trauma) (Fig. C9-95)
   1. Aspect of C1 and dens cut off; C7-T1 not demonstrated
   2. Need to depress shoulders (because chin cannot be adjusted as a result of the trauma)
   3. No evidence of collimation except along anterior, upper margin; central ray centered too posterior, causing upper cervical spine to be cut off; IR placement centered too low
   4. Acceptable exposure factors (poor contrast resulting from using a nongrid technique)
   5. No evidence of anatomic side marker

   Repeatable error(s): 1, 2, and 3

F. Lateral (nontrauma) (Fig. C9-96)
   1. Only six cervical demonstrated vertebrae; slight superimposition of posterior aspect of mandible over anterior arch of C1
   2. Need to depress shoulders more to demonstrate C7-T1; need to extend chin further
   3. Evidence of collimation (but could be tighter); correct central ray centering and IR placement
   4. Radiograph slightly underexposed (difficult to evaluate in this printed version)
   5. No evidence of anatomic side marker

   Repeatable errors: 1 and 2

9

# SELF-TEST

My Score = _____ %

This self-test should be taken only after completing all of the readings, review exercises, and laboratory activities for a particular section. The purpose of this test is not only to provide a good learning exercise but also to serve as a strong indicator of what your final evaluation exam will cover. It is strongly suggested that if you do not get at least a 90% to 95% grade on each self-test, you review those areas in which you missed questions before going to your instructor for the final evaluation exam for this chapter. (There are 116 questions or blanks—each is worth 0.9 point.)

1. At which vertebral level does the solid spinal cord terminate? _____

2. How many segments make up the sacrum in the neonate? _____

3. Which of the following divisions of the spine is described as possessing a primary curve? (There may be more than one correct answer.)

    A. Thoracic        C. Lumbar

    B. Cervical        D. Sacral

4. True/False: The lumbar possesses a concave posterior spinal curvature.

5. An abnormal or exaggerated thoracic curvature with increased convexity is called _____ .

6. An abnormal or exaggerated lateral curvature is called _____ .

7. What is the correct term for the condition involving a "slipped disk"? _____

8. Which foramina are created by the superior and inferior vertebral notches? _____

9. Which joints are found between the superior and inferior articular processes? _____

10. Which one of the following structures makes up the inner aspect of the intervertebral disk?

    A. Annulus fibrosus        C. Annulus pulposus

    B. Nucleus pulposus        D. Nucleus fibrosus

11. True/False: The carotid artery and certain nerves pass through the cervical transverse foramina.

12. True/False: The thoracic spine possesses facets for rib articulations and bifid spinous processes.

13. The intervertebral foramina for the cervical spine lie at a _____ ° angle to the midsagittal plane.

14. Which ligament holds the dens against the anterior arch of C1? _____

15. The large joint space between C1 and C2 is called the _____ .

16. Two partial facets found on the thoracic vertebrae are called _____ .

17. Which of the following thoracic vertebrae do **not** possess a facet for the costotransverse joint? (There may be more than one correct answer.)

    A. T1    B. T7    C. T11    D. T12

18. What are two distinctive features of all cervical vertebrae that make them different from any other vertebra?

    A. _____        B. _____

9

19.   What is the one feature of all thoracic vertebrae that makes them different from all other vertebrae?

_____

20.   Which position of the thoracic spine best demonstrates the intervertebral foramina?

_____

21.   Identify the following structures labeled on Figs. 9-5, 9-6, and 9-7
      (include the specific vertebra of which each structure is a part):

                    *STRUCTURE*                    *VERTEBRA*

*Fig. 9-5*

   A.   _____    _____

   B.   _____    _____

   C.   _____    _____

   D.   _____    _____

   E.   _____    _____

   F.   _____    _____

**Fig. 9-5.** Superior view.

*Fig. 9-6*

   G.   _____    _____

   H.   _____    _____

   I.   _____    _____

   J.   _____    _____

   K.   _____    _____

   L.   _____    _____

**Fig. 9-6.** Posterolateral view, cervical spine.

*Fig. 9-7*

   M.   _____    _____

   N.   _____    _____

   O.   _____    _____

   P.   _____    _____

   Q.   _____    _____

   R.   _____    _____

   S.   Which vertebrae are represented by this drawing?

      _____

   T.   How can these specific vertebrae be identified?

      _____

**Fig. 9-7.** Lateral oblique view.

22. Identify the following structures and vertebrae labeled on this AP "open mouth" cervical spine radiograph (Fig. 9-8):

STRUCTURE          VERTEBRA

A. _____    _____

B. _____    _____

C. _____    _____

D. _____    _____

E. _____    _____

F. _____    _____

G. _____    _____

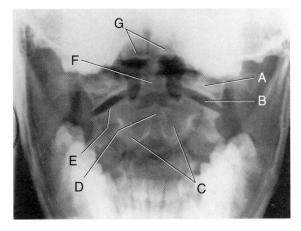

**Fig. 9-8.** AP "open mouth" cervical spine radiograph.

23. Which position or projection of the cervical spine best demonstrates the zygapophyseal joints (between C3 to C7)?

_____

24. Which specific joint spaces are visualized with a left anterior oblique (LAO) projection of the thoracic spine?

_____

25. Match each of the following topographic landmarks to the correct vertebral level (using each choice only once):

_____ 1. Vertebra prominens                              A. T2-3

_____ 2. Jugular notch                                   B. C7-T1

_____ 3. 3 to 4 inches (8 to 10 cm) below jugular notch   C. T7

_____ 4. Gonion                                          D. C3

_____ 5. Sternal angle                                   E. C4-5

_____ 6. Thyroid cartilage                               F. T4-5

26. Which of the following imaging modalities is *not* normally performed to rule out a herniated nucleus pulposus (HNP)?

A. Computed tomography (CT)      C. Magnetic resonance imaging (MRI)

B. Myelography                    D. Nuclear medicine

27. An avulsion fracture of the spinous processes of C6 is called a:

A. Hangman's fracture            C. Jefferson fracture

B. Clay shoveler's fracture      D. Teardrop burst fracture

28. Scheuermann's disease is a form of:

A. Scoliosis and/or kyphosis     C. Arthritis

B. Subluxation                   D. Fracture

29. True/False: HNP most frequently develops at the L2-3 vertebral level.

30. Which two things can be done to minimize the effects of scatter radiation on lateral projections of the thoracic and lumbar spine?

    A. _____          B. _____

31. Which position or projection best demonstrates the zygapophyseal joints between C1 and C2? _____

32. How much and in which direction (caudad or cephalad) should the central ray be angled for each of the following projections?

    A. An AP axial projection of the cervical spine: _____

    B. An anterior oblique projection of the cervical spine: _____

    C. A posterior oblique projection of the cervical spine: _____

33. Which one of the following projections of the cervical spine demonstrates the left intervertebral foramen?

    A. Left posterior oblique (LPO)          C. Lateral projection

    B. Left anterior oblique (LAO)           D. Right anterior oblique (RAO)

34. In addition to using a long SID, list the two positioning maneuvers you can use to lower the shoulders enough to visualize C7 for a lateral projection of the cervical spine.

    A. _____          B. _____

35. Which position or projection demonstrates the lower cervical and upper thoracic spine (C4 to T3) in a lateral perspective?

    _____

36. List the two positions or projections that will project the dens in the center of the foramen magnum.

    A. _____          B. _____

37. A lateral cervical spine radiograph demonstrates that the zygapophyseal joint spaces are not superimposed. Which type of positioning error(s) may lead to this radiographic outcome?

    _____

38. A radiograph of a lateral thoracic spine projection reveals that the intervertebral foramina and intervertebral joint spaces are not clearly demonstrated. Which type of problems can lead to this radiographic outcome?

    _____

39. **Situation:** A patient who was involved in a motor vehicle accident (MVA) 3 days ago is experiencing severe neck pain and comes to the radiology department for a cervical spine series. The patient is not wearing a cervical collar. Should the technologist take a horizontal beam lateral radiograph and have it cleared before proceeding with the study? Explain.

    _____

40. **Situation:** A patient with a possible Jefferson fracture enters the ER. Which specific radiographic position best demonstrates this type of fracture?

    _____

41. What dose range would be received by the breasts of a slightly larger-than-average female during a lateral thoracic spine projection taken at 80 kV and 50 mAs with proper collimation?

    A. 300 to 500 mrad          C. 100 to 200 mrad

    B. 1 to 50 mrad             D. No detectable contribution (NDC)

42. The breast dose used for a posterior oblique thoracic spine projection is approximately _____ the dose used for an anterior oblique projection.

   A. The same as          C. 2 times greater than

   B. One-half of          D. 4 times greater than

43. What skin dose range would be received by an average-size male patient during a lateral thoracic spine projection?

   A. 300 to 400 mrad       C. 1 to 2 rad

   B. 10 to 50 mrad         D. 900 to 1000 mrad

44. The thyroid dose used during a posterior oblique cervical spine projection is approximately _____ the dose used during an anterior oblique projection.

   A. The same as              C. 10 to 15 times greater than

   B. 4 times greater than     D. One-quarter of the amount

45. A radiograph of an AP open mouth projection of the cervical spine demonstrates the upper incisors superimposed over the top of the dens. What specific positioning error is present on this radiograph?

   _____

46. **Situation:** A patient comes to the radiology department for a follow-up study for a clay shoveler's fracture. Which spine projections will best demonstrate this type of fracture?

   _____

47. **Situation:** A patient comes to the radiology department for a follow-up study 6 months after having spinal fusion surgery of the lower cervical spine (C5-C6). The surgeon wants to check for anteroposterior mobility of the fused spine. Beyond the basic cervical spine projections, what additional projections can be taken to assess mobility of the spine?

   _____

48. Which one of the following technical factors is most important in producing a high-quality digital image?

   A. Decrease SID whenever possible      C. Decrease kV as much as possible

   B. Minimize the use of grids           D. Collimate as close as possible

49. For the following critique questions, refer to the AP open mouth radiograph in Fig. C9-91 on p. 320 in the textbook.

   A. Which positioning error(s) is(are) visible on this radiograph? (More than one answer may be selected.)

   (a) All essential anatomic structures are not demonstrated.

   (b) Central ray is centered incorrectly.

   (c) Collimation is not evident.

   (d) Exposure factors are incorrect.

   (e) No anatomic marker is visible on the radiograph.

   (f) Excessive extension of the skull is evident.

   (g) Excessive flexion of the skull is evident.

   B. Which error(s) identified above is(are) considered "repeatable"?

   _____

C.  Which of the following modifications must be made during the repeat exposure? (More than one answer may be selected.)

(a)  Increase collimation.

(b)  Center central ray to femoral neck.

(c)  Decrease exposure factors.

(d)  Increase exposure factors.

(e)  Reposition anatomic marker on IR before exposure.

(f)  Increase skull flexion.

(g)  Increase skull extension.

50.  For the following critique questions, refer to the AP axial cervical spine radiograph in Fig. C9-93 on p. 320 in the textbook.

A.  Which positioning error(s) is(are) visible on this radiograph? More than one answer may be selected.

(a)  All essential anatomic structures are not demonstrated.

(b)  Central ray is centered incorrectly.

(c)  Central ray is angled incorrectly.

(d)  Collimation is not evident.

(e)  Exposure factors are incorrect.

(f)  No anatomic marker is visible on the radiograph.

(g)  Excessive extension of skull is evident.

(h)  Excessive flexion of skull is evident.

B.  Which error(s) identified above is(are) considered "repeatable?"

_____

C.  Which of the following modifications must be made during the repeat exposure? (More than one answer may be selected.)

(a)  Increase collimation.

(b)  Increase central ray cephalic angulation.

(c)  Decrease central ray cephalic angulation.

(d)  Increase skull flexion.

(e)  Increase skull extension.

(f)  Place anatomic marker on IR before exposure.

## CHAPTER 10

# Lumbar Spine, Sacrum, and Coccyx

## CHAPTER OBJECTIVES

After you have successfully completed the activities in this chapter, you will be able to:

_____ 1. On drawings and radiographs, identify specific anatomic structures of the lumbar spine, sacrum, and coccyx.

_____ 2. Identify the anatomic structures that make up the "Scotty dog" sign.

_____ 3. Identify the classification and type of movement of the joints found in the lumbar spine.

_____ 4. List topographic landmarks that can be palpated to locate specific aspects of the lumbar spine, sacrum, and coccyx.

_____ 5. Define specific types of pathologic features of the spine as described in the textbook.

_____ 6. Identify radiographic appearances related to these specific types of pathologic spine features.

_____ 7. Identify basic and special projections of the lumbar spine, sacrum, and coccyx, including the correct size and type of image receptor (IR), central ray location, direction, and angulation of the central ray for each projection.

_____ 8. Identify which structures are best seen with specific projections of the lumbar spine.

_____ 9. List the patient dose ranges for skin, midline, and gonadal doses for specific spine projections.

_____ 10. Identify the approximate difference in patient doses between anteroposterior (AP) compared with posteroanterior (PA) projections and anterior compared with posterior oblique positions of the lumbar spine.

_____ 11. Given various hypothetical situations, identify the correct modification of a position and/or exposure factors to improve the radiographic image.

_____ 12. Given radiographs of specific lumbosacral spine projections or positions, identify positioning and exposure factor errors.

## Positioning and Radiographic Critique

_____ 1. Using a peer, position for basic and special projections of the lumbosacral spine.

_____ 2. Using a lumbar spine radiographic phantom, produce satisfactory radiographs of specific positions (if equipment is available).

_____ 3. Critique and evaluate lumbar spine radiographs based on the four divisions of radiographic criteria: (1) structures shown, (2) position, (3) collimation and central ray, and (4) exposure criteria.

_____ 4. Distinguish between acceptable and unacceptable lumbosacral spine radiographs based on exposure factors, motion, collimation, positioning, or other errors.

## Learning Exercises

Complete the following review exercises after careful study of the associated pages in the textbook as indicated by each exercise. Answers to each review exercise are given at the end of the review exercises.

## Part I: Radiographic Anatomy

1-15

**REVIEW EXERCISE A:** Anatomy of the Lumbar Spine, Sacrum, and Coccyx (see textbook pp. 322-327)

1. A portion of the lamina located between the **superior and inferior** articular processes is called the

   _pars interarticularis._

2. The superior and inferior vertebral notches join together to form the:

   A. Vertebral foramen          C. Pedicle

   (B.) Intervertebral foramina      D. Lamina

3. Which radiographic position best demonstrates the structure identified in the previous question?

   _____ lateral _____

4. Identify the parts of a typical lumbar vertebra as labeled on Fig. 10-1:

   A. ___Pedicle_____

   B. ___Transverse Process_____

   C. ___Superior Articular Process & Facet___

   D. ___Lamina (pars interarticularis)___

   E. ___Spinous Process_____

   F. The central ray projection labeled *F* in this drawing would demonstrate the

   ___Zygapophyseal joint___

   G. The central ray projection labeled *G* would demonstrate the

   ___Intervertebral foramina___

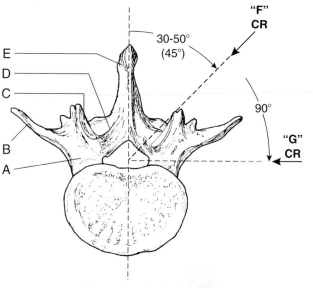

**Fig. 10-1.** Typical L3 vertebra.

5. Would the degree of angle to demonstrate the structures identified in *F* in the previous question be greater or lesser

   for the lower lumbar vertebrae as compared with the upper? ___lesser_____

6. The small foramina found in the sacrum are called ___Pelvic sacral foramina_____ .

7. The anterior and superior aspect of the sacrum that forms the posterior wall of the pelvic inlet is called the

   _____Promontory_____ .

8. What is another term for the sacral horns? _____Cornua_____

9. The sacroiliac joints lie at an oblique angle of __30__° to the coronal plane.

10. What is the formal term for the "tail bone?" _____Coccyx_____

11. What is the name for the upper broad aspect of the coccyx? _____base_____

12. List the structure classification and movement classification and type for the following joints of the vertebrae:

|  | *CLASSIFICATION* | *MOBILITY TYPE* | *MOVEMENT TYPE* |
|---|---|---|---|
| A. Zygapophyseal | Synovial | Diarthrodial | Plane (gliding) |
| B. Intervertebral | Cartilaginous (symphysis) | Ampiarthrodial (slightly moveable) | n/A |

13. Identify the following structures labeled on the radiographs of the lumbar spine (Figs. 10-2 through 10-4):

A. _____Intervertebral disk space L1-2_____

B. _____Spinous process L2_____

C. _____Transverse process L3_____

D. _____Region of lamina (body) L4_____

E. _____Left ala of sacrum_____

F. _____Left Sacroiliac_____ joint

G. _____Body of L1_____

H. _____Pedicles of L2_____

I. _____Intervertebral foramina L3-4_____

J. _____Intervertebral disk space L5-S1_____

K. _____Sacrum_____

**Fig. 10-2.** Anteroposterior.          **Fig. 10-3.** Lateral.

Identify parts of the "Scotty dog" image, which should be visible on an oblique lumbar spine (Figs. 10-4 and 10-5):

L. _____Inferior articular process L3 (leg)_____

M. _____Zygapophyseal joint L4-5_____ joint

N. _____Pars interarticularis L3 (neck)_____

O. _____Pedicle L3 (eye)_____

P. _____Transverse process L3 (nose)_____

Q. _____Superior articular process L3 (ear)_____

**Fig. 10-4.** Oblique.          **Fig. 10-5.** "Scotty dog."

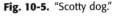

**10**

14. List the specific joints or foramina that are demonstrated with the following lumbar spine positions:

    A. Left posterior oblique (LPO): _____left_____

    B. Right anterior oblique (RAO): _____left_____

    C. Lateral: _intervertebral foramina_

    D. Right posterior oblique (RPO): _right_____

    E. Left anterior oblique (LAO): _right_____

15. The degree of obliquity required for an oblique projection at the T12-L1 level is approximately

    _____50°_____ , whereas the L5-S1 level spine requires a _____30°_____ oblique.

    Therefore, a _____45°_____ oblique is performed for the general lumbar spine.

## Part II: Radiographic Positioning

1-8, 11-23

**REVIEW EXERCISE B:** Topographic Landmarks and Positioning of Lumbar Spine, Sacrum, and Coccyx
(see textbook pp. 328-346)

1. Match each of the following topographical landmarks to the correct vertebral level (using each choice only once):

   _C_ 1. ASIS              _A._ L2-3

   _E_ 2. Xiphoid process    _B._ L4-5

   _A_ 3. Lower costal margin _C._ S1-2

   _B_ 4. Iliac crest        _D._ Tip of coccyx

   _D_ 5. Symphysis pubis    _E._ T9-10

2. True/False: The use of higher kilovoltage (kV) and lower milliampere seconds (mAs) for lumbar spine radiography improves radiographic contrast but increases patient dose.

3. True/False: Placing a lead blocker mat behind the patient for lateral lumbar spine positions improves image quality.

4. True/False: Gonadal shielding should always be used for male and female patients for studies of the lumbar spine, sacrum, and coccyx.

5. True/False: The anteroposterior (AP) projection of the lumbar spine opens the intervertebral joint spaces better than the posteroanterior (PA) projection.

6. True/False: The knees and hips should be extended for an AP projection of the lumbar spine.

7. True/False: An increased source image receptor distance (SID) of 44 or 46 inches (112 to 117 cm) is advantageous for AP and lateral projections of the lumbar spine.

8. True/False: The lead blocker mat and close collimation must not be used when performing digital imaging of the lumbar spine.

9.   Select the imaging modality that best demonstrates each of the following pathologic features or conditions (answers may be used more than once):

   _____   A.   Osteoporosis                                      1.   Magnetic resonance imaging (MRI)

   _____   B.   Soft tissues of lumbar spine                       2.   Computed tomography (CT)

   _____   C.   Structures within subarachnoid space               3.   Myelography

   _____   D.   Inflammatory conditions such as Paget's disease    4.   Bone densitometry

   _____   E.   Compression fractures of the lumbar spine          5.   Nuclear medicine

10.  Match the each of the following pathologic indications to the correct definition or statement (using each choice only once):

   _____   A.   Lateral curvature of the vertebral column          1.   Spina bifida

   _____   B.   Fracture of the vertebral body caused by           2.   Herniated nucleus pulposus (HNP)
                 hyperflexion force
                                                                     3.   Chance fracture
   _____   C.   Congenital defect in which the posterior
                 elements of the vertebrae fail to unite            4.   Spondylolisthesis

   _____   D.   Most common at the L4-5 level and may result       5.   Compression fracture
                 in sciatica
                                                                     6.   Spondylolysis
   _____   E.   Forward displacement of one vertebra onto
                 another vertebra                                    7.   Ankylosing spondylitis

   _____   F.   Inflammatory condition that is most common in      8.   Scoliosis
                 males in their 30s

   _____   G.   Dissolution and separation of the pars interarticularis

   _____   H.   A type of fracture that rarely causes neurologic deficits

11.  With a 35- × 43-cm (14- × 17-inch) IR, the central ray is centered at the level of the ___*iliac crest*___ for

   AP and lateral lumbar spine projections.

12.  Which two structures can be evaluated to determine whether rotation is present on a radiograph of an AP projection of the lumbar spine?

   A.  ___*SI joints equidistant from spine*___   B.  ___*Spinous process should be midline to vertebral column*___

13.  How much obliquity is required to properly visualize the zygapophyseal joints at the L5-S1 level?

   _____*30°*_____

14.  Which specific set of zygapophyseal joints is demonstrated with an LAO position?

   _____*right (upside)*_____

15.  The ___*pedicle*___, which is the eye of the "Scotty dog," should be near the center of the vertebral

   body on a correctly obliqued lumbar spine.

**10**

16. Which positioning error has been committed if the structures described in the previous question are projected too far posterior with a 45° oblique position of the lumbar spine? _excessive obliquity_

17. Which position or projection of the lumbar spine series best demonstrates a possible compression fracture?

_lateral_

18. A patient with a wide pelvis and narrow thorax may require a central ray angle of _5-8_ °

_Caudad_ (**caudad** or **cephalad**) for a lateral position of the lumbar spine.

19. How should the spine of a patient with scoliosis be positioned for a lateral position of the lumbar spine?

_Whichever places the sag or convexity of the spine down_

20. Why should the knees and hips be flexed for an AP lumbar spine projection?

_Straightens the spine, which helps open the intervertebral disk spaces_

21. True/False: The female ovarian dose used for a PA lumbar spine projection is approximately 30% less than the dose used for an AP projection.

22. Where is the central ray centered for a lateral L5-S1 projection of the lumbar spine? _____

_1½" inferior to iliac crest and 2" posterior to ASIS_

23. What type of central ray angulation is required for an AP axial L5-S1 projection on a male patient?

_Cephalad 30° (males) 35° (females)_

24. True/False: A PA or AP projection for a scoliosis series frequently includes one erect and one recumbent position for comparison.

25. True/False: The lower margin of the cassette must include the ~~symphysis pubis~~ for a scoliosis series. _1-2" below crest_

26. True/False: A PA projection for a scoliosis series requires only about one-tenth the dose to the breasts as the AP projection, even if good collimation is used.

27. The typical skin dose range of the lateral projection of a scoliosis series on a small to average female is:

A. 1000 to 1200 mrad   C. 200 to 400 mrad

B. 500 to 700 mrad   D. Less than 100 mrad

28. Which side of the spine should be elevated for the second exposure for the Ferguson scoliosis series (by having patient stand on a block with one foot)? _Convex_

29. During the AP (PA) right and left bending projections of the lumbar spine, the _pelvis_ must remain stationary during positioning.

30. Which projections should be taken to evaluate flexibility following spinal fusion surgery?

_Hyperextension and hyperflexion lateral_

31. How much central ray angulation is required for an AP projection of the sacrum for a typical male patient?

_15° Cephalad_

32. If a patient cannot lie on the back for the AP sacrum because it is too painful, what alternate projection can be

    taken to achieve a similar view of the sacrum? _____ *prone with 15° caudad angle* _____

    _____

33. Where is the central ray centered for an AP projection of the coccyx? _*2" superior to sym. pubis*_

34. True/False: The AP projections of the sacrum and coccyx can be taken as one single projection to decrease gonadal
    dose.                *different CR angles   S- 15° cephalad   C - 10° caudad*

35. Patients should be asked to empty the urinary bladder before performing which projection(s) of the vertebral column?

    _____ *AP sacrum and coccyx* _____

36. In addition to good collimation, what should be done to minimize overall "fogging" on a lateral lumbar spine or

    lateral sacrum and coccyx radiograph? _____ *lead blocker behind patient* _____

                                    *1-4,6,7,10-15*

**REVIEW EXERCISE C: Problem Solving for Technical and Positioning Errors**

1. A radiograph of an AP projection of the lumbar spine reveals that the spinous processes are not midline to the
   vertebral column and distortion of the vertebral bodies is present. Which specific positioning error is present on this

   radiograph? _____ *rotation of the spine* _____

   _____

2. A radiograph of an LPO projection of the lumbar spine reveals that the downside pedicles and zygapophyseal joints
   are projected over the anterior portion of the vertebral bodies. Which specific positioning error is present on this
   radiograph?

   _____ *Insufficient rotation of the spine (should be to midvertebral bodies)* _____

   _____

3. A radiograph of a lateral projection of a female lumbar spine reveals that the mid-to-lower intervertebral joint
   spaces are not open. The technologist supported the midsection of the spine with sponges to straighten the spine.
   What else can be done to open the joint spaces during the repeat exposure?

   _____ *5-8° caudad angle* _____

   _____

4. A radiograph of a lateral L5-S1 projection reveals that the joint space is *not* open. The technologist did support the
   middle aspect of the spine with a sponge. What else can the technologist do to open up the joint space during the
   repeat exposure?

   _____ *Additional support beneath spine or a 5-8°* _____
   _____ *caudad angle* _____

5. A radiograph of an AP axial projection of the coccyx reveals that the distal tip is superimposed over the symphysis
   pubis. What must the technologist do to eliminate this problem during the repeat exposure?

   _____ *An increase in the CR angle to separate the* _____
   _____ *coccyx from the symphysis pubis* _____

**10**

6.  A radiograph of an oblique position of the lumbar spine reveals that the downside pedicle and zygapophyseal joint are posterior in relation to the vertebral body. What modification of the position must be made during the repeat exposure to produce a more diagnostic image?

    _Overrotation- decrease rotation of body_

7.  **Situation:** A patient comes to the radiology department for a follow-up study for a compression fracture of L3. The radiologist requests that collimated projections be taken of L3. Which specific projections and centering would provide a quality study of L3 and the intervertebral joint spaces?

    _AP or PA and collimated lateral    CR 2" above crest._

8.  **Situation:** A young female patient comes to the radiology department for a scoliosis series. She has had repeated radiation exposure over a period of time and is understandably concerned about the radiation. What three things can the technologist do to minimize the dose delivered to the patient's breasts?

    A.  _Use high KU technique_
    B.  _Perform PA rather than AP_
    C.  _Use breast shields_

9.  **Situation:** A patient with an injury to the coccyx enters the emergency room. When attempting the AP projection, the patient complains that it is too uncomfortable to lie on his back. He is unable to stand. What other options are available to complete the study?

    _Perform PA instead and change CR angle to cephalad_

10. **Situation:** A patient with a clinical history of spondylolisthesis at the L5-S1 level comes to the radiology department. Which specific lumbar spine position would be most diagnostic in demonstrating the extent of this condition?

    _Lateral  L5-S1_

11. The AP projection of a scoliosis series of the thoracolumbar spine does not include the iliac crest. Is this an acceptable study? If not, what should the technologist do to correct this problem during the repeat exposure?

    _No it must include at least 2" of crest_

12. **Situation:** A patient comes to the radiology department for a lumbar spine series. He has a clinical history of advanced spondylolysis. Which *specific* projection(s) of the lumbar spine series will best demonstrate this condition?

    _Posterior and anterior obliques_

13. **Situation:** A patient comes to the radiology department with a clinical history of HNP. Which of the following imaging modalities would provide the most diagnostic study for this condition?

    A.  Sonography      C.  Nuclear medicine
    B.  MRI             D.  Radiography

14. **Situation:** A patient comes to the radiology department for a lumbar spine study following spinal fusion surgery. Her surgeon wants a study to assess mobility of the spine at the fusion site. Which radiographic positions would provide this information?

    _Hyperflexion and hyperextension lateral_

15. **Situation:** A patient comes to the radiology department for a lumbar spine series. She has a clinical history of severe kyphosis. How should the lumbar spine series be modified for this patient?

_____Basic lumbar spine projections should be performed erect_____

**REVIEW EXERCISE D:** Critique Radiographs of the Lumbar Spine, Sacrum, and Coccyx (see textbook p. 347)

The following questions relate to the radiographs found at the end of Chapter 10 of the textbook. Evaluate these radiographs for the radiographic criteria categories (_1_ through _5_) that follow. Describe the corrections needed to improve the overall image. The major, or "repeatable," errors are specific errors that indicate the need for a repeat exposure, regardless of the nature of the other errors.

A. **Lateral lumbar spine (Fig. C10-78)**

    1. Structures shown: _____

    2. Part positioning: _____

    3. Collimation and central ray: _____

    4. Exposure criteria: _____

    5. Markers: _____

    Repeatable error(s): _____

B. **AP lumbar spine (Fig. C10-79)**

    1. Structures shown: _____

    2. Part positioning: _____

    3. Collimation and central ray: _____

    4. Exposure criteria: _____

    5. Markers: _____

    Repeatable error(s): _____

C. **Lateral L5-S1 (Fig. C10-80)**

    1. Structures shown: _____

    2. Part positioning: _____

    3. Collimation and central ray: _____

    4. Exposure criteria: _____

    5. Markers: _____

    Repeatable error(s): _____

D.   **Oblique lumbar spine (Fig. C10-81)**

　　1.   Structures shown: _____

　　2.   Part positioning: _____

　　3.   Collimation and central ray: _____

　　4.   Exposure criteria: _____

　　5.   Markers: _____

　　Repeatable error(s): _____

E.   **Oblique lumbar spine (Fig. C10-82)**

　　1.   Structures shown: _____

　　2.   Part positioning: _____

　　3.   Collimation and central ray: _____

　　4.   Exposure criteria: _____

　　5.   Markers: _____

　　Repeatable error(s): _____

## Part III: Laboratory Exercises (see textbook pp. 333-346)

You must gain experience in positioning each part of the lumbar spine, sacrum, and coccyx before performing the following exams on actual patients. You can get experience in positioning and radiographic evaluation of these projections by performing exercises using radiographic phantoms and practicing on other students (although you will not be taking actual exposures).

　　The following suggested activities assume that your teaching institution has an energized lab and radiographic phantoms. If not, perform Laboratory Exercises B and C, the radiographic evaluation and the physical positioning exercises. (Check off each step and projection as you complete it.)

## LABORATORY EXERCISE A: Energized Laboratory

1.   Using the abdomen/lumbosacral radiographic phantom, produce radiographs of the following basic routines:

| _____ | AP lumbar spine | _____ | AP sacrum | _____ | Posterior oblique lumbar spine |
|---|---|---|---|---|---|
| _____ | Lateral lumbar spine | _____ | AP coccyx | _____ | Anterior oblique lumbar spine |
| _____ | Lateral L5-S1 | _____ | Lateral sacrum and coccyx | _____ | AP axial L5-S1 |

## LABORATORY EXERCISE B: Radiographic Evaluation

1.   Evaluate and critique the radiographs produced during the previous experiments, additional radiographs provided by your instructor, or both. Evaluate each radiograph for the following points:

　　_____   Evaluate the completeness of the study. (Are all of the pertinent anatomic structures included on the radiograph?)

_____ Evaluate for positioning or centering errors (e.g., rotation, off centering).

_____ Evaluate for correct exposure factors and possible motion. (Are the density and contrast of the images acceptable?)

_____ Determine whether markers and an acceptable degree of collimation and/or area shielding are visible on the images.

## LABORATORY EXERCISE C: Physical Positioning

On another person, simulate performing all basic and special projections of the lumbar spine, sacrum, and coccyx as follows. (Check off each when completed satisfactorily.) Include the following six steps as described in the textbook.

Step 1. Appropriate size and type of image receptor with correct markers
Step 2. Correct central ray placement and centering of part to central ray and/or IR
Step 3. Accurate collimation
Step 4. Area shielding of patient where advisable
Step 5. Use of proper immobilizing devices when needed
Step 6. Approximate correct exposure factors, breathing instructions where applicable, and "making" exposure

| PROJECTIONS | STEP 1 | STEP 2 | STEP 3 | STEP 4 | STEP 5 | STEP 6 |
|---|---|---|---|---|---|---|
| • AP lumbar spine | ____ | ____ | ____ | ____ | ____ | ____ |
| • Lateral lumbar spine | ____ | ____ | ____ | ____ | ____ | ____ |
| • Lateral L5-S1 | ____ | ____ | ____ | ____ | ____ | ____ |
| • AP sacrum | ____ | ____ | ____ | ____ | ____ | ____ |
| • AP coccyx | ____ | ____ | ____ | ____ | ____ | ____ |
| • Lateral sacrum and coccyx | ____ | ____ | ____ | ____ | ____ | ____ |
| • Posterior oblique lumbar spine | ____ | ____ | ____ | ____ | ____ | ____ |
| • Anterior oblique lumbar spine | ____ | ____ | ____ | ____ | ____ | ____ |
| • AP axial L5-S1 | ____ | ____ | ____ | ____ | ____ | ____ |

Spinal fusion series:

| | | | | | | |
|---|---|---|---|---|---|---|
| • AP (PA) R and L bending | ____ | ____ | ____ | ____ | ____ | ____ |
| • Lateral hyperextension and hyperflexion | ____ | ____ | ____ | ____ | ____ | ____ |

Scoliosis series:

| | | | | | | |
|---|---|---|---|---|---|---|
| • PA (AP) and lateral erect | ____ | ____ | ____ | ____ | ____ | ____ |
| • AP (Ferguson method) | ____ | ____ | ____ | ____ | ____ | ____ |

## *Answers to Review Exercises*

### Review Exercise A: Anatomy of the Lumbar Spine, Sacrum, and Coccyx

1. Pars interarticularis
2. B. Intervertebral foramina
3. Lateral position
4. A. Pedicle
   B. Transverse process
   C. Superior articular process and facet
   D. Lamina
   E. Spinous process
   F. Zygapophyseal joints
   G. Intervertebral foramina
5. Lesser (50° for upper and 30° for lower)
6. Pelvic sacral foramina
7. Promontory
8. Cornu
9. 30°
10. Coccyx
11. Base
12. A. Synovial, diarthrodial, plane, or gliding
    B. Cartilaginous, amphiarthrodial (slightly movable), none
13. A. Intervertebral disk space, L1-2
    B. Spinous process, L2
    C. Transverse process, L3
    D. Region of lamina (body), L4
    E. Left ala of sacrum
    F. Left sacroiliac joint
    G. Body of L1
    H. Pedicles of L2
    I. Intervertebral foramina, L3-4
    J. Intervertebral disk space, L5-S1
    K. Sacrum
    L. Inferior articular process, L3 (leg)
    M. Zygapophyseal joint, L4-5
    N. Pars interarticularis, L3 (neck)
    O. Pedicle, L3 (eye)
    P. Transverse process, L3 (nose)
    Q. Superior articular process, L3 (ear)
14. A. Left zygapophyseal joints
    B. Left zygapophyseal joints
    C. Intervertebral foramina
    D. Right zygapophyseal joints
    E. Right zygapophyseal joints
15. 50°, 30°, 45°

### Review Exercise B: Topographic Landmarks and Positioning of the Lumbar Spine, Sacrum, and Coccyx

1. 1. C
   2. E
   3. A
   4. B
   5. D

2. False
3. True
4. False (not used for females if the shield would obscure essential anatomy)
5. False (PA would open spaces better.)
6. False (should be flexed)
7. True
8. False
9. A. 4
   B. 1
   C. 1
   D. 5
   E. 2
10. A. 8
    B. 3
    C. 1
    D. 2
    E. 4
    F. 7
    G. 6
    H. 5
11. Iliac crest
12. A. Sacroiliac (SI) joints are equidistant from the spine.
    B. Spinous process should be midline to the vertebral column.
13. 30°
14. Right (upside)
15. Pedicle
16. Excessive obliquity
17. Lateral
18. 5 to 8°, caudad
19. With the sag or convexity of the spine closest to the IR
20. Reduces lumbar curvature, which opens the intervertebral disk space
21. True
22. 1½ inches (4 cm) inferior to iliac crest and 2 inches (5 cm) posterior to ASIS
23. 30° cephalad
24. True
25. False (lower margin 1 to 2 inches [3 to 5 cm] below iliac crest)
26. True
27. A. 1000 to 1200 mrad
28. The convex side of the spine
29. Pelvis
30. Hyperextension and hyperflexion projections
31. 15° cephalad
32. A PA (prone) with 15° caudad central ray angle
33. 2 inches (5 cm) superior to the symphysis pubis
34. False (need different central ray angles for AP projections; can combine lateral but not AP projections)

35. AP of sacrum and coccyx
36. Place lead blocker on table top behind patient.

### Review Exercise C: Problem Solving for Technical and Positioning Errors

1. Rotation of the spine
2. Insufficient rotation of the spine (should be to midvertebral bodies).
3. If the patient has a wide pelvis, the central ray can be angled 5° to 8° caudad.
4. Place additional support beneath the spine, or use a 5° to 8° caudad angle.
5. An increase in central ray angle is required to separate the coccyx from the symphysis pubis.
6. Decrease rotation of the body and spine.
7. AP or PA and collimated lateral projections would provide the best view of the L3 region. The central ray should be about 2 inches (5 cm) above the iliac crest.
8. A. Use high kilovoltage technique.
   B. Perform a PA rather than an AP projection.
   C. Use breast shields.
9. Perform a PA rather than an AP projection and reverse the direction of the central ray from caudad to cephalad.
10. A lateral L5-S1 position would demonstrate the degree of forward displacement of L5 onto S1.
11. No, this is not an acceptable AP projection. The lower margin of the IR must extend 1 to 2 inches (3 to 5 cm) below the iliac crest.
12. Although AP and lateral projections of the lumbar spine are helpful, posterior or anterior oblique positions will best demonstrate advanced signs of spondylolysis.
13. B. MRI
14. Hyperflexion and hyperextension lateral positions
15. Basic lumbar spine projections should be performed erect

### Review Exercise D: Critique Radiographs of the Lumbar Spine, Sacrum, and Coccyx

A. Lateral lumbar spine (Fig. C10-78)
   1. Posterior elements of upper lumbar spine cut off
   2. Patient too far posterior

**10**

3. Evident and acceptable collimation (could be collimated a little more tightly if centering were correct); central ray centering too anterior, causing posterior elements to become cut off
4. Acceptable but slightly underexposed exposure factors
5. Anatomic side marker cut off
Repeatable errors: 1, 2, and 3

B. AP lumbar spine (Fig. C10-79)
1. Metallic artifacts obscuring aspects of lumbar spine
2. Part positioning acceptable but centered slightly to left
3. Acceptable collimation; acceptable central ray centering and IR placement
4. Overexposed exposure factors
5. No evidence of anatomic side marker
Repeatable errors: 1 and 4

C. Lateral L5-S1 (Fig. C10-80)
1. All pertinent anatomic structures included
2. Excellent part and central ray centering
3. Additional collimation needed; S1 joint space not open; may need waist support or central ray caudal angle
4. Underexposed L5-S1 joint space region
5. Evidence of anatomic side marker (better to place up and posterior to spine)
Repeatable errors: 3 and 4

D. Oblique lumbar spine (Fig. C10-81)
1. Posterior elements of upper lumbar spine cut off
2. Overrotated upper aspect of lumbar spine (eye of "Scotty dog" [pedicles] posterior and not centered to body)
3. Evidence of collimation; central ray centered too anterior; posterior elements of lumbar spine to become cut off
4. Acceptable exposure factors
5. Evidence of anatomic side marker
Repeatable errors: 1, 2, and 3

E. Oblique lumbar spine (Fig. C10-82)
1. Entire lumbar spine demonstrated
2. Underrotated lumbar spine (eye of "Scotty dog" [pedicles] too anterior)
3. Collimation too loose and not evident (should be visible on sides); central ray centering and IR placement correct
4. Acceptable but slightly overexposed exposure factors
5. No evidence of anatomic side marker
Repeatable error: 2

# SELF-TEST

My Score = _____ %

This self-test should be taken only after completing all of the readings, review exercises, and laboratory activities for a particular section. The purpose of this test is not only to provide a good learning exercise but also to serve as a strong indicator of what your final evaluation exam will cover. It is strongly suggested that if you do not get at least a 90% to 95% grade on each self-test, you review those areas in which you missed questions before going to your instructor for the final evaluation exam for this chapter. (There are 70 questions in this chapter—each is worth 1.4 points.)

1. Compared with the spinous processes of the cervical and thoracic spine, the lumbar spinous processes are:

    A. Smaller                C. Larger and more blunt

    B. Pointed downward more     D. Absent

2. The anterior ridge of the upper sacrum is called the:

    A. Median sacral crest     C. Promontory

    B. Cornua                  D. Sacral horns

3. Each sacroiliac joint is obliqued posteriorly _____°.

    A. 20     C. 45

    B. 30     D. 50

4. The angle of the midlumbar spine zygapophyseal joints in relation to the midsagittal plane is _____°.

5. Where is the pars interarticularis found?

    A. Superior and inferior aspect of the pedicle     C. Between the superior and inferior articular processes

    B. Between the intervertebral disk and vertebra     D. Between the lamina and body spinous processes

6. Identify the labeled parts of the sacrum and coccyx on the following drawings (Figs. 10-6 and 10-7):

    A. _____

    B. _____

    C. _____

    D. _____

    E. _____

    F. _____

    G. _____

    H. _____

    I. _____

    J. _____

    K. _____

    L. _____

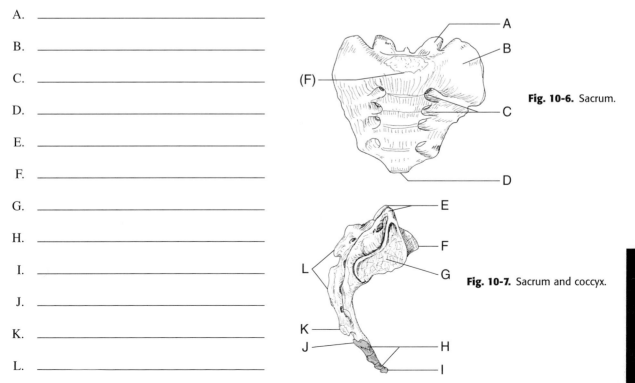

**Fig. 10-6.** Sacrum.

**Fig. 10-7.** Sacrum and coccyx.

**10**

7.  Identify the labeled parts on these radiographs of
    individual vertebrae (Figs. 10-8 and 10-9).

    A. _____

    B. _____

    C. _____

    D. _____

    E. _____

    F. _____

    G. _____

    H. _____

    I. _____

    J. _____

**Fig. 10-8.** Individual vertebra,
A-F.

**Fig. 10-9.** Individual vertebra, G-J.

8.  What are the characteristics of the vertebra in Fig. 10-9 that identify it as a lumbar vertebra rather than a thoracic?

    _____

9.  The zygapophyseal joints of the lumbar spine are classified as _____ joints with

    _____ type of joint movement.

10. List the correct terms of the lumbar vertebra that correspond to the following
    labeled parts of the "Scotty dog" as seen on an oblique radiograph of the
    lumbar spine (Fig. 10-10).

    A. _____

    B. _____

    C. _____

    D. _____

    E. _____

    F. _____ joint

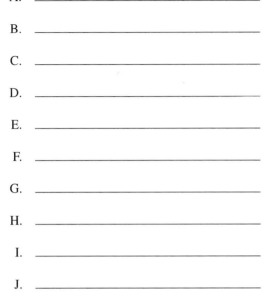

**Fig. 10-10.** Oblique lumbar spine.

11. The ear and front leg of the "Scotty dog" make up the _____ joint, best seen in the
    oblique position.

12. Which one of the following topographic landmarks corresponds to the L2-3 level?

    A.  Xiphoid process          C.  Iliac crest

    B.  Lower costal margin       D.  ASIS

**10**

13. True/False: It is possible to shield females for an AP projection of the sacrum or coccyx if the gonadal shields are correctly placed.

14. True/False: The female gonadal dose is approximately that of the midline dose and is almost the same for either AP or PA projections of the lumbar spine.

15. Why should the knees and hips be flexed for an AP projection of the lumbar spine? _____

_____

16. True/False: A lead blocker mat for lateral positions of the lumbar spine should not be used with digital imaging.

17. True/False: The efficiency of CT and MRI of the spine is reducing the number of myelograms being performed.

18. Anterior wedging and loss of vertebral body height are characteristic of:

    A. Chance fracture          C. Compression fracture

    B. Spina bifida             D. Spondylolysis

19. Which one of the following conditions is often diagnosed by prenatal ultrasound?

    A. Scoliosis                C. Spondylolisthesis

    B. Spina bifida             D. Ankylosing spondylitis

20. Which one of the following conditions usually requires an increase in manual exposure factors?

    A. Ankylosing spondylitis   C. Spina bifida

    B. Spondylolysis            D. Spondylolisthesis

21. Where is the central ray centered for an AP projection of the lumbar spine with a 30 × 35 cm (11 × 14 inch) IR?

_____

22. Which set of zygapophyseal joints of the lumbar spine is best demonstrated with an LAO position? _____

_____

23. How much rotation of the spine is required to demonstrate the zygapophyseal joint space between L1-2?

_____

24. Describe the body build that may require central ray angulation to open the intervertebral joint spaces with a lateral projection of the lumbar spine, even if the patient has some support under the waist.

_____

25. What type of central ray angulation should be used for the lateral L5-S1 projection if the waist is not supported?

    A. Central ray perpendicular to IR      C. 10° to 15° cephalad

    B. 5° to 8° caudad                      D. 3° to 5° cephalad

26. What type of central ray angulation should be used for an AP axial projection for L5-S1 on a female patient?

    A. 35° cephalad          C. 5° to 8° caudad

    B. 30° cephalad          D. Central ray perpendicular to IR

27. Where is the central ray centered for an AP axial projection for L5-S1?

_____

**10**

28. True/False: The center ionization chamber should be used when utilizing automatic exposure control (AEC) for either a lateral lumbar spine or a lateral L5-S1 projection.

29. Which projection or method is designed to demonstrate the degree of scoliosis deformity between the primary and compensatory curves as part of a scoliosis study? _____

_____

30. Which projections are designed to measure anteroposterior movement at the site of a spinal fusion?

_____

31. Where is the central ray centered for an AP projection of the sacrum? _____

_____

32. What two things can be done to reduce the high amounts of scatter reaching the IR during a lateral projection of the sacrum and coccyx?

    A. _____    B. _____

33. Why should a single, lateral projection of the sacrum and coccyx be performed rather than separate laterals of the

    sacrum and coccyx? _____

    _____

34. The skin dose on a lateral sacrum and/or coccyx projection on an average-size patient is in the _____ range.

    A.  200 to 500 mrad          C.      1000 to 1500 mrad

    B.  500 to 700 mrad          D.      1500 to 2000 mrad

35. A radiograph of an AP projection of the lumbar spine reveals that the sacroiliac (SI) joints are *not* equidistant from the spine. The right ala of the sacrum appears larger, and the left SI joint is more open than the left. Which specific positioning error is evident on this radiograph?

    _____

36. A radiograph of an LPO projection of the lumbar spine reveals that the downside pedicles are projected toward the posterior aspect of the vertebral bodies. What must be done to correct this error during the repeat exposure?

    _____

37. An AP projection of the sacrum reveals that the sacrum is foreshortened and the foramina are not open. What

    positioning error led to this radiographic outcome? _____

    _____

38. **Situation:** A patient with a possible compression fracture of L3 enters the emergency room. Which projection(s) of

    the lumbar spine best demonstrate(s) the extent of this injury? _____

    _____

**10**

39.  **Situation:** A patient with a clinical history of spondylolisthesis of the L5-S1 region comes to the radiology department. What basic (i.e., routine) and special (i.e., optional) projections should be included in this study? (HINT: If the

obliques are included, how much spine rotation should be used?)  _____

_____

40.  For the following critique questions, refer to the oblique lumbar spine radiograph (Fig. C10-81 on p. 347) in your textbook:

A.  Which positioning error(s) is(are) visible on this radiograph? (More than one answer may be selected.)

(a)  All essential anatomic structures are not demonstrated.

(b)  Central ray is centered incorrectly.

(c)  Collimation is not evident.

(d)  Exposure factors are incorrect.

(e)  No anatomic marker is visible on the radiograph.

(f)  Excessive obliquity of the spine is evident.

(g)  Insufficient obliquity of the spine is evident.

B.  Which error(s) identified above is(are) considered "repeatable"?

_____

C.  Which of the following modifications must be made during the repeat exposure? (More than one answer may be selected.)

(a)  Center central ray to long aspect of spine.

(b)  Use closer collimation.

(c)  Decrease exposure factors.

(d)  Increase exposure factors.

(e)  Place anatomic side marker on IR before exposure.

(f)  Decrease obliquity of lumbar spine.

(g)  Increase obliquity of lumbar spine.

## CHAPTER 11

# Bony Thorax—Sternum and Ribs

After you have successfully completed the activities in this chapter, you will be able to:

_____ 1. Using drawings and radiographs, identify specific anatomic structures of the sternum and ribs.

_____ 2. Classify ribs as either true, false, or floating ribs.

_____ 3. Classify specific joints in the bony thorax according to their structural classification, mobility classification, and movement type.

_____ 4. Define specific types of pathologic features of the bony thorax as described in the textbook.

_____ 5. Identify basic and special projections of the ribs and sternum, including the correct size and type of image receptor (IR) and the location, direction, and angulation of the central ray for each position.

_____ 6. Identify which structures are best seen with specific projections of the ribs and sternum.

_____ 7. Identify the technical considerations important in radiography of the ribs and sternum, including breathing instructions, general body position, kilovoltage range, and other imaging options.

_____ 8. Identify patient dose ranges for skin, midline, thyroid, and breast for specific projection of the ribs and sternum.

_____ 9. Given various hypothetical situations, identify the correct modification of a position and/or exposure factors to improve the radiographic image.

_____ 10. Given radiographs of specific bony thorax projections or positions, identify specific positioning and exposure factor errors.

## Positioning and Radiographic Critique

_____ 1. Using a peer, position for basic and special projections of the bony thorax.

_____ 2. Using a chest radiographic phantom, produce satisfactory radiographs of specific positions (if equipment is available).

_____ 3. Critique and evaluate cranial radiographs based on the four divisions of radiographic criteria: (1) structures shown, (2) position, (3) collimation and central ray, and (4) exposure criteria.

_____ 4. Distinguish between acceptable and unacceptable bony thorax radiographs based on exposure factors, motion, collimation, positioning, or other errors.

## Learning Exercises

The following review exercises should be completed only after careful study of the associated pages in the textbook as indicated by each exercise. Answers to each review exercise are given at the end of the review exercises.

## Part I: Radiographic Anatomy

**REVIEW EXERCISE A:** Anatomy of Bony Thorax, Sternum, and Ribs (see textbook pp. 350-352)

1. List the three structures that make up the bony thorax:

   A. _Sternum_          B. _12 pairs of ribs_        C. _thoracic vertebrae_

2. Identify the parts of the sternum and ribs labeled in Fig. 11-1.

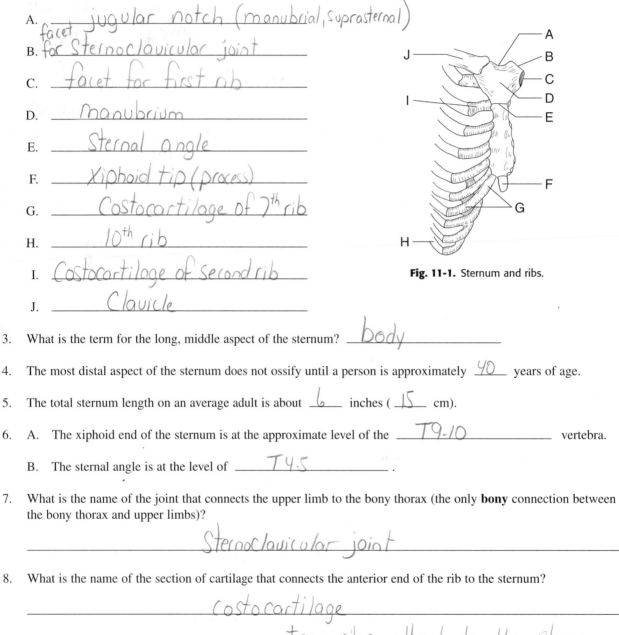

   A. _facet jugular notch (manubrial, suprasternal)_
   B. _for Sternoclavicular joint_
   C. _facet for first rib_
   D. _Manubrium_
   E. _Sternal angle_
   F. _Xiphoid tip (process)_
   G. _Costocartilage of 7th rib_
   H. _10th rib_
   I. _Costocartilage of second rib_
   J. _Clavicle_

**Fig. 11-1.** Sternum and ribs.

3. What is the term for the long, middle aspect of the sternum? _body_

4. The most distal aspect of the sternum does not ossify until a person is approximately _40_ years of age.

5. The total sternum length on an average adult is about _6_ inches ( _15_ cm).

6. A. The xiphoid end of the sternum is at the approximate level of the _T9-10_ vertebra.

   B. The sternal angle is at the level of _T4.5_ .

7. What is the name of the joint that connects the upper limb to the bony thorax (the only **bony** connection between the bony thorax and upper limbs)?
   _Sternoclavicular joint_

8. What is the name of the section of cartilage that connects the anterior end of the rib to the sternum?
   _Costocartilage_

9. What distinguishes a true rib from a false rib? _True ribs attach to the sternum by their own costocartilage / false connected by costocartilage of 7th rib_

10. (True)/False: The eleventh and twelfth ribs are classified as false *and* floating ribs.

11. True/False: The ~~anterior~~ *posterior* end of the ribs is called the vertebral end.

12. Which aspect of the ribs articulates with the transverse process of the thoracic vertebrae?

    A. Head              C. Neck

    B. Costal angle     (D.) Tubercle

13. List the three structures found within the costal groove of each rib:

    A. ___artery___          B. ___nerve___          C. ___vein___

14. Answer the following questions as you study Fig. 11-2.

    A. Which end of the ribs is most superior—the posterior vertebral ends or the anterior sternal ends?

       ___posterior vertebral___

    B. Approximately how much difference in height is there between these two ends of the ribs?

       ___3-5 inches___

    C. Which ribs articulate with the upper lateral aspect of the manubrium of the sternum?

       ___first (anterior sternal end)___

    D. The bony thorax is widest at the lateral margins of

       which ribs? ___8 or 9___

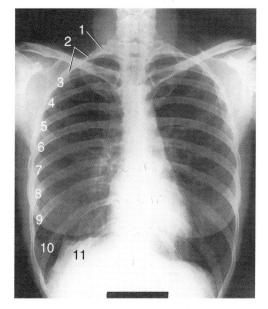

**Fig. 11-2.** Rib radiograph.

    E. How many posterior ribs are shown above the diaphragm? (HINT: Recall from Chapter 3 that a **minimum** of 10 posterior ribs must be seen on an average inspiration posteroanterior [PA] chest projection.)

       ___11___

15. Match each of the following joints with the correct movement type:

    A. Movable—diarthrodial (plane or gliding)     B. Immovable—synarthrodial

    _B_  1. First sternocostal  *first rib to manubrium*

    _A_  2. First through twelfth costovertebral joints

    _B_  3. First through tenth costochondral unions (between costocartilage and ribs)   *rib/ cart*

    _A_  4. First through tenth costotransverse joints (between ribs and transverse processes of T vertebrae)

    _A_  5. Second through seventh sternocostal joints (between second through seventh ribs and sternum)

    _A_  6. Sixth through tenth interchondral joints (between anterior sixth through tenth costal cartilage)   *not connected*

16. The joints from the previous question that have diarthrodial movement are classified as ___synovial___.

**11**

17. Classify the following groups of ribs (labeled on the diagram as *A*, *B*, and *C*) and identify the number of the ribs in each category (Fig. 11-3):

    A. _1-7___ True ribs_____

    B. _8-12__ false ribs (do not have their own costocartilage)

    C. _11-12_ floating ribs_____

18. What is unique about the ribs in category *A* in the previous question?

    _they each attach to sternum with their own costocartilage_

19. What is unique about the ribs in category *C* in the previous question?

    _they do not have costocartilage / do not_
    _connect to anything_

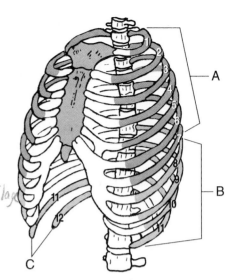

**Fig. 11-3.** Rib groups.

20. Identify the labeled parts of this posterior view of a typical rib (Fig. 11-4):

    A. ___Vertebral end (posterior)___

    B. _____tubercles_____

    C. _____angle_____

    D. ____Costal groove_____

    E. ___Sternal end (anterior)_____

    F. _____neck_____

    G. _____head_____

**Fig. 11-4.** Posterior view of a typical rib.

## Part II: Radiographic Positioning

**REVIEW EXERCISE B:** Positioning of the Ribs and Sternum (see textbook pp. 353-364)

1. ⟨True⟩/False: It is virtually impossible to visualize the sternum with a direct PA or anteroposterior (AP) projection.

2. True/⟨False⟩: A large, "deep-chested" (hypersthenic) patient requires ~~more~~ ^less^ obliquity for a frontal view of the sternum as compared with a "thin chested" (asthenic) patient.

3. How much rotation should be used for the oblique position of the sternum for a large, "deep-chested" patient?

    _____15°_____

4. List the ideal ranges (high or low) for the following exposure factors as they apply to an oblique position of the sternum (breathing technique):

    A. Kilovoltage range: ____60-70_____

    B. Milliamperage: _____low_____

    C. Exposure time: _high  3-4 seconds_

5. What is the advantage of performing a breathing technique for radiography of the sternum?

    _____ blurs lung markings and ribs _____

6. What is the primary reason that a source image receptor distance (SID) of less than 40 inches (100 cm) should *not*

    be used for sternum radiography? _____ increased pt. dose _____

7. What other imaging option is available to study the sternum if routine RAO and lateral radiographs do not provide

    sufficient information? _____ CT or nuclear medicine _____

8. Identify the preferred positioning factors to demonstrate an injury to the ribs found **below** the diaphragm:

    A. General body position (**erect** or **recumbent**): _____ recumbent _____

    B. Breathing instructions (**inspiration** or **expiration**): _____ expiration _____

    C. Recommended kilovoltage range: _____ medium 75-85 _____

9. An injury to the region of the eighth or ninth rib would require the _____ above _____ (**above** or
    **below**) diaphragm technique.

10. To properly elongate and visualize the axillary aspect of the ribs, the patient's spine should be rotated

    _____ away from _____ (**toward** or **away from**) the area of interest.

11. Which projections (AP or PA and anterior or posterior oblique) should be performed for an injury to the **anterior**

    aspect of the ribs? _____ PA and anterior obl. (affected side closest to IR) _____

12. Which two rib projections should be performed for an injury to the **right posterior** ribs?

    _____ AP and RPO (shift spine away from area of interest) _____

13. How can the site of injury be marked for a rib series? _____ metallic "BB" over site of injury _____

14. If the physician suspects a pneumothorax or hemothorax has occurred as a result of a rib fracture, which additional
    radiographic projection(s) should be performed in addition to the routine rib projections?

    _____ erect PA and lateral chest _____

15. A flail chest is defined as a(an):

    A. Asthenic body habitus

    B. Pulmonary injury caused by blunt trauma to two or more ribs

    C. Chronic obstructive pulmonary disease (COPD; e.g., emphysema)

    D. Cardiac injury caused by blunt trauma

16. Osteolytic metastases of the ribs produce which of the following radiographic appearances?

    A. Irregular bony margins            C. Sharp lucent lines through the ribs

    B. Increased bony density of the ribs     D. Smooth lucent "holes" in the rib

17. Which of the following definitions applies to pectus excavatum?

    A. Multiple fractures of the sternum with fragments in the pericardium

    B. Abnormally prominent lower aspect of sternum

    C. Depressed sternum due to congenital defect

    D. Separation between ribs and sternum due to trauma

18. A proliferative bony lesion of increased density is generally termed:

    A. Osteoblastic    C. Osteolytic

    B. Osteoporotic    D. Osteostenotic

19. True/False: MRI provides a more diagnostic image of rib metastases as compared with a nuclear medicine scan.

20. True/False: Patients can develop osteomyelitis as a postoperative complication following open heart surgery.

21. Which is preferred for a study of the sternum—RAO or LAO? _RAO_

    Why? _It places the sternum over the heart to provide a more uniform background for added visibility_

22. Where is the central ray centered for the oblique and lateral projections of the sternum?

    _Center of sternum (midway between jugular notch and xiphoid)_

23. What other position can be performed if the patient cannot assume a prone position for the RAO sternum?

    _LPO_

24. What is the recommended SID for a lateral projection of the sternum? _60-72"_

    Why? _reduces magnification created by the long OID_

25. Which of the following criteria apply to a radiograph for an evaluation of the oblique sternum?

    A. The entire sternum should be adjacent to the spine and adjacent to the heart shadow.

    B. The entire sternum should lie over the heart shadow and be adjacent to the spine.

    C. The left sternoclavicular joint should be adjacent to the spinal column.

    D. The second rib should lie directly over the manubrium of the sternum.

26. Where is the central ray centered for a PA projection of the sternoclavicular joints?

    A. Level of T7          C. At the vertebra prominens

    B. Level of T2-3        D. Level of xiphoid process

27. What type of breathing instructions should be given to the patient for a PA projection of the sternoclavicular joints?

    A. Suspend respiration on inspiration.    C. Suspended breathing is not necessary.

    B. Use a breathing technique.

28. How much rotation of the thorax is recommended for an anterior oblique of the sternoclavicular joints?

    _____

29. Which specific oblique position best demonstrates the **left** sternoclavicular joint next to the spine?

    _____

30. What are the three points that must be included in the patient's clinical history prior to a rib series?

    A. _Nature of trauma or complaint_

    B. _Location of rib pain or injury_

    C. _Whether the patient has been coughing up blood_

31. Where is the central ray centered for an AP projection of the ribs for an injury located above the diaphragm?

    _3-4" below jugular notch (T7)_

32. Which two specific oblique positions can be used to demonstrate the **left** axillary portion of the ribs?

    _RAO or LPO elongates the left axillary ribs (shifts spine away from injury site)_

33. Which two specific projections or positions should be performed for an injury to the right anterior ribs?

    _PA and LAO_

34. How many degrees of rotation are needed for a routine oblique projection of the ribs? _45°_

35. Both the patient thyroid dose and the breast dose for a correctly collimated PA sternoclavicular (SC) joint

    projection are in the _____ range.

    (A) 1 to 5 mrad         C. 300 to 400 mrad

    B. 25 to 100 mrad       D. 500 to 1000 mrad

36. True/False: The thyroid dose for an anterior oblique rib projection is only about 5% of what it would be for a posterior oblique rib projection.

37. True/False: The breast dose for an anterior oblique rib projection is only about 5% of what it would be for a posterior oblique rib projection.

38. True/False: The amount of gonadal dose given for rib projections is less than 1 mrad.

## REVIEW EXERCISE C: Problem Solving for Technical and Positioning Errors (see textbook pp. 350-364)

1. A radiograph of an RAO sternum reveals that part of the sternum is superimposed over the thoracic spine. Which specific positioning error is visible on this radiograph?

    _Underrotation of the patient_

2. A radiograph of an RAO sternum reveals that the sternum is difficult to visualize because of excessive density. The following factors were used for this image: 75 kV, 25 mA, 3-second exposure, 40 inch (100 cm) SID, Bucky, and 100-speed screens. Which one of these factors should be modified during the repeat exposure to produce a more diagnostic image?

    _lower kV to 65 for higher contrast and to prevent overpenetration of the sternum_

3. A radiograph of an RAO sternum reveals that the sternum is poorly visualized because of excessive lung markings superimposed over the sternum. The following factors were used for this image: 65 kV, 200 mA, 1¼-second exposure, 40 inch (100 cm) SID, Bucky, and 100-speed screens. Which of these factors can be altered to increase the visibility of the sternum?

    _Increase exposure time and shorten mA to allow for greater blurring of the lung markings_

4. A radiograph of a lateral projection of the sternum reveals that the patient's breasts are obscuring the sternum. What can be done to minimize the breast artifact over the sternum?

*have pt bring breasts to the side*

5. Repeat PA projections of the sternoclavicular joints do not clearly demonstrate them. What other imaging modality may produce a more diagnostic image of these joints?

*CT*

6. **Situation:** A patient with trauma to the sternum and the left sternoclavicular joint region enters the emergency room. In addition to the sternum routine, the ER physician asks for a specific projection to better demonstrate the left sternoclavicular joint. Describe the positioning routine, including the breathing instructions that you would use. (HINT: Three projections are required.)

*15-20° RAO sternum w/br.tech , lateral sternum on inspiration , and 15-20° LAO of SC Joint with suspended respiration*

7. A radiograph of the upper ribs demonstrates that the diaphragm is superimposed over the eighth ribs, which is in the area of interest. The following factors were used for the initial exposure: 65 kV, 400 mA, 1/40 second, 400-speed screens, grid, suspended respiration on expiration, erect position, 40 inch (102 cm) SID. Which one of these factors can be modified to increase the visibility of the area of interest?

*Suspend on inspiration to move diaphragm down*

8. **Situation:** A patient enters the emergency room on a backboard after being involved in a motor vehicle accident. Because of the condition of the patient, the physician orders a portable study of the sternum in the ER. Which two projections of the sternum would be most diagnostic yet minimize movement of the patient? (See Chapter 19 in the textbook for a demonstration.)

*LPO and horizontal beam lateral (Can use 15-20° mediolateral angle if pt cannot obl)*

9. **Situation:** A patient with trauma to the right upper anterior ribs enters the ER. He is able to sit in erect position. Which positioning routine of the ribs should be performed? (Include general body position, breathing instructions, and specific projections or positions performed.)

*PA-inspiration (above diaphragm), LAO(or RPO) with inspiration*

10. **Situation:** A patient with trauma to the left lower anterior ribs enters the ER. Which positioning routine of the ribs should be performed? (Include general body position, breathing instructions, and specific positions performed.)

*Recumbent PA (below diaphragm), RAO or (LPO) with expiration*

11. **Situation:** An elderly patient comes to the radiology department for a complete rib series with an emphasis on the posterior ribs. She has advanced osteoporosis and has difficulty moving and lying down. Her physician wants both upper and lower ribs examined. What type of positions should be performed? How would you adjust technical factors for this patient?

*Erect for all AP and obl. (RPO & LPO) Lower kV due to osteoporosis*

12. **Situation:** A patient enters the ER with blunt trauma to the chest. He is restricted on a backboard. The ER physician suspects a flail chest. Beyond the initial chest projections, what positioning routine would confirm the diagnosis of flail chest?

*Limited rib series*

**REVIEW EXERCISE D:** Critique Radiographs of the Bony Thorax (see textbook p. 366)

The following questions relate to the radiographs found at the end of Chapter 11 of the textbook. Evaluate these radiographs for the radiographic criteria categories (*1* through *5*) that follow. Describe the corrections needed to improve the overall image. The major, or "repeatable," errors are specific errors that indicate the need for a repeat exposure, regardless of the nature of the other errors.

A.   **Ribs above diaphragm (Fig. C11-43)**

NOTE: This radiograph was included to keep you alert and to present a challenge to even the most advanced student or technologist. To critique and evaluate this may require more information about this patient than was presented in the textbook. This patient was brought to the radiology department from the county morgue to be radiographed so that the cause of death could be determined. This was a reported drowning victim whose body had been in the water for several days. Note the air in the lungs, which may suggest that the cause of death was not drowning. No specific critique questions and answers are included for this unique radiograph; continue to the following radiograph.

B.   **Oblique sternum (Fig. C11-44)**

   1.   Structures shown: _____

   2.   Part positioning: _____

   3.   Collimation and central ray: _____

   4.   Exposure criteria: _____

   5.   Markers: _____

   Repeatable error(s): _____

C.   **Ribs below diaphragm (Fig. C11-45)**

   1.   Structures shown: _____

   2.   Part positioning: _____

   3.   Collimation and central ray: _____

   4.   Exposure criteria: _____

   5.   Markers: _____

   Repeatable error(s): _____

D.   **Lateral sternum (Fig. C11-46)**

   1.   Structures shown: _____

   2.   Part positioning: _____

   3.   Collimation and central ray: _____

   4.   Exposure criteria: _____

   5.   Markers: _____

   Repeatable error(s): _____

**11**

## Part III: Laboratory Activities (see textbook pp. 358-364)

You must gain experience in positioning each part of the sternum and ribs before performing the following exams on actual patients. You can get experience in positioning and radiographic evaluation of these projections by performing exercises using radiographic phantoms and practicing on other students (although you will not be taking actual exposures).

The following suggested activities assume that your teaching institution has an energized lab and radiographic phantoms. If not, perform Laboratory Exercises B and C, the radiographic evaluation and the physical positioning exercises. (Check off each step and projection as you complete it.)

## LABORATORY EXERCISE A: Energized Laboratory

1. Using the chest radiographic phantom, produce radiographs of the following basic routines:

   _____ RAO sternum

   _____ PA sternoclavicular joints

   _____ AP (PA) ribs

   _____ AP (PA) ribs, above and below diaphragm

   _____ Lateral sternum

   _____ RAO (LAO) sternoclavicular joints

   _____ Posterior and anterior oblique ribs, above diaphragm

   _____ Horizontal beam lateral sternum

## LABORATORY EXERCISE B: Radiographic Evaluation

1. Evaluate and critique the radiographs produced above, additional radiographs provided by your instructor, or both. Evaluate each radiograph for the following points:

   _____ Evaluate the completeness of the study. (Are all of the pertinent anatomic structures included on the radiograph?)

   _____ Evaluate for positioning or centering errors (e.g., rotation, off centering).

   _____ Evaluate for correct exposure factors and possible motion. (Are the density and contrast of the images acceptable?)

   _____ Determine whether markers and an acceptable degree of collimation and/or area shielding are visible on the images.

## LABORATORY EXERCISE C: Physical Positioning

On another person, simulate performing all basic and special projections of the sternum and ribs as follows. Include the six steps listed below and described in the textbook. (Check off each step when completed satisfactorily.)

Step 1. Appropriate size and type of image receptor with correct markers
Step 2. Correct central ray placement and centering of part to central ray and/or image receptor
Step 3. Accurate collimation
Step 4. Area shielding of patient where advisable
Step 5. Use of proper immobilizing devices when needed
Step 6. Approximate correct exposure factors, breathing instructions where applicable, and "making" exposure

## PROJECTIONS

| | STEP 1 | STEP 2 | STEP 3 | STEP 4 | STEP 5 | STEP 6 |
|---|---|---|---|---|---|---|
| • RAO sternum | ___ | ___ | ___ | ___ | ___ | ___ |
| • Erect lateral sternum | ___ | ___ | ___ | ___ | ___ | ___ |
| • Recumbent left posterior oblique (LPO) sternum | ___ | ___ | ___ | ___ | ___ | ___ |
| • Horizontal beam lateral sternum | ___ | ___ | ___ | ___ | ___ | ___ |
| • PA sternoclavicular joints | ___ | ___ | ___ | ___ | ___ | ___ |
| • Oblique sternoclavicular joints | ___ | ___ | ___ | ___ | ___ | ___ |
| • Rib routine for injury to right upper anterior ribs | ___ | ___ | ___ | ___ | ___ | ___ |
| • Rib routine for injury to left lower posterior ribs | ___ | ___ | ___ | ___ | ___ | ___ |

*Optional exercise if the school or hospital has a tomography unit:*

| | | | | | | |
|---|---|---|---|---|---|---|
| • Linear tomogram of the sternum | ___ | ___ | ___ | ___ | ___ | ___ |

# Answers to Review Exercises

## REVIEW EXERCISE A: Anatomy of the Bony Thorax, Sternum, and Ribs

1. A. Sternum
   B. Thoracic vertebra
   C. 12 pairs of ribs
2. A. Jugular (suprasternal) notch
   B. Facet for sternoclavicular joint
   C. Facet for first rib
   D. Manubrium
   E. Sternal angle
   F. Xiphoid process
   G. Costocartilage of seventh rib (last of "true" ribs)
   H. Tenth rib
   I. Costocartilage of second rib
   J. Clavicle
3. Body
4. 40
5. 6 inches (15 cm)
6. A. T9 or 10
   B. T4-5
7. Sternoclavicular joint
8. Costocartilage
9. True ribs connect to the sternum by their own costocartilage. False ribs are connected to the sternum via the costocartilage of the seventh rib.
10. True
11. False (called the sternal end)
12. D. Tubercle
13. A. Artery
    B. Vein
    C. Nerve
14. A. Posterior vertebral ends
    B. 3 to 5 inches (7.5 to 12.5 cm)
    C. First (anterior sternal end)
    D. Eighth or ninth
    E. 11
15. 1. B
    2. A
    3. B
    4. A
    5. A
    6. A
16. Synovial
17. A. True ribs, 1 through 7
    B. False ribs, 8 through 12
    C. Floating ribs, 11 through 12
18. Each rib attaches to the sternum by its own costocartilage.
19. They do not connect to anything anteriorly (thus the term "floating" ribs).
20. A. Vertebral end (posterior)
    B. Tubercles (for articulation with vertebrae)
    C. Axillary or angle portion of rib
    D. Costal groove
    E. Sternal end (anterior)
    F. Neck
    G. Head

## Review Exercise B: Positioning of the Ribs and Sternum

1. True
2. False (less obliquity)
3. Approximately 15°
4. A. Low (60 to 70)
   B. Low
   C. High (3 to 4 seconds) with breathing technique
5. It blurs lung markings and ribs, which improves the visibility of the sternum.
6. Increase in patient dose, especially skin dose
7. CT or nuclear medicine
8. A. Recumbent
   B. Expiration
   C. Medium (75 to 85)
9. Above
10. Away from
11. PA and anterior obliques (Placing the area of interest closest to the IR is one recommended routine.)
12. AP and RPO (to shift spine away from area of interest)
13. By taping a small, metallic "BB" over the site of the injury
14. Erect PA and lateral chest
15. B
16. A
17. C
18. A
19. False
20. True
21. RAO; it places the sternum over the heart to provide a uniform background for added visibility of the sternum.
22. Midsternum (midway between jugular notch and xiphoid)
23. LPO (oblique supine position)
24. 60 to 72 inches (152 to 183 cm); reduces magnification created by the long object image receptor distance (OID)
25. B. The entire sternum should lie over the heart shadow adjacent to the spine.
26. B. Level of T2-3
27. A. Suspend respiration on inspiration.
28. 15°
29. LAO
30. A. The nature of the trauma or patient complaint
    B. The location of the rib pain or injury
    C. Whether or not the patient has been coughing up blood
31. 3 to 4 inches (8 to 10 cm) below the jugular notch, level of T7
32. RAO or LPO elongates the left axillary ribs (and shifts the spine away from the injury site)
33. PA and LAO (to shift spine away from injury site)
34. 45°
35. A. 1 to 5 mrad
36. False (only about one-third, or 33%)
37. True (Note: A greater difference in breast dose exists for posterior versus anterior rib projections than for thyroid doses because of the more anterior surface placement of the breasts compared with the thyroid.)
38. True. The gonadal dose is so low that it is not listed on the dose charts for rib projections.

## Review Exercise C: Problem Solving for Technical and Positioning Errors

1. Underrotation of the patient
2. Lower the kilovoltage to 65 for higher contrast and to prevent overpenetration of the sternum.
3. Increase the exposure time (and lower the milliamperage) to allow for greater blurring of the lung markings.
4. Have the patient bring the breasts to the side; hold them in this position with a wide bandage.
5. CT
6. 15° to 20° RAO sternum with breathing technique; lateral sternum on inspiration; and 15° to 20° LAO of sternoclavicular joint with suspended inspiration
7. Suspend respiration during inspiration to move the diaphragms below the eighth ribs.
8. LPO and horizontal beam lateral projections (may use 15° to 20° mediolateral central angle if patient cannot be in oblique position)
9. Erect PA and LAO (or RPO) position with suspended **inspiration**
10. Recumbent PA (or AP if the patient cannot assume prone position) and LPO (or RAO) positions with suspended **expiration**
11. Because of patient condition, it is best to perform all positions erect and initiate exposure on full inspiration for upper ribs and full expiration for lower ribs. AP projections

and both oblique positions (RPO and LPO) must be performed. It is recommended that kV (manual technique employed) for all projections be lowered because of the advanced osteoporosis.

12. A limited rib series will indicate which ribs are fractured (and whether this has led to flail chest). Since the patient is restricted to a backboard, the oblique positions may not be possible.

## Review Exercise D: Critique Radiographs of the Bony Thorax

A. Ribs above diaphragm (Fig. C11-43)—See explanation on p. 251.

B. Oblique sternum (Fig. C11-44)
1. All pertinent anatomic structures included
2. Sternum is overrotated; sternum away from the spine and rotated beyond heart shadow and distorted (NOTE: Because of additional patient dose, some departments may choose not to repeat this projection since the outline of the sternum is visible.)
3. Collimation not completely evident; central ray centering and IR placement correct
4. Acceptable exposure factors and processing
5. No evidence of anatomic side marker
Repeatable errors: 2

C. Ribs below diaphragm (Fig. C11-45)
1. Right lower ribs cut off; only lower three pair of ribs demonstrated, indicating diaphragm is too low from poor expiration
2. No elevation of diaphragm; need to take exposure during expiration with the patient in a recumbent position to raise the diaphragm to the highest level
3. No evidence of collimation; acceptable central ray centering, but IR should have been placed crosswise to prevent lateral margins of ribs from being cut off
4. Acceptable exposure factors and processing
5. Anatomic side marker evident but placed a little low and almost off the radiograph
Repeatable errors: 1 and 3

D. Lateral sternum (Fig. C11-46)
1. Lower aspect of sternum cut off
2. Acceptable part positioning
3. No evidence of collimation; central ray centering and IR placement too high, causing lower sternum to be cut off
4. Acceptable exposure factors
5. No evidence of markers
Repeatable errors: 1 and 3

# SELF-TEST

This self-test should be taken only after completing all of the readings, review exercises, and laboratory activities for a particular section. The purpose of this test is not only to provide a good learning exercise but also to serve as a strong indicator of what your final evaluation exam will cover. It is strongly suggested that if you do not get at least a 90% to 95% grade on each self-test, you review those areas in which you missed questions before going to your instructor for the final evaluation exam for this chapter. (There are 63 questions or blanks—each is worth 1.6 points.)

1.  List the three parts of the sternum:

    A.  _____

    B.  _____

    C.  _____

2.  What is the most distal aspect of the sternum? _____

3.  What is the name of the palpable junction between the upper and midportion of the sternum?

    _____

4.  Which aspect of the sternum possesses the jugular notch?

    A.  Body              C.  Xiphoid process

    B.  Sternal angle     D.  Manubrium

5.  What distinguishes a true rib from a false rib?

    A.  A true rib attaches directly to the sternum with it own costocartilage.

    B.  A true rib possesses a costovertebral and a costotransverse joint.

    C.  A false rib does not possess a head.

    D.  A false rib is primarily composed of cartilage.

6.  What distinguishes a floating rib from a false rib?

    A.  A floating rib is found only at the T1, T10, and T11 levels.

    B.  A floating rib does not possess a head.

    C.  A floating rib has no costal groove.

    D.  A floating rib does not possess costocartilage.

7.  The fifth rib is an example of a _____ (**true rib** or **false rib**).

8.  Which part of the sternum do the second ribs articulate?

    A.  Midbody           C.  Middle manubrium

    B.  Upper manubrium   D.  Sternal angle

9.  Which of the following structures is(are) found in the costal groove of each rib?

    A.  Nerve      C.  Vein

    B.  Artery     D.  All of the above

**11**

10. Match each of the following joints with the correct type of movement:

_____ 1. Sternoclavicular        A. Plane (gliding)–diarthrodial

_____ 2. Costovertebral joint    B. Immovable—synarthrodial

_____ 3. First sternocostal joint

_____ 4. Eighth interchondral joint

_____ 5. Third costochondral union

11. Identify the structures labeled on the following radiographs of the sternum (Figs. 11-5 and 11-6).

*Fig. 11-5*

A. _____

B. _____ (Joint)

C. _____

D. _____

E. _____

F. _____

G. _____

**Fig. 11-5.** The sternum, A-G.

**Fig. 11-6.** The sternum, H-L.

*Fig. 11-6*

H. _____

I. _____

J. _____

K. _____

L. _____

12. List the correct positioning considerations for a study of the ribs above the diaphragm:

A. Breathing instructions: _____

B. Kilovoltage range: _____

C. General body position: _____

13. What is the SID for radiography of the sternum? (NOTE: This is a radiation safety concern.)

_____

14. Which one of the following breathing instructions should be employed for an RAO position of the sternum to maximize visibility of it?

    A. Suspended inspiration   C. Suspended expiration

    B. Breathing technique     D. Valsalva maneuver

15. List the two factors to be considered when determining which specific projections to include in the rib routine as described in the textbook.

    A. _____

    B. _____

16. List two chest pathologic conditions that may result from a rib injury and require a PA and lateral chest projections to be included with the rib routine.

    A. _____    B. _____

17. A. What is the average degree of rotation for an RAO position of the sternum?

    _____

    B. Does an asthenic patient require a little more or a little less obliquity than a hypersthenic patient?

    _____

18. For which of the following conditions of the bony thorax are nuclear medicine bone scans *not* normally performed?

    A. Possible fractures     C. History of multiple myeloma

    B. Osteoporosis         D. Osteomyelitis

19. Pathology of the sternum is most commonly due to:

    A. Metastases     C. Infection

    B. Osteoporosis    D. Blunt trauma

20. What is the average breast dose range for each of the following projections?

    A. A posterior oblique rib projection: _____

    B. An anterior oblique rib projection: _____

21. What other position can be used for the sternum if the patient cannot assume the recumbent RAO position?

    A. LAO   C. LPO

    B. RPO   D. Left lateral decubitus

22. How should the arms be positioned for an erect lateral projection of the sternum?

    A. Raised over the head    C. Depressed by holding 5 to 10 lb in each hand

    B. Drawn back          D. Extended in front of the thorax

23. Which radiographic sign can be evaluated to determine whether rotation is present on a PA projection of the sternoclavicular joints?

_____

24. How much rotation of the thorax is required for the anterior oblique projection of the sternoclavicular joints?

_____

25. Where is the central ray centered for an AP projection of the ribs below the diaphragm?

_____

26. What range of kilovoltage should be used for ribs above the diaphragm?

   A.  55 to 65 kV        C.  80 to 90 kV

   B.  65 to 75 kV        D.  90 to 100 kV

27. Which one of the following positions or projections will best demonstrate the right axillary ribs?

   A.  LAO        C.  RAO

   B.  LPO        D.  PA

28. A radiograph of an RAO projection of the sternum reveals that the width of the sternum is foreshortened and the sternum is shifted away from the spine and out of the heart shadow. The patient has a large "barrel" chest. The technologist performed the RAO with 20° to 25° of rotation and used a breathing technique. Which positioning error led to this radiographic outcome?

_____

29. A radiograph of a lateral sternum reveals that anterior ribs are superimposed over the sternum. Which specific positioning error led to this radiographic outcome?

_____

30. **Situation:** A patient with an injury to the **right lower posterior ribs** comes to the emergency room. She is unable to stand. List the positioning routine that would be performed for this patient. Include breathing instructions.

   A.  Positions performed: _____

   B.  Breathing instructions: _____

31. **Situation:** A patient with an injury to the **left upper anterior ribs** comes to the ER. He is unable to stand but can lie on his abdomen. List the positioning routine that would be used for this patient. Include breathing instructions.

   A.  Positions performed: _____

   B.  Breathing instructions: _____

32. **Situation:** A routine chest study reveals a possible lesion near the right sternoclavicular joint. A PA projection of the sternoclavicular joints is taken, but the area of interest is superimposed over the spine. What specific position can be used to better demonstrate this region?

_____

33. **Situation:** A patient is brought into the ER with multiple injuries due to an MVA. The patient can move but cannot stand or lie prone because of his injuries. A sternum study is ordered. What positions should be performed for this patient?

_____

34. **Situation:** A patient comes to the ER with multiple rib fractures. The ER physician suspects a flail chest. The patient is able to stand and move. Beyond a rib series, what projections should be taken for this patient?

_____

35. True/False: The automatic exposure control (AEC) system is recommended for sternum and rib routines if the center chamber is used.

36. True/False: A breathing technique is recommended for studies of the sternoclavicular joints.

37. For the following critique questions, refer to the oblique sternum radiograph in Fig. C11-44 on p. 366 in your textbook.

   A. Which positioning error(s) is(are) visible on this radiograph? (More than one answer may be selected.)

     (a) All essential anatomic structures are not demonstrated.

     (b) Central ray is centered incorrectly.

     (c) Collimation is not evident.

     (d) Exposure factors are incorrect.

     (e) No anatomic marker is visible on the radiograph.

     (f) Excessive rotation of the sternum is evident.

     (g) Insufficient rotation of the sternum is evident.

   B. Which error(s) identified above is(are) considered "repeatable"? _____

   C. Which of the following modifications must be made during the repeat exposure? (More than one answer may be selected.)

     (a) Center central ray to middle aspect of sternum.

     (b) Increase collimation.

     (c) Decrease exposure factors.

     (d) Increase exposure factors.

     (e) Place anatomic side marker on IR before exposure.

     (f) Decrease rotation of body.

     (g) Increase rotation of body.

## CHAPTER 12

# Skull and Cranial Bones

After you have successfully completed the activities in this chapter, you will be able to:

_____ 1. List the eight cranial bones and describe their features, related structures, location, and function.

_____ 2. Using drawings and/or radiographs, identify specific structures of the eight cranial bones.

_____ 3. Define specific terminology, reference points, positioning lines, and topographic landmarks of the cranium.

_____ 4. Identify specific radiographic and topographic landmarks of the cranium.

_____ 5. List the location, joint classification, and related terminology for the sutures and joints of the cranium.

_____ 6. List the differences among the three shape and size (morphology) classifications of the skull and their implications for radiography of the cranium.

_____ 7. Identify alternative imaging modalities that best demonstrate specific conditions or disease processes of the cranium and brain.

_____ 8. Match specific pathologic indications of the cranium to the correct definition or statements.

_____ 9. List the three main portions of the temporal bones.

_____ 10. Identify specific structures of the external, middle, and internal ear.

_____ 11. Using drawings, identify the three divisions of the ear and the structures found in each division.

_____ 12. Match specific pathologic indications of the temporal bone to the correct definition.

_____ 13. Using radiographs, identify specific structures of the temporal bone.

_____ 14. Identify the correct size and type of image receptor and central ray location, direction, and angle for basic and special projections of the cranium.

_____ 15. Identify which structures are best seen with specific projections of the cranium.

_____ 16. Identify basic and special projections of the temporal bones and list the correct size and type of image receptor, central ray location, direction, and angulation for each projection.

_____ 17. List the patient dose ranges for skin, midline, and thyroid for each basic and special projection of the cranium and mastoids.

_____ 18. Identify the difference in dose ranges for the thyroid region for frontal projections (anteroposterior [AP]) compared with posteroanterior (PA) projections of the cranium (such as PA axial or PA Caldwell versus AP axial projections).

_____ 19. Given various hypothetical situations, identify the correct modification of a position and/or exposure factors to improve the radiographic image.

## Positioning and Radiographic Critique

_____ 1. Using a peer, position for basic and special projections of the cranium.

_____ 2. Using a cranial radiographic phantom, produce satisfactory radiographs of specific positions (if equipment is available).

_____    3.  Critique and evaluate cranial radiographs based on the four divisions of radiographic criteria: (1) structures shown, (2) position, (3) collimation and central ray, and (4) exposure criteria.

_____    4.  Distinguish between acceptable and unacceptable cranial radiographs based on exposure factors, motion, collimation, positioning, or other errors.

## Learning Exercises

The following review exercises should be completed only after careful study of the associated pages in the textbook as indicated by each exercise. Answers to each review exercise are given at the end of the review exercises.

## Part I: Radiographic Anatomy

All

**REVIEW EXERCISE A:** Anatomy and Pathology of the Cranium (see textbook pp. 369-379)

1.  Fill in the total number of bones:

   A.  Cranium _____ 8 _____         B.  Facial bones ___ 14 _____

2.  List the four cranial bones that form the calvaria (skull cap):

   A.  ___ Frontal _____       C.  ___ Right parietal _____

   B.  ___ Occipital _____       D.  ___ Left parietal _____

3.  List the four cranial bones that form the floor of the cranium:

   A.  ___ Right temporal _____       C.  ___ Sphenoid _____

   B.  ___ Left temporal _____       D.  ___ Ethmoid _____

4.  Identify the cranial bones labeled on Figs. 12-1 and 12-2 (NOTE: All eight cranial bones, including each paired bone, are visible in at least one of the following drawings):

   A.  ___ Frontal _____

   B.  ___ Right parietal _____

   C.  ___ Right temporal _____

   D.  ___ Sphenoid _____

   E.  ___ Ethmoid _____

   F.  ___ Left Temporal _____

   G.  ___ Left Parietal _____

   H.  ___ Occipital _____

**Fig. 12-1.** Frontal view.

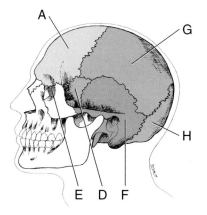

**Fig. 12-2.** Lateral view.

5.  Identify all eight cranial bones on the two superior-view drawings
    (Figs. 12-3 and 12-4):

    A.  _Frontal_

    B.  _Ethmoid_

    C.  _Sphenoid_

    D.  _Left temporal_

    E.  _Left parietal_

    F.  _Occipital_

    G.  _Right parietal_

    H.  _Right temporal_

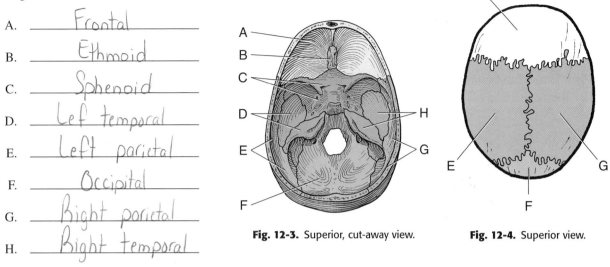

**Fig. 12-3.** Superior, cut-away view.    **Fig. 12-4.** Superior view.

**12**

6.  Identify the labeled parts on the three views of the ethmoid bone
    (Figs. 12-5 and 12-6):

    A.  _Crista galli_

    B.  _Cribriform plate_

    C.  _Perpendicular plate_

    D.  _Lateral labyrinth (mass)_

    E.  _Middle nasal concha (turbinate)_

**Fig. 12-5.** Medial sectional view.

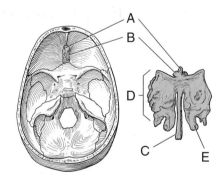

**Fig. 12-6.** Superior *(left)* and coronal sectional *(right)* views.

7.  The small horizontal plate of the ethmoid seen in the above drawings is called the

    _Cribriform plate_                                                                .

8.  The vertical plate of the ethmoid bone forming the upper portion of the bony nasal septum is the

    _perpendicular plate_                                                             .

**12**

9.  Identify the labeled parts on the four views of the sphenoid in Figs. 12-7 through 12-10 (NOTE: Most of the parts are identified on more than one drawing):

A. _Anterior clinoid process_

B. _Lesser wing_

C. _Greater wing_

D. _Sella turcica_

E. _Dorsum sellae_

F. _Posterior clinoid process_

G. _Clivus_

*Foramina (H-L)*

H. _Foramen rotundum_

I. _Foramen ovale_

J. _Foramen Spinosum_

K. _Foramen magnum_

L. _Optic foramen_

M. _Lateral pterygoid process (plate)_

N. _Pterygoid hamulus_

O. _Medial pterygoid process (plate)_

P. _Superior orbital fissure_

Q. _Body of sphenoid (sinus)_

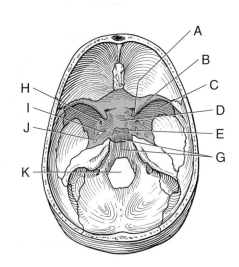

**Fig. 12-7.** Sphenoid, superior view.

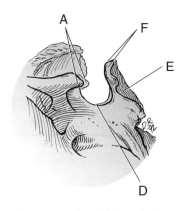

**Fig. 12-8.** Sphenoid, lateral view.

**Fig. 12-9.** Sphenoid, superior view.

**Fig. 12-10.** Sphenoid, medial sectional view.

10. A structure found in the middle of the sphenoid bone that surrounds the pituitary gland is the *Sella turcica* .

11. The posterior aspect of the sella turcica is called the *dorsum sellae* .

12. Which structure of the sphenoid bone allows for the passage of the optic nerve and is the actual opening into the orbit? *optic foramen*

13. Which structures of the sphenoid bone help form part of the lateral walls of the nasal cavities?

*medial and lateral pterygoid processes*

14. Which radiographic cranial position best demonstrates the sella turcica? *lateral*

15. Which aspect of the frontal bone forms the superior aspect of the orbit? *Orbital or horizontal portion*

16. Identify the four major sutures and the six associated asterions and fontanels labeled on these drawings of an adult cranium and an infant cranium (Figs. 12-11 to 12-14):

*Sutures*

A. *Coronal*

B. *Squamosal*

C. *Lambdoidal*

D. *Sagittal*

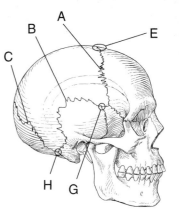

**Fig. 12-11.** Adult cranium, lateral view.

*Asterions*

E. *Bregma*

F. *Lambda*

G. Right and left *pterion*

H. Right and left *asterion*

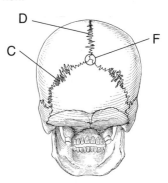

**Fig. 12-12.** Posterior view.

*Fontanels:*         *Associated adult asterion:*

I. *Anterior* ( *bregma* )

J. *Posterior* ( *lambda* )

K. Right and left *Sphenoid* ( *pterion* )

L. Right and left *Mastoid* ( *asterion* )

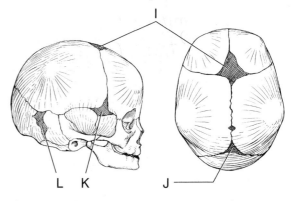

**Fig. 12-13.** Infant cranium, lateral view.     **Fig. 12-14.** Infant cranium, superior view.

12

17. Cranial sutures are classified as being _Synarthroidal_ joints.

18. Small irregular bones that sometimes develop in adult skull sutures are called _Sutural_ or _Wormian_ bones and are most frequently found in the _lamdoidal_ suture.

19. Which term describes the superior rim of the orbit? (Include the abbreviation also.) _Supraorbital margin (Som)_

20. What is the name of the notch that separates the orbital plates from each other? _ethmoidal_

21. Which cranial bones form the upper lateral walls of the calvarium? _R & L parietal_

22. Which cranial bone contains the foramen magnum? _occipital_

23. A small prominence located on the squamous portion of the occipital bone is called the _external occipital protuberance or inion_.

24. What is the name of the oval processes found on the occipital bone that help form the occipito-atlantal joint? _occipital condyles or lateral condylar portions_

25. List the three aspects of the temporal bones:

    A. _Squamous_    B. _petrous_    C. _mastoid_

26. True/False: The mastoid portion of the temporal bone is the densest of the three aspects of the temporal bone.

27. Which external landmark corresponds with the level of the petrous ridge? _TEA_

28. Which opening in the temporal bone serves as a passageway for nerves of hearing and equilibrium? _Internal acoustic meatus_

29. Identify the following cranial structures labeled on Figs. 12-15 and 12-16:

    *Fig. 12-15*

    A. _Supraorbital margin (Som) Right_
    B. _Crista galli_
    C. _Sagittal_ (suture)
    D. _Lamdoidal_ (suture)
    E. _Petrous ridge_

**Fig. 12-15.** Cranial structures, posteroanterior (PA) Caldwell projection.

*Fig. 12-16*

A. _____ EAM _____

B. ___ Mastoid portion of temporal bone ___

C. _____ Occipital bone _____

D. _____ Lamdoidal _____ (suture)

E. _____ Clivus _____

F. _____ Dorsum sellae _____

G. ___ Posterior clinoid processes ___

H. ___ Anterior clinoid processes ___

I. _____ Vertex of skull _____

J. _____ Coronal _____ (suture)

K. _____ Frontal bone _____

L. ___ Orbital plates of frontal bone ___

M. _____ Cribriform plate _____

N. _____ Sella turcica _____

O. ___ Body of sphenoid bone : Sphenoid sinus ___

1-21

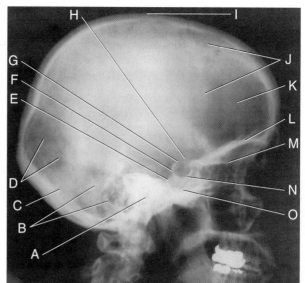

**Fig. 12-16.** Cranial structures, lateral projection.

12

**REVIEW EXERCISE B:** Specific Anatomy and Pathology of the Temporal Bone (see textbook pp. 376-379)

1. List the three aspects of the temporal bone:

   A. ___ Squamous ___   B. ___ Mastoid ___   C. ___ Petrous ___

2. Which aspect of the temporal bone is considered the densest?  ___ Petrous portion ___

3. Which structure makes up the cartilaginous, external ear?  ___ auricle or pinna ___

4. How long is the average external acoustic meatus (EAM)? ___ 2.5 cm ___

5. Which small membrane marks the beginning of the middle ear? ___ Tympanic membrane (eardrum) ___

6. What is the collective term for the small bones of the middle ear? ___ auditory ossicles ___

7. Which structure allows for communication between the nasopharynx and middle ear? ___ Eustachian tube ___

8. What is the major function of the structure described in question 7? ___ Equalize pressure (atmospheric) ___

9. Which structure serves as an opening between the mastoid portion of the temporal bone and the middle ear?

   _____ Aditus _____

10.   What is the name of the thin plate of bone that separates the mastoid air cells from the brain?  _tegmen Tympani_

11.   Which one of the auditory ossicles picks up sound vibrations from the tympanic membrane?

_____Malleus_____

12.   Which one of the auditory ossicles is considered to be the smallest?  ____Stapes_____

13.   Which one of the auditory ossicles resembles a premolar tooth?  ____Incus_____

14.   What is the name of the small membrane that connects the middle to the inner ear?  _Oval window_____

15.   Which two sensory functions occur within the inner ear?

A.  _____hearing_____   B.  _____equilibrium_____

16.   What is the name of the small membrane that will move outward to transmit impulses to the auditory nerve, thus

creating the sense of hearing?  ____round or cochlear window_____

17.   (True)/False: The cochlea is a closed system relating to the sense of hearing.

18.   Identify the structures labeled on Fig. 12-17:

A.  _Malleus (hammer)_____

B.  _Incus (anvil)_____

C.  _Stapes (stirup)_____

D.  _Oval window_____

E.  _Cochlea_____

F.  _Round window_____

G.  _Eustachian tube_____

H.  _Tympanic Cavity_____

I.  _Tympanic membrane_____

J.  _EAm_____

**Fig. 12-17.** Structures of the middle and internal ear.

19.   Match each of the following pathologic indications for the temporal bone to the correct definition or description
      (using each choice only once):

_5_   A.  Neoplasia          1.  Bacterial infection of the mastoid process

_3_   B.  Otosclerosis        2.  Growth arising from a mucous membrane

_1_   C.  Mastoiditis         3.  Hereditary disease involving excessive bone formation of middle and inner ear

_6_   D.  Acoustic neuroma    4.  Benign, cystlike mass or tumor of the middle ear

_2_   E.  Polyp               5.  New and abnormal growth

_4_   F.  Cholesteatoma       6.  Benign tumor of the auditory nerve sheath

20.    Which one of the following radiographic appearances pertains to an acoustic neuroma?

    (A.)  Expansion of the internal acoustic canal      C.    Increased density in the sinus

    B.   Bone destruction within the middle ear      D.   Sinus mucosal thickening

21.    Which one of the following imaging modalities best demonstrates otosclerosis?

    A.  MRI      C.  Conventional radiography

    (B.)  CT      D.  Ultrasound

## Part II: Radiographic Positioning

*1-6*

**REVIEW EXERCISE C:** Skull Morphology, Topography, and Positioning of the Cranium (see textbook pp. 380-395)

1.    List the three classifications of the skull; then match them with the correct shape description listed on the right:

                  *CLASSIFICATION*                          *SHAPE DESCRIPTION*

    A.    *Dolicocephalic*                    a.    Width less than 75% of length

    B.    *Brachycephalic*                   b.    Width 80% or more than length

    C.    *Mesocephalic*                    c.    Width between 75% and 80% of length

2.    Central ray angles and degree of rotation stated for basic skull positions are based on the

    *mesocephalic* (average) skull, which has an angle of *47* ° between the midsagittal plane and

    the long axis of the petrous bone.

3.    The long, narrow-shaped skull has an angle of approximately *40* ° between the midsagittal plane and the long

    axis of the petrous bone.

4.    True/(False) Two other terms for the *infra*orbitomeatal line (OML) are Reid's base line and the anthropologic base line.

5.    There is a *2-8* ° difference between the orbitomeatal and infraorbitomeatal lines, and *2-8* ° between the

    orbitomeatal and glabellomeatal lines.

**12**

6. Match each of the following cranial landmarks and positioning lines with the correct definition (using each choice only once):

___G___ 1. Lateral junction of the eyelid

___E___ 2. Posterior angle of the jaw

___J___ 3. A line between the infraorbital margin and EAM

___N___ 4. The most prominent point of the external occipital protuberance

___H___ 5. A line between the glabella and alveolar process of the maxilla

___K___ 6. A line between the mental point and EAM

___D___ 7. A depression at the bridge of the nose

___F___ 8. The small cartilaginous flap covering the ear opening

___B___ 9. Corresponds to the highest level of the facial bone mass

___I___ 10. A line between the midlateral orbital margin and the EAM

___O___ 11. The center point of the EAM

___L___ 12. A positioning line that is primarily used for the modified Waters projection

___C___ 13. A line used in positioning to ensure that the skull is in a true lateral position

___A___ 14. Corresponds to the level of the petrous ridge

___M___ 15. A smooth, slightly depressed area between the eyebrows

A. TEA

B. Supraorbital groove

C. Interpupillary line

D. Nasion

E. Gonion

F. Tragus

G. Outer canthus

H. Glabelloalveolar line

I. OML

J. Infraorbitomeatal line (IOML)

K. Mentomeatal line

L. Lips-meatal line

M. Glabella

N. Inion

O. Auricular point

7. What is the average kilovoltage range for skull radiography? __medium   75-85__

8. True/False: According to HEW Report 76-8031, the patient receives no detectable gonadal exposure during skull radiography when accurate collimation is used.

9. True/False: The AP axial (Towne) skull results in about 10 times more dose to the thyroid than a PA axial (Haas) projection.

10. The thyroid dose for a submentovertex (SMV) projection of the skull is in the _____ range (which is the highest thyroid dose of any skull projection).

   A. 10 to 50 mrad    C. 200 to 300 mrad

   B. 50 to 100 mrad   D. 500 to 600 mrad

11. List the five most common errors made during skull radiography:

   A. __Rotation__          C. __Excessive flexion__     E. __Incorrect CR angle__

   B. __Tilt__              D. __Excessive extension__

12.  Of the five causes listed in the previous question, which two are the most common?

A.  _____Rotation_____        B.  _____Tilt_____

13.  True/False: Adults with osteoporosis may require a 25% to 30% reduction in milliampere seconds (mAs) during skull projections.

14.  Which one of the following imaging modalities is the most common neuroimaging procedure performed for the cranium?

(A.)  Computed tomography (CT)        C.  Magnetic resonance imaging (MRI)

B.  Ultrasound        D.  Nuclear medicine

15.  Which of the following imaging modalities is usually performed on neonates with a possible intracranial hemorrhage?

A.  CT        C.  MRI

(B.)  Ultrasound        D.  Nuclear medicine

16.  Which of the following imaging modalities is most commonly performed to evaluate patients for Alzheimer's disease?

A.  CT        C.  MRI

B.  Ultrasound        (D.)  Nuclear medicine

17.  Match each of the following pathologic indications to the correct definition or statement (using each choice only once):

_3_  A.  Fracture that may produce an air-fluid level in the sphenoid sinus

_5_  B.  Destructive lesion with irregular margins

_6_  C.  Also called a "ping pong" fracture

_1_  D.  Proliferative bony lesion of increased density

_2_  E.  A tumor that may produce erosion of the dorsum sellae

_4_  F.  Also known as *osteitis deformans*

_7_  G.  A bone tumor that originates in the bone marrow

1.  Osteoblastic neoplasm

2.  Pituitary adenoma

3.  Basal skull fracture

4.  Paget's disease

5.  Osteolytic neoplasm

6.  Depressed skull fracture

7.  Multiple myeloma

18.  Which one of the following pathologic indications may require an increase in manual exposure factors?

(A.)  Paget's disease        C.  Multiple myeloma

B.  Metastatic neoplasm        D.  Basal skull fracture

19.  Which cranial bone is best demonstrated with an AP axial (Towne method) projection of the skull?

_____Occipital_____

20.  When using a 30° caudad angle for the AP axial (Towne) projection of the skull, which positioning line should be perpendicular to the image receptor?

(A.)  OML        C.  GAL

B.  IOML        D.  AML

21. A properly positioned AP axial (Towne) projection should place the dorsum sellae into the middle aspect of the:

    A. Orbits     C. Foramen magnum

    B. Clivus     D. Anterior arch of C1

22. A lack of symmetry of the petrous ridges indicates which of the following problems with a radiograph of an AP axial projection?

    A. Tilt               C. Flexion or extension

    B. Central ray angle     D. Rotation

23. If the patient cannot flex the head adequately for the AP axial (Towne) projection, the technologist could place the

    _____IOmL_____ perpendicular to the image receptor and angle the central ray _37_ ° caudad.

24. What evidence on an AP axial (Towne) radiograph indicates whether the correct central ray angle and correct head

    flexion were used? _Dorsum selbe and posterior Clinoids in shadow of foramen magnum_

25. What central ray angle should be used for the PA axial (Haas method) projection for the cranium?

    _____25° Cephalad to omL_____

26. Where is the central ray centered for a lateral projection of the skull? _2" Superior to EAm_

27. Which specific positioning error is present if the mandibular rami are *not* superimposed on a lateral skull radiograph?

    A. Tilt          C. Overflexion of head and neck

    B. Rotation     D. Incorrect central ray angle

28. Where will the petrous ridges be projected with a 15° PA axial (Caldwell) projection of the cranium?

    _____Into lower ⅓ of the orbits_____

29. Which specific positioning error is present if the petrous ridges are projected **higher** in the orbits than expected for

    a 15° PA axial projection? _Excessive flexion or insufficient CR angle_

30. Which projection of the cranium produces an image of the frontal bone with little or no distortion?

    _____PA 0° CR_____

31. With a possible trauma patient, what must be determined before performing the SMV projection of the skull?

    _____Cervical fx or subluxation_____

32. Where is the central ray centered for a lateral projection of the sella turcica? _¾" anterior & ¾" superior to EAm_

33. Which skull positioning line is placed parallel to the plane of the IR for the SMV projection?

    A. OML     C. AML

    B. IOML     D. GML

34. Which one of the following AP axial projections best visualizes the anterior clinoids and projects the dorsum sella just above the foramen magnum?

    A. 30° caudal to IOML     C. 30° caudal to OML

    B. 37° caudal to IOML     D. 45° caudal to OML

35.   Which one of the following projections best demonstrates the sella turcica in profile?

    A.   AP axial      C.   15° PA axial

    B.   SMV       (D.)  Lateral

36.   Which one of the following projections best demonstrates the foramen rotundum?

    A.   SMV       (C.)  30° PA axial

    B.   25° to 30° AP axial    D.   Lateral

37.   Which one of the following projections best demonstrates the clivus?

    A.   AP axial      (C.)  Lateral

    B.   15° PA      D.   SMV

## REVIEW EXERCISE D: Positioning of the Temporal Bone (see textbook pp. 396-398)

1.   Why are the auricles taped forward for lateral projections of the temporal bone?

    _____

2.   True/False: Temporal bone studies require that both sides be radiographed for comparison purposes.

3.   Which two projections of the mastoid routine provide a relative lateral perspective of the mastoid air cells?

    A.   _____    B.   _____

4.   Which positioning line must be perpendicular to the image receptor to prevent incorrect tilting of the skull for the

    axiolateral oblique (modified Law) projection? _____

5.   The axiolateral oblique (modified Law) projection of the mastoids requires a _____ ° caudad CR angle and a

    _____ ° rotation of the skull toward the image receptor.

6.   A.   What is the proper method name for the posterior profile projection for mastoids? _____

    B.   The petrous pyramid should be _____ (**parallel** or **perpendicular**) to the IR with the
        posterior profile projection for the mastoids.

    C.   For this projection the head is rotated _____ ° and the CR angled _____ °

        _____ (**caudad** or **cephalad**), which visualizes the

        _____ (**upside** or **downside**) mastoids.

7.   Which of the following projections provides a comparative, bilateral view of both right and left mastoids with a
    single exposure?

    A.   Posterior profile      C.   AP axial

    B.   Axiolateral oblique    D.   Anterior profile

8.   What CR angulation must be utilized for the axiolateral (Schuller) method for mastoids?

    A.   15° caudad      C.   Perpendicular beam

    B.   12° cephalad    D.   25 to 30° caudad

9.   Where is the CR centered for an anterior profile (Arcelin method) projection of the mastoids?

    _____

**12**

**REVIEW EXERCISE E:** Problem Solving for Technical and Positioning Errors (see textbook pp. 388-398)

1.  A radiograph of an AP axial projection of the cranium reveals that the right petrous ridge is wider than the left side. Which **specific** positioning error is present on this radiograph?

    _rotation of the skull to the left_

2.  A radiograph of a 15° PA axial (Caldwell) projection of the cranium indicates that the petrous ridges are projected at the inferior orbital margin. Which positioning error(s) led to this radiographic outcome?

    _excessive extension or excessive CR Angle_

3.  A radiograph of a 15° PA axial (Caldwell) projection indicates that the distance between the midlateral borders of the orbit and lateral margin of the skull is not equal. Which positioning error led to this radiographic outcome?

    _rotation of the skull_

4.  A radiograph of an SMV projection of the skull reveals that the mandibular condyles are within the petrous bone. Which specific positioning error led to this problem?

    _Insufficient extension of the skull or CR not perp. to IOML_

5.  A radiograph of a lateral projection of the skull reveals that the orbital plates are not superimposed (one orbital plate is slightly superior to the other). Which specific positioning error led to this radiographic outcome?

    _Tilt_

6.  A lateral skull radiograph demonstrates one mandibular ramus about 0.5 cm more anterior than the other. Which positioning error occurred?

    _Rotation_

7.  An AP axial (Towne) radiograph demonstrates the dorsum sellae projected above or superior to, rather than within, the foramen magnum. Which positioning error occurred?

    _Underangulation_

8.  **Situation:** A patient comes to the radiology department with a possible tumor of the pituitary gland. Which projection of the cranium best demonstrates any bony involvement of the sella turcica?

    _Collimated lateral of sella turcica_

9.  **Situation:** A patient with a possible linear fracture of the right parietal bone enters the emergency room. Which single projection of the skull best demonstrates this fracture?

    _Right lateral of skull_

10. **Situation:** A patient comes to the radiology department for a skull series, but the patient cannot assume the correct position for either version of the AP axial Towne projection because of a very short neck and severe spinal kyphosis. What can the technologist do to demonstrate the occipital bone?

    _PA Axial or Haas method_

11. **Situation:** A patient with a possible basal skull fracture enters the emergency room. Which specific position may provide radiographic evidence of this fracture?

    _Horizontal beam lateral (air-fluid levels)_

12. **Situation:** A neonate has a clinical history of craniosynostosis. Because of the age of the patient, the physician does not order a radiographic procedure of the cranium. What other imaging modality can be performed to evaluate the patient for this condition?

_____

13. A radiograph of an axiolateral oblique (modified Law) projection for mastoids reveals that the external ear has cast a shadow over the mastoid air cells. What can be done to avoid this problem during the repeat exposure?

_____

14. A radiograph of an AP axial projection for mastoids reveals that the petrous ridges are not symmetrical (equal size). What specific positioning error is present on this radiograph?

_____

15. A radiograph of a Stenvers method for mastoids reveals that the petrous bone appears to be foreshortened. The patient's skull was classified as being dolichocephalic. What must be done to create a better profile image of the mastoids?

_____

16. **Situation:** A patient comes to the radiology department for a mastoid series. He cannot lie prone on the table or stand erect. He must remain supine. Which projections of the mastoid routine can be performed on this patient?

_____

17. **Situation:** A patient with a clinical history of acoustic neuroma comes to the radiology department. Which imaging modality(ies) can be performed for this type of pathology?

_____

**REVIEW EXERCISE F:** Critique Radiographs of the Cranium (see textbook p. 399)

The following questions relate to the radiographs found at the end of Chapter 12 of the textbook. Evaluate these radiographs for the radiographic criteria categories (*1* through *5*) that follow. Describe the corrections needed to improve the overall image. The major, or "repeatable," errors are specific errors that indicate the need for a repeat exposure, regardless of the nature of the other errors.

A.  **Lateral skull: 4-year-old (Fig. C12-83)**

1. Structures shown: _____

2. Part positioning: _____

3. Collimation and central ray: _____

4. Exposure criteria: _____

5. Markers: _____

Repeatable error(s): _____

B.  **Lateral skull: 54-year-old, posttraumatic injury (Fig. C12-84)**

1.  Structures shown: _____

2.  Part positioning: _____

3.  Collimation and central ray: _____

4.  Exposure criteria: _____

5.  Markers: _____

Repeatable error(s): _____

C.  **AP axial: Towne skull (Fig. C12-85)**

1.  Structures shown: _____

2.  Part positioning: _____

3.  Collimation and central ray: _____

4.  Exposure criteria: _____

5.  Markers: _____

Repeatable error(s): _____

D.  **AP or PA skull (Fig. C12-86)**
How can you determine whether this was a PA or an AP projection? _____

1.  Structures shown: _____

2.  Part positioning: _____

3.  Collimation and central ray: _____

4.  Exposure criteria: _____

5.  Markers: _____

Repeatable error(s): _____

E.  **AP or PA skull (Fig. C12-87)**
Is this an AP or a PA skull? (Compare with Fig. C12-86, looking at the size of the orbits.) _____

1.  Structures shown: _____

2.  Part positioning: _____

3.  Collimation and central ray: _____

4.  Exposure criteria: _____

5.  Markers: _____

Repeatable error(s): _____

**Part III: Laboratory Exercises** (see textbook pp. 387-395)

You must gain experience in positioning each part of the cranium before performing the following exams on actual patients. You can get experience in positioning and radiographic evaluation of these projections by performing exercises using radiographic phantoms and practicing on other students (although you will not be taking actual exposures).

The following suggested activities assume that your teaching institution has an energized lab and radiographic phantoms. If not, perform Laboratory Exercises B and C, the radiographic evaluation and the physical positioning exercises. (Check off each step and projection as you complete it.)

## LABORATORY EXERCISE A: Energized Laboratory

1. Using the skull radiographic phantom, produce radiographs of the following basic routines:

_____ 15° PA axial skull       _____ PA axial (Haas)       _____ AP axial sella turcica

_____ Lateral skull            _____ SMV                   _____ Lateral sella turcica

_____ AP axial skull

## LABORATORY EXERCISE B: Radiographic Evaluation

1. Evaluate and critique the radiographs produced above, additional radiographs provided by your instructor, or both. Evaluate each radiograph for the following points:

_____ Evaluate the completeness of the study. (Are all of the pertinent anatomic structures included on the radiograph?)

_____ Evaluate for positioning or centering errors (e.g., rotation, off centering).

_____ Evaluate for correct exposure factors and possible motion. (Are the density and contrast of the images acceptable?)

_____ Determine whether markers and an acceptable degree of collimation and/or area shielding are visible on the images.

## LABORATORY EXERCISE C: Physical Positioning

On another person, simulate performing all basic and special projections of the sternum and ribs as follows. Include the six steps listed below and described in the textbook. (Check off each step when completed satisfactorily.)

Step 1. Appropriate size and type of image receptor with correct markers
Step 2. Correct central ray placement and centering of part to central ray and/or image receptor
Step 3. Accurate collimation
Step 4. Area shielding of patient where advisable
Step 5. Use of proper immobilizing devices when needed
Step 6. Approximate correct exposure factors, breathing instructions where applicable, and "making" exposure

| PROJECTIONS | STEP 1 | STEP 2 | STEP 3 | STEP 4 | STEP 5 | STEP 6 |
|---|---|---|---|---|---|---|
| *Skull series: basic* | | | | | | |
| • AP axial (Towne) | ____ | ____ | ____ | ____ | ____ | ____ |
| • Lateral skull | ____ | ____ | ____ | ____ | ____ | ____ |
| • PA 15° axial (Caldwell) | ____ | ____ | ____ | ____ | ____ | ____ |
| *Skull series: special* | | | | | | |
| • PA axial (Haas) | ____ | ____ | ____ | ____ | ____ | ____ |
| • SMV | ____ | ____ | ____ | ____ | ____ | ____ |
| *Sella turcica: basic* | | | | | | |
| • Lateral | ____ | ____ | ____ | ____ | ____ | ____ |
| • AP axial (Towne) | ____ | ____ | ____ | ____ | ____ | ____ |

**12**

## *Answers to Review Exercises*

### Review Exercise A: Anatomy of the Cranium

1. A. 8
   B. 14
2. A. Frontal
   B. Right parietal
   C. Left parietal
   D. Occipital
3. A. Right temporal
   B. Left temporal
   C. Sphenoid
   D. Ethmoid
4. A. Frontal
   B. Right parietal
   C. Right temporal
   D. Sphenoid
   E. Ethmoid
   F. Left temporal
   G. Left parietal
   H. Occipital
5. A. Frontal
   B. Ethmoid
   C. Sphenoid
   D. Left temporal
   E. Left parietal
   F. Occipital
   G. Right parietal
   H. Right temporal
6. A. Crista galli
   B. Cribriform plate
   C. Perpendicular plate
   D. Lateral labyrinth (mass)
   E. Middle nasal conchae (turbinate)
7. Cribriform plate
8. Perpendicular plate
9. A. Anterior clinoid processes
   B. Lesser wing
   C. Greater wing
   D. Sella turcica
   E. Dorsum sellae
   F. Posterior clinoid process
   G. Clivis
   H. Foramen rotundum
   I. Foramen ovale
   J. Foramen spinosum
   K. Jugular foramen
   L. Optic foramen
   M. Lateral pterygoid process (plate)
   N. Pterygoid hamulus
   O. Medial pterygoid process (plate)
   P. Superior orbital fissure
   Q. Body of sphenoid (sinus)
10. Sella turcica
11. Dorsum sellae
12. Optic foramen
13. Medial and lateral pterygoid processes
14. Lateral
15. Orbital or horizontal portion
16. A. Coronal
    B. Squamosal
    C. Lambdoidal
    D. Sagittal
    E. Bregma
    F. Lambda
    G. Pterion
    H. Asterion
    I. Anterior (bregma)
    J. Posterior (lambda)
    K. Sphenoid (pterion)
    L. Mastoid (asterion)
17. Fibrous or synarthrodial
18. Sutural or wormian; lambdoidal
19. Supraorbital margin (SOM)
20. Ethmoidal notch
21. Right and left parietals
22. Occipital
23. External occipital protuberance, or inion
24. Occipital condyles, or lateral condylar portions
25. A. Squamous
    B. Mastoid
    C. Petrous
26. False (petrous portion)
27. Top of the ear attachment (TEA)
28. Internal acoustic meatus
29. *Fig. 12-15*
    A. Supraorbital margins of right orbit
    B. Crista galli of ethmoid
    C. Sagittal suture—posterior skull
    D. Lambdoidal suture—posterior skull
    E. Petrous ridge
    *Fig. 12-16*
    A. External acoustic meatus (EAM)
    B. Mastoid portion of temporal bone
    C. Occipital bone
    D. Lambdoidal suture
    E. Clivus
    F. Dorsum sellae
    G. Posterior clinoid processes
    H. Anterior clinoid processes
    I. Vertex of skull
    J. Coronal suture
    K. Frontal bone
    L. Orbital plates of frontal bone
    M. Cribriform plate
    N. Sella turcica
    O. Body of sphenoid bone: sphenoid sinus

### Review Exercise B: Specific Anatomy and Pathology of the Temporal Bone

1. A. Squamous
   B. Mastoid
   C. Petrous
2. Petrous portion
3. Auricle or pinna
4. 1 inch (or 2.5 cm)
5. Tympanic membrane (eardrum)
6. Auditory ossicles
7. Eustachian or auditory tube
8. To equalize the atmospheric pressure within the middle ear
9. Aditus
10. Tegmen tympani
11. Malleus
12. Stapes
13. Incus
14. Oval or vestibular window
15. A. Hearing
    B. Equilibrium
16. Round or cochlear window
17. True
18. A. Malleus
    B. Incus
    C. Stapes
    D. Oval window
    E. Cochlea
    F. Round window
    G. Eustachian tube
    H. Tympanic cavity
    I. Tympanic membrane
    J. EAM or canal
19. A. 5
    B. 3
    C. 1
    D. 6
    E. 2
    F. 4
20. A. Expansion of the internal acoustic canal
21. B. CT

### Review Exercise C: Skull Morphology, Topography, and Positioning of the Cranium

1. A. Mesocephalic (c)
   B. Brachycephalic (b)
   C. Dolichocephalic (a)
2. Mesocephalic, 47
3. ±40
4. False (These are other terms for the *infraorbitomeatal* line.)
5. 7° to 8°; 7° to 8° (same degrees of difference)

12

6. 1. G
   2. E
   3. J
   4. N
   5. H
   6. K
   7. D
   8. F
   9. B
   10. I
   11. O
   12. L
   13. C
   14. A
   15. M
7. 75 to 85 kV
8. True
9. True
10. C. 200 to 300 mrad
11. A. Rotation
    B. Tilt
    C. Excessive flexion
    D. Excessive extension
    E. Incorrect central ray angulation
12. A. Rotation
    B. Tilt
13. True
14. A. Computed tomography (CT)
15. B. Ultrasound
16. D. Nuclear medicine
17. A. 3
    B. 5
    C. 6
    D. 1
    E. 2
    F. 4
    G. 7
18. A. Paget's disease
19. Occipital
20. A. OML
21. C. Foramen magnum
22. D. Rotation
23. IOML; 37
24. Dorsum sellae and posterior clinoids should be projected into the foramen magnum.
25. 25° cephalad
26. 2 inches (5 cm) above the EAM
27. B. Rotation
28. In the lower one-third of the orbits
29. Excessive flexion or insufficient central ray angle
30. 0° posteroanterior (PA)
31. Rule out any possible cervical fractures or subluxation.
32. ½ inch (2 cm) anterior and ½ inch (2 cm) superior to the EAM
33. B. IOML
34. A. 30° caudal to IOML
35. D. Lateral
36. C. 30° PA axial
37. C. Lateral

## Review Exercise D: Positioning of the Temporal Bone

1. To prevent shadows from the cartilaginous ear superimposing the mastoid air cells
2. True
3. A. Axiolateral oblique (modified Law) projection
   B. Axiolateral oblique (Schuller) projection
4. Interpupillary
5. 15, 15
6. A. Stenvers
   B. Parallel
   C. 45, 12, cephalad, downside
7. C. AP axial
8. D. 25° to 30° caudad
9. 1 inch (2.5 cm) anterior and ¾ inch (2 cm) superior to elevated EAM

## Review Exercise E: Problem Solving for Technical and Positioning Errors

1. Rotation of skull present; rotation of skull toward left
2. Excessive extension or excessive caudad central ray angle—projects the petrous ridges lower than expected (should be in the lower third of the orbit)
3. Rotation of the skull
4. Insufficient extension of the skull, or central ray was not perpendicular to IOML
5. Skull tilt
6. Skull rotation
7. Central ray angled less than 37° to the IOML, or less than 30° to the OML (would be caused by 30° angle to IOML)
8. Collimated, lateral projection of the sella turcica
9. Right lateral projection of the skull
10. Should perform the PA axial projection or Haas method
11. Horizontal beam lateral position—will demonstrate a possible air-fluid level in the sphenoid sinus
12. Ultrasound—a noninvasive means of evaluating the newborn's cranium
13. Tape the patient's auricle forward to prevent it from superimposing the mastoids.
14. Rotation of the head
15. A dolichocephalic skull requires more rotation of the skull as compared with an average-shaped skull (mesocephalic). The 45° rotation for the Stenvers needs to be increased to at least 50° for the dolichocephalic skull.

16. AP axial (Towne) and anterior profile oblique (Arcelin) projections could be performed without turning the patient from the supine position.
17. Either MRI or CT can be performed.

## Review Exercise F: Critique Radiographs of the Cranium

A. Lateral skull: 4-year-old (Fig. C12-83)
   1. Foreign bodies (earrings) obscuring essential anatomic structures
   2. Correct part positioning, but patient's hand seen supporting mandible; can use positioning sponge if needed to support skull
   3. No evidence of collimation; correct central ray and IR placement
   4. Appears underexposed on this printed copy (may be a repeatable error if actual radiograph also appears this light)
   5. No evidence of anatomic side marker
   Repeatable errors: 1 and possibly 4
B. Lateral skull: 54-year-old, post-traumatic injury (Fig. C12-84)
   1. Vertex of the skull just slightly cut off (may be repeatable error because of proximity to the site of trauma)
   2. Tilted and rotated skull (separation of the orbital plates from the tilt; separation of the greater wings of the sphenoid, the rami of the mandible, and the EAMs—all indicating rotation)
   3. No evidence of collimation; slightly high central ray centering if the photo borders are also the collimation borders, which would add to the tilt appearance
   4. Acceptable exposure factors
   5. No evidence of anatomic side marker
   Repeatable errors: 1 and 2
C. AP axial: Towne skull (C12-85)
   1. Entire occipital bone and foramen magnum demonstrated
   2. Correct part positioning
   3. No evidence of collimation; overangled central ray; anterior arch of C1 projected into the foramen magnum rather than the dorsum sellae
   4. Acceptable but slightly underexposed exposure factors
   5. No evidence of anatomic side marker
   Repeatable errors: 3

D. AP or PA skull (Fig. C12-86)
AP projection, as indicated by the large size of the orbits, which was caused by magnification from increased OID (can compare with radiograph that follows)
  1. All pertinent anatomic structures demonstrated but with some foreshortening of frontal bone
  2. Petrous ridges not in the lower third of orbits; position requires more flexion or less central ray angle as an AP; skull slightly rotated (note distance between orbits and lateral margins of skull)
  3. No evidence of collimation; less central ray angle needed (see previous answer; can also compare with correctly angled central ray on PA radiograph in Fig. C12-87)
  4. Acceptable exposure factors
  5. No evidence of anatomic side marker

Repeatable errors: 2 and 3

E. AP or PA skull (Fig. C12-87)
PA 15° Caldwell projection
  1. All pertinent anatomic structures not demonstrated; patient ID marker and side marker obscuring skull
  2. Correct part positioning
  3. Evidence of collimation (circular cone); size of cassette too small for the skull; correct central ray placement and angle (petrous ridges in lower third of orbit)
  4. Acceptable exposure factors
  5. Evidence of anatomic side marker, but placed over skull; patient ID marker over upper right cranium—both repeatable errors

Repeatable errors: 1 and 5

**12**

# SELF-TEST

My Score = _____ %

This self-test should be taken only after completing all of the readings, review exercises, and laboratory activities for a particular section. The purpose of this test is not only to provide a good learning exercise but also to serve as a strong indicator of what your final unit evaluation exam will cover. It is strongly suggested that if you do not get at least a 90% to 95% grade on each self-test, you review those areas in which you missed questions before going to your instructor for the final unit evaluation exam. (There are 125 questions or blanks—each is worth 0.8 point.)

1. Which one of the following bones is not part of the floor of the cranium?

    A. Temporal     B. Ethmoid     C. Occipital     D. Sphenoid

2. Which aspect of the frontal bone is thin-walled and forms the forehead?

    A. Orbital          B. Horizontal     C. Squamous     D. Superciliary margin

3. Which four cranial bones articulate with the frontal bone?

    A. _____     C. _____

    B. _____     D. _____

4. Which structures are found at the widest aspect of the skull? _____

5. What is the name of a prominent landmark (or "bump") found on the external surface of the occipital bone?

    _____

6. List the number of individual bones that articulate with the following cranial bones:

    A. Parietal bone: _____

    B. Occipital bone: _____

    C. Temporal bone: _____

    D. Sphenoid: _____

    E. Ethmoid: _____

7. What is the thickest and densest structure in the cranium? _____

8. True/False: The hypophysis is another term for the pituitary gland.

9. True/False: The sphenoid bone articulates with all the other cranial bones.

10. The shallow depression just posterior to the base of the dorsum sellae and anterior to the foramen magnum is the

    _____ .

11. What is the name of the paired collections of bone found inferior to the cribriform plate that contain numerous air

    cells and help form the lateral walls of the nasal cavity? _____

12. Which small section of bone is located superior to the cribriform plate? _____

13.   What is the formal term for the left sphenoid fontanel in the adult? _____

14.   What is the name of the cranial suture formed by the inferior junction of the parietals to the temporal bones?

_____

15.   What are the two terms for the small, irregular bones found in the adult skull sutures?

_____

16.   Match each of the following structures to its related cranial bone:

_____   1.   Pterygoid hamulus          A.   Occipital

_____   2.   Anterior clinoid processes   B.   Frontal

_____   3.   Glabella                   C.   Sphenoid

_____   4.   Foramen ovale              D.   Ethmoid

_____   5.   Perpendicular plate         E.   Temporal

_____   6.   Superior nasal conchae      F.   Parietal

_____   7.   Foramen magnum

_____   8.   Cribriform plate

_____   9.   Zygomatic process

_____   10.  Lateral condylar portions

_____   11.  Superciliary arch

_____   12.  EAM

_____   13.  Inion

_____   14.  Sella turcica

_____   15.  Petrous ridge

17.   Identify the cranial structures, sutures, and regions labeled on the following radiographs (Figs. 12-18 and 12-19):

*Fig. 12-18*

   *STRUCTURE*                  *BONE(S)*

   A.   _____

   B.   _____

   C.   _____

   D.   _____ (suture)

   E.   _____

   F.   _____

**Fig. 12-18.** PA Caldwell cranium.

*Fig. 12-19*

G. _____

H. _____

I. _____

J. _____

K. _____

L. _____

M. _____

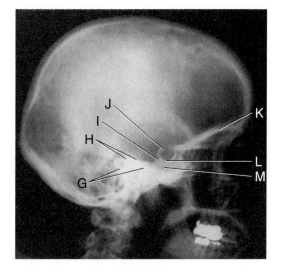

**Fig. 12-19.** Lateral cranium.

18. Which one of the following skull classifications applies to a skull with an angle of 54° between the midsagittal plane and the long axis of the pars petrosa?

    A. Mesocephalic          C. Brachycephalic

    B. Dolichocephalic       D. None of the above

19. Which of the above classifications is considered the average-shape skull? _____

20. Identify the labeled landmarks and positioning lines used in skull and facial bone positioning, as shown in Fig. 12-20 (including abbreviations):

    A. _____

    B. _____

    C. _____

    D. _____

    E. _____

    F. _____

    G. _____

    H. _____

    I. _____

    J. _____

    K. _____

    L. _____

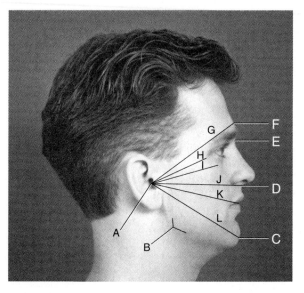

**Fig. 12-20.** Skull and facial bone landmarks and positioning lines.

21. The center point of structure *A* as used for the positioning lines in the previous question is called the

    _____ .

22.  Which one of the following terms is defined as the large cartilaginous aspect of the external ear?

A.  Pinna          C.  Glabella

B.  Tragus         D.  Acanthion

23.  Reid's base line is more commonly referred to as:

A.  GML            C.  OML

B.  IOML           D.  GAL

24.  How much of a difference in degrees is there between the OML and IOML?

A.  10°            C.  3°

B.  7° to 8°       D.  None (they represent the same positioning line)

25.  Which one of the following positioning errors frequently results in a repeat exposure of a cranial position?

A.  Rotation                       C.  Slight flexion

B.  Incorrect central ray placement    D.  None of the above

26.  Match each of the following pathologic indications to the correct definition or description (using each choice only once):

_____  A.  Bone tumor originating in the bone marrow                         1.  Linear fracture

_____  B.  Fracture evident by sphenoid sinus effusion                       2.  Paget's disease

_____  C.  Condition that begins with bony destruction followed by bony repair   3.  Depressed fracture

_____  D.  Destructive lesion with irregular margins                         4.  Osteolytic neoplasm

_____  E.  Fracture of the skull with jagged or irregular lucent line        5.  Multiple myeloma

_____  F.  Tangential view may be helpful to determine extent or degree of this   6.  Basal fracture
            fracture

27.  Which one of the following pathologic indications may require a decrease in manual exposure factors?

A.  Pituitary adenoma          C.  Paget's disease

B.  Linear skull fracture      D.  Multiple myeloma

28.  Which one of the following imaging modalities may be used to examine a possible cranial bleed caused by trauma?

A.  CT          C.  Ultrasound

B.  MRI         D.  Nuclear medicine

29.  Which one of the following imaging modalities provides an excellent distinction between normal and abnormal brain tissue?

A.  CT          C.  Ultrasound

B.  MRI         D.  Nuclear medicine

30.  Which aspect of the temporal bone is considered to be thinnest? _____

31.  Which aspect of the temporal bone contains the organs of hearing and balance?

_____

32. The correct term for the eardrum is the

_____ .

33. Which one of the following middle ear structures is considered to be most lateral?

    A.  Malleus      C.  Stapes

    B.  Incus        D.  Oval window

34. Which structure helps equalize atmospheric pressure in the middle ear?

_____

35. What passes through the internal acoustic meatus?

_____

36. The aditus is an opening between the _____ and the _____ portion of the temporal bone.

37. An infection of the mastoid air cells, if untreated, can lead to a serious infection of the brain called

_____ .

38. Which auditory ossicle attaches to the oval window?

    A.  Malleus      C.  Stapes

    B.  Incus        D.  None

39. The internal ear is divided into the osseous or bony labyrinth and the _____ labyrinth.

40. List the three divisions of the bony labyrinth of the inner ear:

    A. _____    B. _____    C. _____

41. Identify the structures labeled on Fig. 12-21:

    A. _____

    B. _____

    C. _____

    D. _____

    E. _____

    F. _____

    G. _____

    H. _____

    I. _____

**Fig. 12-21.** Three divisions of the ear.

42. A benign, cystlike mass of the middle ear is a(n):

    A.  Acoustic neuroma      C.  Cholesteatoma

    B.  Osteomyelitis         D.  Acoustic sarcoma

43.  True/False: Otosclerosis is a hereditary disease.

44.  Which two projections of the cranium project the dorsum sellae within the foramen magnum?

A.  _____

B.  _____

45.  A.  What central ray angle is used for the AP axial projection (Towne method) with the IOML perpendicular to the

image receptor?  _____

B.  What is the central ray angle for this same projection with a perpendicular OML?  _____

46.  Where is the central ray centered for a lateral projection of the cranium?  _____

47.  To prevent tilting of the skull for the lateral projection of the cranium, the  _____ line is placed perpendicular to the image receptor.

48.  Where should the petrous ridges be located (on the image) for a well-positioned, 25° caudad PA axial (Haas

method) projection?  _____

49.  Where is the central ray centered for an SMV projection of the skull?

_____

50.  A.  How much is the central ray angled to the IOML for an AP axial projection of the sella turcica when the

posterior clinoid processes are of primary interest?  _____

B.  How much is the central ray angled to the IOML when the anterior clinoid processes are of primary interest?

_____

51.  A radiograph of an AP axial projection for the cranium reveals that the dorsum sellae is projected just above rather than into the foramen magnum. What must be modified during the repeat exposure to correct this problem?

_____

52.  A radiograph of a lateral projection of the cranium reveals that the mandibular rami are *not* superimposed. What type of positioning error is present on this radiograph?

_____

53.  A radiograph of a 15° caudad PA axial projection of the cranium reveals that the petrous ridges are at the level of the supraorbital margin. Without changing the central ray angle, how must the head position be modified during the repeat exposure to produce a more acceptable image?

_____

_____

54.  **Situation:** A patient with a possible basilar skull fracture enters the emergency room. The physician wants a projection to demonstrate a possible sphenoid sinus effusion. Which projection of the cranium would be best for this situation?

_____

**12**

55. **Situation:** The same patient in the previous situation also requires a frontal projection of the skull. The physician wants the projection to demonstrate the frontal bone and place the petrous ridges in the lower one-third of the orbits, but it has not been determined whether the patient's cervical spine has been fractured, so the patient cannot be moved from a supine position. What should the technologist do to obtain this image?

_____

_____

56. **Situation:** A patient comes to the radiology department for a skull series. Because of the size of the patient's shoulders, he is unable to flex his neck sufficiently to place the OML perpendicular to the IR for the AP axial projection. His head cannot be raised because of possible cervical trauma. What other options does the technologist have to obtain an acceptable AP axial projection?

_____

_____

57. A radiograph of an axiolateral (Schuller) projection of the mastoid air cells reveals that the opposite, or upside, mastoid is projected on the mastoid of interest. What specific positioning error may have led to this radiographic outcome?

_____

58. A radiograph of an AP axial (Towne) projection for mastoids reveals that the dorsum sellae is projected above the foramen magnum. Also, the petrous pyramids appear foreshortened. What modification is needed to correct these errors present on the initial radiograph?

_____

59. **Situation:** A patient comes to the radiology department for a mastoid series. The positioning routine includes a posterior profile (Stenvers) projection. Classification of the skull reveals that the patient has a brachycephalic skull. What specific degree of rotation is needed for the posterior profile projection for this patient?

_____

60. For the following critique questions, refer to the radiograph of the lateral skull shown in Fig. C12-84 (p. 399 in your textbook).

    A.  Which positioning error(s) is(are) visible on this radiograph? (More than one answer may be selected.)

        (a)  All essential anatomic structures are not demonstrated.

        (b)  Central ray is centered incorrectly.

        (c)  Collimation is not evident.

        (d)  Exposure factors are incorrect.

        (e)  No anatomic marker is visible on the radiograph.

        (f)  Tilt of skull is evident.

        (g)  Rotation of skull is evident.

        (h)  Excessive flexion and extension are evident.

    B.  Which error(s) identified above is(are) considered "repeatable"? _____

C.  Which of the following modifications must be made during the repeat exposure? (More than one answer may be selected.)

    (a)  Increase collimation.

    (b)  Center central ray correctly.

    (c)  Decrease exposure factors.

    (d)  Increase exposure factors.

    (e)  Place anatomic marker on image receptor before exposure.

    (f)  Adjust skull to place midsagittal plane parallel to plane of image receptor to eliminate rotation and tilt.

    (g)  Adjust skull to eliminate excessive flexion and extension.

61.  For the following critique questions, refer to the radiograph of the AP skull position shown in Fig. C12-86 on p. 399 in your textbook.

A.  Which positioning error(s) is(are) visible on this radiograph? (More than one answer may be selected.)

    (a)  All essential anatomic structures are not demonstrated.

    (b)  Central ray is centered incorrectly.

    (c)  Collimation is not evident.

    (d)  Exposure factors are incorrect.

    (e)  No anatomic marker is visible on the radiograph.

    (f)  Central ray is angled insufficiently.

    (g)  No anatomic marker is visible on the radiograph.

    (h)  Tilt of skull is evident.

    (i)  Rotation of skull is evident.

B.  Which error(s) identified above is(are) considered "repeatable"? (NOTE: Petrous ridges should be in the lower third of the orbits.)  _____

C.  Which of the following modifications must be made during the repeat exposure? (More than one answer may be selected.)

    (a)  Increase collimation.

    (b)  Center central ray correctly.

    (c)  Decrease exposure factors.

    (d)  Increase exposure factors.

    (e)  Place anatomic marker on image receptor before exposure.

    (f)  Align midsagittal plane perpendicular to the image receptor to eliminate rotation and tilt.

    (g)  Decrease central ray angle or increase flexion.

    (h)  Increase central ray angle or increase extension.

## CHAPTER 13

# Facial Bones and Paranasal Sinuses

After you have successfully completed the activities in this chapter, you will be able to:

_____ 1. List the specific features, characteristics, location, and functions of the fourteen facial bones.

_____ 2. List the seven cranial and facial bones that make up the bony orbit.

_____ 3. Using drawings and/or radiographs, identify specific structures of the facial bone region.

_____ 4. Explain the advantages of performing facial bone projections erect.

_____ 5. Identify alternative imaging modalities that best demonstrate specific facial bone and paranasal sinus pathology.

_____ 6. Identify specific types of fractures of the facial bone region.

_____ 7. List the location, function, and characteristics of the four groups of paranasal sinuses.

_____ 8. Using drawings and radiographs, identify specific paranasal sinuses.

_____ 9. Match specific pathologic indications of the paranasal sinuses to the correct definition.

_____ 10. Identify basic and special projections of the facial bones and list the correct size of image receptor, as well as the location, direction, and angulation of the central ray for each projection.

_____ 11. List which structures are best seen with basic and special projections of the facial bones.

_____ 12. Identify the basic operational and positioning considerations when performing a mandible study using the Panorex unit.

_____ 13. Identify basic and special projections of the paranasal sinuses and list the correct size and type of image receptor, as well as the location, direction, and angulation of the central ray for each position.

_____ 14. List patient dose ranges for skin, midline, and thyroid doses for specific projections of the facial bones and paranasal sinuses.

_____ 15. Given various hypothetical situations, identify the correct modification of a position and/or exposure factors to improve the radiographic image.

_____ 16. Given radiographs of specific facial and paranasal sinus projections/positions, identify specific errors in positioning and exposure factors.

## Positioning and Radiographic Critique

_____ 1. Using a peer, position for basic and special projections of the facial bones and sinuses.

_____ 2. Using a cranial radiographic phantom, produce satisfactory radiographs of specific positions (if equipment is available).

_____ 3. Critique and evaluate facial bone radiographs based on the four divisions of radiographic criteria: (1) structures shown, (2) position, (3) collimation and central ray, and (4) exposure criteria.

_____ 4. Distinguish between acceptable and unacceptable cranial radiographs resulting from exposure factors, motion, collimation, positioning, or other errors.

## Learning Exercises

The following review exercises should be completed only after careful study of the associated pages in the textbook as indicated by each exercise. Answers to each review exercise are given at the end of the review exercises.

## Part I: Radiographic Anatomy

**REVIEW EXERCISE A:** Radiographic Anatomy of the Facial Bones (see textbook pp. 402-407)     _1-25_

1.   Which of the following bones is not a facial bone?

   (A)   Middle nasal conchae          C.   Lacrimal bone

   B.   Vomer                    D.   Mandible

2.   What is the largest immovable bone of the face? _maxillary_

3.   List the four processes of the maxilla:

   A.   _Frontal_              C.   _Alveolar_

   B.   _Zygomatic_            D.   _Palatine_

4.   Which one of the above-mentioned processes is considered most superior? _Frontal_

5.   Which soft tissue landmark is found at the base of the anterior nasal spine? _acanthion_

6.   Which facial bones form the posterior aspect of the hard palate? _Palatine_

7.   Which two cranial bones articulate with the maxilla? _frontal & ethmoid_

8.   Which facial bones are sometimes called the "cheek bones"? _zygoma_

9.   Which of the following bones does not articulate with the zygomatic bone?

   A.   Temporal      C.   Frontal

   B.   Maxilla      (D)   Sphenoid

10.   Which facial bone is associated with the tear ducts? _lacrimal_

11.   The purpose of the _nasal conchae_, or _turbinates_, is to divide the nasal cavity into compartments and circulate air coming into the nasal cavities. (Include both terms for these bones.)

12.   True/False: The majority of the nose is formed by the right and left nasal bones.

13.   A deviated nasal septum is most likely to occur at the junction between _Septal cartilage_

   and _Vomer_ .

14.    Match each of the following mandibular terms to the correct definition or description (using each choice only once):

___3___    A.   Gonion                    1.   Vertical portion of mandible

___8___    B.   Mandibular notch          2.   The chin

___6___    C.   Body                      3.   Mandibular angle

___7___    D.   Condyloid process        4.   The point of union between both halves of the mandible

___5___    E.   Coronoid process         5.   Bony process located anterior to mandibular notch

___1___    F.   Ramus                    6.   Horizontal portion of mandible

___2___    G.   Mentum                   7.   Posterior process of upper ramus

___4___    H.   Symphysis menti          8.   U-shaped notch

15.    Identify the labeled facial bones visible on Figs. 13-1 and 13-2:

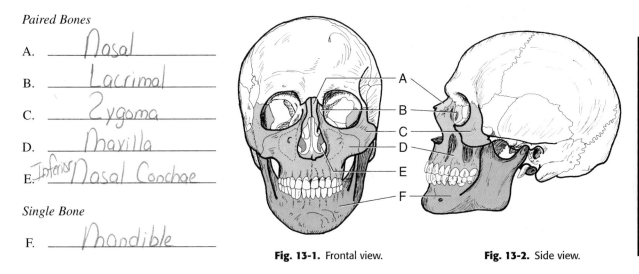

*Paired Bones*

A.   _Nasal_

B.   _Lacrimal_

C.   _Zygoma_

D.   _Maxilla_

E.   Inferior _Nasal Conchae_

*Single Bone*

F.   _Mandible_

**Fig. 13-1.** Frontal view.          **Fig. 13-2.** Side view.

16.    The one single facial bone and the one pair of facial bones not visible from the exterior and not demonstrated on the above drawings are the _____Vomer_____ and _Palatine bones_ , respectively. (These are demonstrated on special view drawings in the following questions.)

17.    Identify the labeled structures (and the facial bones of which they are a part) on this inferior surface view of the maxillae (Fig. 13-3):

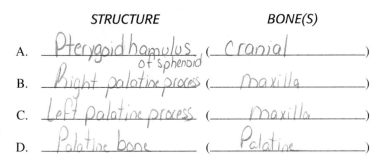

| STRUCTURE | BONE(S) |
|---|---|
| A.   _Pterygoid hamulus of sphenoid_ | ( _Cranial_ ) |
| B.   _Right palatine process_ | ( _maxilla_ ) |
| C.   _Left palatine process_ | ( _maxilla_ ) |
| D.   _Palatine bone_ | ( _Palatine_ ) |

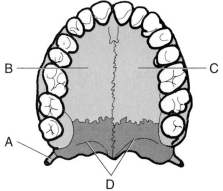

**Fig. 13-3.** Inferior surface view of the maxillae.

18.   List the three structures that form the nasal septum as shown on Fig. 13-4:

A.   _Perpendicular plate of ethmoid_

B.   _Vomer_

C.   _Septal Cartilage_

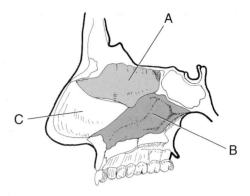

**Fig. 13-4.** Nasal septum.

19.   Identify the parts of the mandible and skull as labeled on Figs. 13-5 and 13-6:

A.   _Condyle_

B.   _Neck_

C.   _Ramus_

D.   _Gonion (Angle)_

E.   _Body_

F.   _Mental foramen_

G.   _Mentum_

H.   _Alveolar process_

I.   _Coronoid process_

J.   _Mandibular notch_

K.   (Cranial bone)   _Temporal_

L.   (Joint)   _Temporomandibular TMJ_

M.   (Key landmark)   _EAM_

N.   (Landmark)   _Mastoid process_

**Fig. 13-5.** Mandible.

**Fig. 13-6.** Lateral skull and mandible.

13

20.  Identify the seven bones that form the orbit and indicate whether
     they are cranial or facial bones (Fig. 13-7):

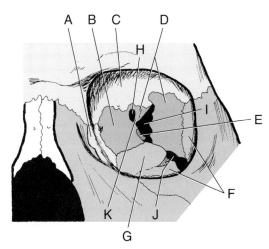

**Fig. 13-7.** Slightly oblique frontal view of orbit, A-K.

|        | *BONE* | *CRANIAL OR FACIAL?* |
|--------|--------|----------------------|
| A.     | Lacrimal | ( facial ) |
| B.     | Ethmoid | ( Cranial ) |
| C.     | Frontal | ( Cranial ) |
| D.     | Sphenoid | ( Cranial ) |
| E.     | Palatine | ( facial ) |
| F.     | Zygomatic | ( facial ) |
| G.     | Maxilla | ( facial ) |

21.  Identify the three foramina found within the orbits as labeled on Fig. 13-7:

H.  ___Optic foramen___

I.  ___Superior orbital fissure___

J.  ___Inferior orbital fissure___

Small section of bone:

K.  ___Sphenoid strut___

22.  From anterior to posterior, the cone-shaped orbits project upward at an angle of __30__ ° and toward the

     midsagittal plane at an angle of __32__ °.

23.  Which facial bone opening has the maxillary branch of the fifth cranial nerve passing through it?

___Inferior orbital fissure___

24.  Which one of the facial bone openings is formed by a cleft between the greater and lesser wings of the sphenoid
     bone?

     (A.)  Superior orbital fissure          C.   Inferior orbital fissure

     B.   Optic foramen                      D.   Optic canal

25.  What is another term for the second cranial nerve?

     A.   Olfactory nerve        C.   Maxillary nerve

     (B.)  Optic nerve            D.   Trigeminal nerve

1-10

**REVIEW EXERCISE B:** Radiographic Anatomy of the Paranasal Sinuses (see textbook pp. 408-410)

1.  What is the older term for the maxillary sinuses?  ___Antrum of Highmore___

2.  An infection of the teeth may travel upward and involve the ___Maxillary___ sinus.

3.  Specifically, where are the frontal sinuses located? ___Between inner and outer tables of the skull; posterior to glabella___

4.  The frontal sinuses rarely become aerated before the age of ___6___.

13

5.  Which specific aspect of the ethmoid bone contains the ethmoid sinuses? _lateral masses or labyrinths_

6.  The drainage pathway for the paranasal sinuses is called the:

    A.  Uncinate process          C.  Paranasal meatus

    B.  Osteomeatal complex       D.  Lateral masses

7.  Which sinus will be projected through the open mouth with a PA axial transoral projection? _sphenoid_

8.  Identify the sinuses, structures, or bones labeled on Fig. 13-8:

    A.  _Nasal cavity (fossae)_

    B.  _Maxillary Sinus_

    C.  _Right temporal bone_

    D.  _Frontal Sinus_

    E.  _Ethmoid Sinus_

    F.  _Sphenoid Sinus_

    G.  _Maxillary Sinus_

    H.  _Ethmoid Sinus_

    I.  _Frontal Sinus_

    J.  _Left temporal bone_

    K.  _Mastoid portion of temporal_

    L.  _Sphenoid Sinus_

    M.  _Alveolar process (roots)_

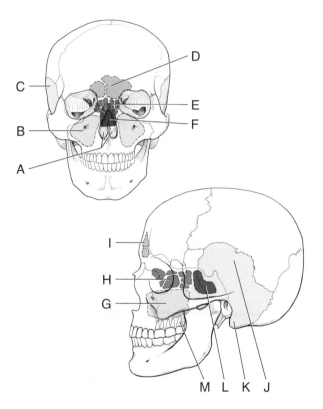

**Fig. 13-8.** Frontal and lateral views.

9.  Identify the following paranasal sinuses labeled on Figs. 13-9 and 13-10:

    *Fig. 13-9*

    A.  _Sphenoid_

    B.  _Maxillary_

    C.  _Ethmoid_

    D.  _Frontal_

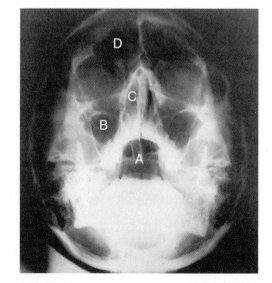

**Fig. 13-9.** Paranasal sinuses. PA axial transoral projection.

*Fig. 13-10*

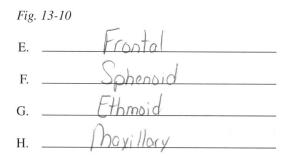

E. _____Frontal_____

F. _____Sphenoid_____

G. _____Ethmoid_____

H. _____Maxillary_____

**Fig. 13-10.** Paranasal sinuses. Lateral projection.

10. What is the name of the passageway between the maxillary sinuses and the middle nasal meatus?

_____Infundibulum_____

## Part II: Radiographic Positioning

**REVIEW EXERCISE C:** Positioning of the Facial Bones, Nasal Bones, Zygomatic Arches, and Optic Foramina and Orbits (see textbook pp. 415-442)

1. True/False: Facial bone studies should always be performed recumbent whenever possible.

2. True/False: The common basic PA axial projection for facial bones requires a 15° caudad angle of the central ray, which projects the dense petrous ridges into the lower one-third of the orbits.

3. True/False: An increase in mAs of 25% to 30% (using manual techniques) is often required for the geriatric patient with advanced osteoporosis.

4. True/False: CT is useful for facial bone studies because it allows for visualization of bony structures as well as related soft tissues of the facial bones.

5. True/False: Nuclear medicine is not helpful in diagnosing occult facial bone fractures.

6. True/False: MRI is an excellent imaging modality for the detection of small metal foreign bodies in the eye.

7. What is the name of the fracture that results from a direct blow to the orbit leading to a disruption of the inferior

   orbital margin? _____

8. A "free-floating" zygomatic bone is the frequent result of a _____ fracture.

9. What is the major disadvantage of performing a straight PA projection for facial bones, with no CR angulation or neck extension, as compared with other PA facial bone projections?

   _____

10. Where is the CR centered for a lateral position for facial bones?

   A. Outer canthus        C. Zygoma

   B. Acanthion            D. Nasion

**13**

11. What is the proper method name for the parietoacanthial projection of the facial bones? _____

12. Which facial bone structures are best seen with a parietoacanthial projection?

_____

13. What CR angle must be used to project the petrous ridges just below the orbital floor with the PA axial (Caldwell method) projection?

   A.  None. CR is perpendicular.         C.  20°

   B.  30°                                 D.  45°

14. Which structures specifically are visualized better on the modified parietoacanthial (Waters) projection as compared

   with the basic Waters projection? _____

15. Give two reasons why projections of the facial bones are performed PA rather than AP when possible:

   A.  _____         B.  _____

16. What are two positioning differences between the lateral projection of the cranium and the lateral projection for the facial bones?

   A.  _____

   B.  _____

17. The parietoacanthial (Waters) projection for the facial bones will have the _____ line

   perpendicular to the image receptor, which places the orbitomeatal line (OML) at a _____° angle to the tabletop and image receptor.

18. Where does the CR exit for a parietoacanthial (Waters) projection of the facial bones?

_____

19. Where does the CR exit for a 15° PA axial (Caldwell) projection for facial bones?

_____

20. The modified parietoacanthial (modified Waters) projection requires that the _____ line is

   perpendicular to the image receptor, which places the OML at a _____° angle to the tabletop and image receptor.

21. True/False: Lateral projections for nasal bones generally are taken bilaterally for comparison.

22. True/False: The tangential projection for a unilateral zygomatic arch requires that the skull be rotated and tilted 15° **away from** the affected side.

23. True/False: Both oblique inferosuperior (tangential) projections for the zygomatic arch are generally taken for comparison.

24. True/False: The gonadal and/or thyroid dose for all facial bone projections is NDC (no discernible contribution).

25. For a PA Waters projection, the petrous ridges should be projected directly below the _____

   and projected into the lower half of the maxillary sinuses or below the _____ for a modified Waters projection.

26.   For the superoinferior projection of the nasal bones, the image receptor is placed perpendicular to the

      _____ line. (Include the full name and abbreviation.)

27.   Which specific facial bone structures (other than the mandible) are best demonstrated with the submentovertex

      (SMV) projection if the correct exposure factors are used (soft tissue technique)? _____

28.   Where is the CR centered for an AP axial projection for the zygomatic arches?

      _____

29.   List the proper method name and the common descriptive name for the parieto-orbital projection for the optic
      foramen.

      A.   _____          B.   _____

30.   The three aspects of the face that should be in contact with the head unit or tabletop when beginning positioning for

      the parieto-orbital projection are the (A)  _____ , _____ , and

      _____ . The final angle between the midsagittal plane and the IR should be (B)

      _____ , with the (C) _____ line perpendicular to the IR. This

      places the optic foramen in the (D) _____ quadrant of the orbit.

31.   Match each of the following structures to the facial bone projection that **best** demonstrates the structure(s) (using
      each choice only once):

      _E_   1.   Floor of orbits (blowout fractures)              A.   Lateral (nasal bones)

      _C_   2.   Optic foramen                                    B.   Parietoacanthial projection

      _F_   3.   View of single zygomatic arch                    C.   Parieto-orbital projection

      _A_   4.   Profile image of nasal bones and nasal septum    D.   Submentovertex (SMV) projection

      _D_   5.   Bilateral zygomatic arches                       E.   Modified Waters method

      _B_   6.   Inferior orbital rim, maxillae, nasal septum,    F.   Oblique inferosuperior projection
                 nasal spine, zygomatic bone and arches

**REVIEW EXERCISE D:** Positioning of the Mandible and Temporomandibular Joints (TMJ) (see textbook pp.
429-437)

1.   Which projection for the mandible results in a thyroid dose that is four or five times greater than the thyroid dose

     for any other projection described in this chapter? _____SMV_____

2.   Which projection of the mandible will project the opposite half of the mandible away from the side of interest?

     _____Axiolateral_____

3.   What must be done to prevent the ramus of the mandible from being superimposed over the cervical spine with an

     axiolateral projection of the mandible? _____extend the neck_____

13

4. How much skull rotation toward the image receptor is required with an axiolateral projection for demonstrating each of the following?

   A. Body of the mandible: _____ 30° _____

   B. Mentum region: _____ 45° _____

   C. Ramus region: _____ true lateral _____

   D. General survey of the mandible: _____ 10°-15° _____

   E. What CR angle is needed for all of these projections? _____ 25° Cephalad _____

5. What specific positioning error has been committed if both sides of the mandible are superimposed with an axiolateral projection?

   _____ Insufficient CR angle _____

6. Where should the CR exit for a **PA axial** projection of the mandible? _____ Acanthion _____

7. Which skull positioning line is placed perpendicular to the image receptor for a PA or PA axial projection of the mandible?

   _____ OML _____

8. True/False: For a true frontal view of the mandibular body (if this is the area of interest), the AML should be perpendicular to the image receptor.

9. True/False: The CR should be angled 20° to 25° cephalad ~~caudad~~ for the PA axial projection of the mandible.

10. Which aspect of the mandible is best visualized with an AP axial projection? Condyloid processes

11. A. What CR angle is required for the AP axial projection of the mandible if the OML is placed perpendicular to the image receptor? 35-40° Caudad

    B. If the infraorbitomeatal line (IOML) is perpendicular, what CR angle is needed? _____ 42-47° Caudad

12. Where is the CR centered, and where will it pass through, for an AP axial projection of the mandible?

    Glabella, midway between EAM's and angles of mandible

13. Which projection of the mandible will demonstrate the entire mandible, including the coronoid and condyloid processes?

    _____ SMV _____

14. Which imaging system provides a single, frontal perspective of the entire mandible? _____ Panorex _____

15. What device provides inherent collimation during a Panorex procedure? Vertical slit diaphragm

16. Which cranial line is placed parallel to the floor for a Panorex of the mandible? _____ IOML _____

17. What type of image receptor must be used with Panorex? 9x12 Curved nongrid

18. True/False: The modified Law method provides a bilateral and functional study of the TMJ.

19. True/False: The mandibular condyles move anteriorly as the mouth is opened.

20.    Which projection of the TMJ requires that the skull be kept in a true lateral position?

    A.  Modified Law    C.  Axiolateral oblique projection

    B.  Schuller    D.  Modified Towne

21.    The axiolateral (Schuller method) projection for the TMJ requires a CR angle of _____25-30_____ °

    ____Caudad____ (**caudad** or **cephalad**).

22.    The axiolateral oblique projection of the TMJ is commonly referred to as the (A) _Law_ *Modified* method, which requires a

    (B) _15_ ° head rotation from lateral and a (C) _15_ ° caudad CR angle.

23.    Which projection best visualizes the condyloid processes and the temporomandibular fossae?

    ____AP Axial Modified Towne w/ 40° caudad angle____

24.    Aligning the ____midsagittal____ plane perpendicular to the IR will prevent rotation of either a PA or
    AP axial mandible.

## REVIEW EXERCISE E: Positioning of the Paranasal Sinuses (see textbook pp. 438-442)

1.    What kV range should be used for sinus radiography? _____

2.    To demonstrate any possible air or fluid levels within the sinuses, it is important to:

    A.  _____

    B.  _____

3.    True/False: Ultrasound exams of the maxillary sinuses to rule out sinusitis are possible.

4.    True/False: Magnetic resonance imaging is the preferred modality to study soft tissue changes and masses within
    the sinuses.

5.    True/False: Secondary osteomyelitis is often due to tumor invasion.

6.    List the four most commonly performed basic or routine projections for paranasal sinuses:

    A.  _____    C.  _____

    B.  _____    D.  _____

7.    Which single projection for a paranasal sinus routine provides an image of all four sinus groups? _____

8.    If the patient cannot stand for the lateral projection of the paranasal sinuses, it should be taken:

    _____

9.    Which paranasal sinuses are best demonstrated with a PA (Caldwell) projection? _____

10.    To avoid angling the CR for the erect PA Caldwell sinus projection, the head should be adjusted so that the OML is

    _____° from horizontal.

**13**

11.  A.   Which group of paranasal sinuses is best demonstrated with a parietoacanthial (Water) projection?

     _____

     B.   The OML forms a _____° angle with the image receptor with this projection.

12.  Which positioning line is placed perpendicular to the image receptor for a parietoacanthial projection?

     _____

13.  Where are the petrous ridges located on a well-positioned parietoacanthial projection?

     _____

14.  Which paranasal sinuses are demonstrated with an SMV projection of the paranasal sinuses?

     _____

15.  Where should the CR exit for both the PA parietoacanthial (Waters) and the PA transoral (open-mouth Waters)

     projection? _____

16.  What is the one major difference in positioning between the parietoacanthial and PA axial transoral projections?

     _____

17.  Which sinuses are projected thorough the oral cavity with the PA axial transoral projection? _____

18.  Match each of the following sinus projections with the anatomy best seen (using each choice only once):

     _____  1.  Lateral                    A.  Sphenoid sinus in oral cavity

     _____  2.  Parietoacanthial            B.  Inferosuperior view of sphenoid and ethmoid sinus

     _____  3.  PA Caldwell                 C.  All four paranasal sinuses demonstrated

     _____  4.  PA transoral                D.  Best view of maxillary sinuses

     _____  5.  SMV for sinuses             E.  Best view of frontal and ethmoid sinuses

**REVIEW EXERCISE F: Problem Solving for Technical and Positioning Errors (see textbook pp. 419-442)**

1.  A radiograph of a lateral projection of the facial bones reveals that the mandibular rami are not superimposed. What positioning error led to this radiographic outcome?

    _____

2.  A radiograph of a parietoacanthial (Waters) projection reveals that the petrous ridges are projected within the maxillary sinuses. Is this an acceptable image? If not, what must be done to improve the image during the repeat exposure?

    _____

3.  A radiograph of a parietoacanthial (Waters) projection reveals that the distance between the lateral margins of the orbits and the lateral aspect of the skull is not equal. What type of positioning error led to this radiographic outcome?

    _____

4.   A radiograph of a 30° PA axial projection of the facial bones reveals that the petrous ridges are projected at the level of the inferior orbital margins. Is this an acceptable image for this projection? If not, what must be done to improve the quality of the image during the repeat exposure?

_____

5.   A radiograph of a superoinferior projection of the nasal bones reveals that the glabella is superimposed over the nasal bones. What positioning error led to this radiographic outcome, and how can it be corrected during the repeat exposure?

_____ excessive flexion _____

_____ GAL Perp to IR _____

6.   A lateral radiograph of the facial bones demonstrates that the gonions (angles) of the mandible are not superimposed; one is about 1 cm superior to the other. How would this be corrected on a repeat exposure?

_____

7.   A radiograph of a parieto-orbital (Rhese) projection reveals that the optic foramen is located in the upper outer quadrant of the orbit. Is this an acceptable image for this projection? If not, what must be done to correct this problem during the repeat exposure?

_____

_____

8.   A radiograph of an axiolateral projection of the mandible reveals that the body of the mandible is severely foreshortened. The body of the mandible is the area of interest. What positioning error led to this radiographic outcome?

_____ Insufficient rotation of the head toward the IR. _____

_____

9.   **Situation:** A patient with a possible fracture of the nasal bones enters the emergency room. The physician is concerned about deviation of the bony nasal septum along with possible nasal bones fracture. What radiographic routine would be best for this situation?

_____ PA Waters and Bil laterals _____

_____

_____

10.  **Situation:** A patient with a possible blowout fracture of the right orbit enters the emergency room. In addition to the basic facial bone routine, what single projection would best demonstrate this type of injury?

_____

11.  **Situation:** A patient with a possible fracture of the left zygomatic arch enters the emergency room. Neither the AP axial nor the SMV projection demonstrates the left side well. The radiologist is indecisive as to whether this zygomatic arch is fractured. What other projections can the technologist provide to better define this area?

_____

**13**

12. **Situation:** As part of a study of the zygomatic arches, the technologist attempts to perform the SMV position. Because of the size of the patient's shoulders, he is unable to flex the neck adequately to place the IOML parallel to the image receptor. What other options does the technologist have to produce an acceptable SMV projection?

_____

13. A radiograph of a PA (Caldwell) projection for sinuses reveals that the petrous ridges are projected into the lower half of the orbits and obscuring the ethmoid sinuses. The technologist used a horizontal x-ray beam for the projection. The skull was positioned to place the OML at a 15° angle from the horizontal plane. What positioning modification is needed to correct this problem during the repeat exposure?

_____

14. A radiograph of a parietoacanthial projection reveals that the distance between the midsagittal plane and the outer orbital margin is not equal. What positioning error is present on this radiograph?

_____

15. A radiograph of an SMV projection for sinuses reveals that the distance between the mandibular condyles and lateral border of the skull is not equal. What specific positioning error is present on this radiograph?

_____

16. A radiograph of a PA transoral projection reveals that the sphenoid sinus is superimposed over the upper teeth and the nasal cavity. How must the position be modified to avoid this problem during the repeat exposure?

_____

17. A radiograph of a parietoacanthial projection reveals that the petrous ridges are projected just below the maxillary sinuses. What positioning error (if any) is present?

_____

18. **Situation:** A patient with a clinical history of sinusitis comes to the radiology department for a sinus study. The patient is quadriplegic and cannot be placed erect. Which single projection will demonstrate any possible air-fluid levels in the sinuses?

_____

19. **Situation:** A patient comes to the radiology department to rule out a possible polyp within the sphenoid sinus. What routine and/or special projection would provide the best overall assessment of the sinuses for this patient?

_____

20. **Situation:** A patient comes to the radiology department with a clinical history of a deviated bony nasal septum. Which facial bone projections will best demonstrate the degree of deviation? (More than one correct answer is possible.)

_____PA, PA Axial, and parietoocanthial_____

_____

**REVIEW EXERCISE G:** Critique Radiographs of the Facial Bones (see textbook p. 443)

The following questions relate to the radiographs found at the end of Chapter 13 of the textbook. Evaluate these radiographs for the radiographic criteria categories (_1_ through _5_) that follow. Describe the corrections needed to improve the overall image. The major, or "repeatable," error(s) are specific errors that indicate the need for a repeat exposure, regardless of the nature or degree of the other errors.

A. **Parietoacanthial (Waters) projection (Fig. C13-135)**
Description of possible error:

1.  Structures shown: _____

2.  Part positioning: _____

3.  Collimation and central ray: _____

4.  Exposure criteria: _____

5.  Markers: _____

Repeatable error(s): _____

B. **SMV mandible (Fig. C13-136)**
Description of possible error:

1.  Structures shown: _____

2.  Part positioning: _____

3.  Collimation and central ray: _____

4.  Exposure criteria: _____

5.  Markers: _____

Repeatable error(s): _____

C. **Optic foramina, Rhese method (Fig. C13-137)**
Description of possible error:

1.  Structures shown: _____

2.  Part positioning: _____

3.  Collimation and central ray: _____

4.  Exposure criteria: _____

5.  Markers: _____

Repeatable error(s): _____

D. **Optic foramina, Rhese method (Fig. C13-138)**
Description of possible error:

1.  Structures shown: _____

2.  Part positioning: _____

3.  Collimation and central ray: _____

4.  Exposure criteria: _____

5.  Markers: _____

Repeatable error(s): _____

**13**

E. **Lateral facial bones (Fig. C13-139)**
Description of possible error:

1. Structures shown: _____

2. Part positioning: _____

3. Collimation and central ray: _____

4. Exposure criteria: _____

5. Markers: _____

Repeatable error(s): _____

## REVIEW EXERCISE H: Critique Radiographs of the Paranasal Sinuses (see textbook p. 444)

The following questions relate to the radiographs found at the end of Chapter 13 of the textbook. Evaluate these radiographs for positioning accuracy as well as exposure factors, collimation, and correct use of anatomical markers. Describe the corrections needed to improve the overall image. The major, or "repeatable," error(s) imply that these specific errors require a repeat exposure be taken regardless of the nature or degree of the other errors. Answers to each critique are given at the end of the laboratory activities.

A. **Parietoacanthial transoral (open-mouth Waters) (Fig. C13-140)**
Description of possible error:

1. Structures shown: _____

2. Part positioning: _____

3. Collimation and central ray: _____

4. Exposure criteria: _____

5. Markers: _____

Repeatable error(s): _____

B. **Parietoacanthial (Waters) (Fig. C13-141)**
Description of possible error:

1. Structures shown: _____

2. Part positioning: _____

3. Collimation and central ray: _____

4. Exposure criteria: _____

5. Markers: _____

Repeatable error(s): _____

13

**C. Submentovertex (SMV) (Fig. C13-142)**
Description of possible error:

1. Structures shown: _____

2. Part positioning: _____

3. Collimation and central ray: _____

4. Exposure criteria: _____

5. Markers: _____

Repeatable error(s): _____

**D. Submentovertex (SMV) (Fig. C13-143)**
Description of possible error:

1. Structures shown: _____

2. Part positioning: _____

3. Collimation and central ray: _____

4. Exposure criteria: _____

5. Markers: _____

Repeatable error(s): _____

## Part III: Laboratory Exercises (see textbook pp. 419-437)

You must gain experience in positioning each part of the facial bones before performing the following exams on actual patients. You can get experience in positioning and radiographic evaluation of these projections by performing exercises using radiographic phantoms and practicing on other students (although you will not be taking actual exposures).

The following suggested activities assume that your teaching institution has an energized lab and radiographic phantoms. If not, perform Laboratory Exercises B and C, the radiographic evaluation and the physical positioning activities. (Check off each step and projection as you complete it.)

**LABORATORY EXERCISE A:** Energized Laboratory

1. Using the skull radiographic phantom, produce radiographs of the following basic routines:

| *Facial bones* | *Zygomatic arches* | *Temporomandibular joints* |
|---|---|---|
| _____ Parietoacanthial (Waters) | _____ Submentovertex (SMV) | _____ Modified Law |
| _____ Modified Waters | _____ Oblique tangential | _____ Schuller method |
| _____ Lateral | _____ AP axial | _____ AP axial |
| _____ 15° PA axial (Caldwell) | | |

| *Nasal bones* | *Mandible* | *Optic foramina* |
|---|---|---|
| _____ Lateral | _____ Axiolateral | _____ Parieto-orbital (Rhese) |
| _____ Superoinferior (tangential) | _____ PA | |
| _____ SMV | _____ AP axial | |

2. Using the skull radiographic phantom, produce radiographs of the following basic routines:

*Sinuses*

_____ Parietoacanthial (Waters)

_____ Lateral

_____ PA

_____ Submentovertex (SMV)

## LABORATORY EXERCISE B: Radiographic Evaluation

1. Evaluate and critique the radiographs produced during the previous experiments, additional radiographs provided by your instructor, or both. Evaluate each radiograph for the following points:

_____ Evaluate the completeness of the study. (Are all pertinent anatomic structures included on the radiograph?)

_____ Evaluate for positioning or centering errors (e.g., rotation, off centering).

_____ Evaluate for correct exposure factors and possible motion. (Are the density and contrast of the images acceptable?)

_____ Determine whether markers and an acceptable degree of collimation and/or area shielding are visible on the images.

## LABORATORY EXERCISE C: Physical Positioning

On another person, simulate performing all basic and special projections of the facial bones as follows. Include the six steps listed below and described in the textbook. (Check off each step when completed satisfactorily.)

Step 1. Appropriate size and type of image receptor (IR) with correct markers
Step 2. Correct CR placement and centering of part to CR and/or IR
Step 3. Accurate collimation
Step 4. Area shielding of patient where advisable
Step 5. Use of proper immobilizing devices when needed
Step 6. Approximate correct exposure factors, breathing instructions where applicable, and "making" exposure

| PROJECTIONS | STEP 1 | STEP 2 | STEP 3 | STEP 4 | STEP 5 | STEP 6 |
|---|---|---|---|---|---|---|
| ***Facial bones*** | | | | | | |
| • Parietoacanthial (Waters) | ___ | ___ | ___ | ___ | ___ | ___ |
| • Modified parietoacanthial | ___ | ___ | ___ | ___ | ___ | ___ |
| • Lateral facial bones | ___ | ___ | ___ | ___ | ___ | ___ |
| • 15° PA axial (Caldwell) | ___ | ___ | ___ | ___ | ___ | ___ |
| ***Nasal bones*** | | | | | | |
| • Laterals | ___ | ___ | ___ | ___ | ___ | ___ |
| • Superoinferior nasal bones | ___ | ___ | ___ | ___ | ___ | ___ |
| ***Zygomatic arches*** | | | | | | |
| • Submentovertex (SMV) | ___ | ___ | ___ | ___ | ___ | ___ |
| • Oblique tangential | ___ | ___ | ___ | ___ | ___ | ___ |
| • AP axial | ___ | ___ | ___ | ___ | ___ | ___ |
| ***Optic foramina*** | | | | | | |
| • Parieto-orbital (Rhese) | ___ | ___ | ___ | ___ | ___ | ___ |
| ***Mandible*** | | | | | | |
| • PA | ___ | ___ | ___ | ___ | ___ | ___ |
| • AP axial | ___ | ___ | ___ | ___ | ___ | ___ |
| • Axiolateral (general survey) | ___ | ___ | ___ | ___ | ___ | ___ |
| ***Temporomandibular joints*** | | | | | | |
| • Modified Law | ___ | ___ | ___ | ___ | ___ | ___ |
| • Schuller method | ___ | ___ | ___ | ___ | ___ | ___ |
| • AP axial | ___ | ___ | ___ | ___ | ___ | ___ |
| ***Paranasal sinus projections*** | | | | | | |
| • Parietoacanthial (Waters) | ___ | ___ | ___ | ___ | ___ | ___ |
| • Lateral | ___ | ___ | ___ | ___ | ___ | ___ |
| • PA | ___ | ___ | ___ | ___ | ___ | ___ |
| • Submentovertex (SMV) | ___ | ___ | ___ | ___ | ___ | ___ |
| • Parietoacanthial transoral (open-mouth Waters) | ___ | ___ | ___ | ___ | ___ | ___ |

**13**

# Answers to Review Exercises

## Review Exercise A: Radiographic Anatomy of the Facial Bones

1. A. Middle nasal conchae
2. Maxilla
3. A. Frontal process
   B. Zygomatic process
   C. Alveolar process
   D. Palatine process
4. Frontal process
5. Acanthion
6. Horizontal portion of the palatine bones
7. Frontal and ethmoid
8. Zygomatic or malar bones
9. D. Sphenoid
10. Lacrimal bones
11. Conchae, turbinates
12. False (Most of the nose is made up of cartilage.)
13. Septal cartilage, vomer (pushed laterally to one side)
14. A. 3
    B. 8
    C. 6
    D. 7
    E. 5
    F. 1
    G. 2
    H. 4
15. A. Nasal bones
    B. Lacrimal bones
    C. Zygomatic bones
    D. Maxillary bones
    E. Inferior nasal conchae
    F. Mandible
16. Vomer and palatine bones
17. A. Pterygoid hamulus, sphenoid
    B. Right palatine process, left maxilla
    C. Left palatine process, left maxilla
    D. Horizontal portions, right and left palatine bones
18. A. Perpendicular plate of ethmoid
    B. Vomer
    C. Septal cartilage
19. A. Condyle
    B. Neck
    C. Ramus
    D. Gonion or mandibular angle
    E. Body
    F. Mental foramen
    G. Mentum or mental protuberance
    H. Alveolar process
    I. Coronoid process
    J. Mandibular notch
    K. Temporal bone
    L. Temporomandibular joint (TMJ)

M. External auditory meatus (EAM)
N. Mastoid process
20. A. Lacrimal (facial)
    B. Ethmoid (cranial)
    C. Frontal (cranial)
    D. Sphenoid (cranial)
    E. Palatine (facial)
    F. Zygomatic (facial)
    G. Maxilla (facial)
21. H. Optic foramen
    I. Superior orbital fissure
    J. Inferior orbital fissure
    K. Sphenoid strut
22. 30, 37
23. Inferior orbital fissure
24. A. Superior orbital fissure
25. B. Optic nerve

## Review Exercise B: Radiographic Anatomy of the Paranasal Sinuses

1. Antrum of Highmore
2. Maxillary
3. Between the inner and outer tables of the skull, posterior to the glabella
4. 6 years
5. Lateral masses or labyrinths
6. B. Osteomeatal complex
7. Sphenoid sinus
8. A. Nasal cavity (fossae)
   B. Maxillary sinuses
   C. Right temporal bone (squamous portion)
   D. Frontal sinuses
   E. Ethmoid sinuses
   F. Sphenoid sinuses
   G. Maxillary sinuses
   H. Ethmoid sinuses
   I. Frontal sinuses
   J. Squamous portion of left temporal bone
   K. Mastoid portion of left temporal bone
   L. Sphenoid sinus
   M. Roots of upper teeth (alveolar process
*Fig. 13-9*
9. A. Sphenoid sinus
   B. Maxillary sinuses
   C. Ethmoid sinuses
   D. Frontal sinus
*Fig. 13-10*
   E. Frontal sinuses
   F. Sphenoid sinus
   G. Ethmoid sinuses
   H. Maxillary sinuses
10. Infundibulum

## Review Exercise C: Positioning of the Facial Bones

1. False (may also be performed erect)
2. True
3. False (decrease of 25%-30%)
4. True
5. False (It *is* used for this.)
6. False (Strong magnets in MRI prohibit this.)
7. Blowout fracture
8. Tripod
9. Dense petrous pyramids superimpose the orbits, obscuring facial bone structures.
10. C. Zygoma
11. Waters method
12. Orbits including infraorbital rims, bony nasal septum, maxillae, zygomatic bones and arches
13. B. 30°
14. Orbital rims and orbital floors
15. A. Reduces OID of facial bones
    B. Reduces exposure to anterior facial bones and neck structures such as thyroid glands
16. A. IR is placed lengthwise for facial bones but crosswise for the cranium.
    B. CR is centered to the zygoma for facial bones and 2 inches (5 cm) above the EAM for the cranium.
17. Mentomeatal; 37
18. Acanthion
19. Nasion
20. Lips–meatal; 55
21. True
22. False (toward the affected side)
23. True
24. False (Thyroid gland dose is significant.)
25. Maxillary sinuses; inferior orbital rims
26. Glabelloalveolar (GAL)
27. Zygomatic arches
28. 1 inch (2.5 cm) superior to glabella to pass through midarches
29. A. Rhese method
    B. Three-point landing
30. A. Cheek, nose, chin
    B. 53°
    C. Acanthiomeatal
    D. Lower outer
31. 1. E
    2. C
    3. F
    4. A
    5. D
    6. B

**13**

## Review Exercise D: Positioning of the Mandible and Temporomandibular Joints (TMJ)

1. Submentovertex (SMV)
2. Axiolateral
3. Extend the chin
4. A. 30°
   B. 45°
   C. 0°, true lateral
   D. 10°-15°
   E. 25° cephalad
5. Insufficient cephalic CR angle
6. Acanthion (at lips for PA projection)
7. Orbitomeatal line (OML)
8. True
9. False (cephalad)
10. Condyloid process
11. A. 35°-40° caudad
    B. 42°-47°
12. Glabella, to pass through midway between EAM and angle of mandible
13. SMV projection
14. Panoramic tomography (Panorex)
15. Narrow, vertical slit diaphragm
16. Infraorbitomeatal line (IOML)
17. Curved, nongrid cassette
18. True
19. True
20. B. Schuller
21. 25-30; caudad
22. A. Modified Law
    B. 15
    C. 15
23. Modified Towne with 40° caudad angle (see Note on p. 435 in textbook)
24. Midsagittal

## Review Exercise E: Positioning of the Paranasal Sinuses

1. 70-80 kV
2. A. Perform positions erect when possible
   B. Use horizontal x-ray beam
3. True
4. True
5. False
6. A. Lateral
   B. PA Caldwell
   C. Parietoacanthial (Waters)
   D. SMV
7. Lateral
8. Cross-table with horizontal x-ray beam
9. Frontal and anterior ethmoid
10. 15 degrees
11. A. Maxillary
    B. 37
12. Mentomeatal line (MML)
13. Just below the maxillary sinuses
14. Sphenoid, ethmoid, and maxillary sinuses

15. Level of the acanthion
16. The mouth (oral cavity) is open with the PA transoral projection.
17. Sphenoid sinuses
18. 1. C
    2. D
    3. E
    4. A
    5. B

## Review Exercise F: Problem Solving for Technical and Positioning Errors

1. Rotation of the head
2. No. The petrous ridges should be projected just below the maxillary sinuses. The patient's head needs to be extended more.
3. Rotation of the head
4. Yes, this image meets the evaluation criteria for a 30° PA axial projection.
5. Excessive flexion of the head and neck or incorrect CR angle will project the glabella into the nasal bones. The CR must be aligned with the glabelloalveolar line.
6. The head was tilted. Ensure that the IPL is perpendicular to the image receptor.
7. No. Increase extension of the head and neck. The AML should be placed perpendicular to the IR to ensure that the optic foramen is open and is projected into the lower outer quadrant of the orbit (head rotation is correct).
8. Insufficient rotation of the head toward the IR. The head should be rotated 30° toward the IR to prevent foreshortening of the body.
9. PA Waters and R and L laterals. The PA Waters or the optional PA axial would demonstrate any possible septal deviation. The lateral projections would demonstrate any possible fracture of the nasal bones or anterior nasal spine. (The superoinferior projection would provide an axial perspective but is considered an optional projection in most departments and not part of the routine unless specifically requested.)
10. Modified parietoacanthial (modified Waters) projection
11. Perform the oblique inferosuperior (tangential) projections. These projections are most ideal to demonstrate a depressed fracture of the zygomatic arch. (Bilateral projections are generally taken for comparison.)
12. Angle CR to place it perpendicular to the IOML. If possible, angle image

receptor to maintain a perpendicular relationship between the CR and image receptor.
13. The head and neck need to be extended more to project the petrous ridges below the ethmoid sinuses.
14. Rotation of the head
15. Tilt of the head
16. Increase extension of the head and neck to project the entire sphenoid sinus through the oral cavity.
17. None. The petrous ridges should be below the floors of the maxillary sinuses on a well-positioned parietoacanthial projection.
18. The most diagnostic projection is the horizontal beam lateral projection to demonstrate any air-fluid levels.
19. The PA transoral special projection in addition to the routine four sinuses projection series (the lateral, PA Caldwell, parietoacanthial, and SMV)
20. PA, PA axial, and parietoacanthial projections will demonstrate a possible bony nasal septal deviation.

## Review Exercise G: Critique Radiographs of the Facial Bones

A. PA Waters (C13-135)
   1. Pertinent anatomy is all included but not well demonstrated due to positioning and exposure errors.
   2. Skull is underextended. This led to the petrous ridges being projected into the lower maxillary sinuses. Also, skull appears to be rotated.
   3. Collimation is not evident. CR and image receptor appears correct.
   4. Facial bone region appears to be overexposed with very poor contrast.
   5. Anatomic side marker is not evident.
   Repeatable error(s): 2 and 4
B. SMV mandible (C13-136)
   1. Pertinent anatomy is included but not well demonstrated due to positioning error.
   2. Skull is underextended and/or CR angle is incorrect. (IOML was not parallel to IR and not perpendicular to CR.) Mandible is foreshortened and rami projected into temporal bone.
   3. Collimation is not evident. CR centering and IR placement is correct.

4. Image appears to be slightly underexposed.
5. Anatomic side marker is not evident.

Repeatable error(s): 2 (possibly 4)

C. Optic foramina, Rhese method (C13-137)
1. Optic foramen is included but is slightly distorted.
2. Skull is rotated excessively toward a PA. (The skull is rotated more than 53° from the lateral position. This led to the optic foramen being projected into the middle lower aspect of the orbit.)
3. Collimation is not evident. CR and IR placement are correct.
4. Exposure factors are acceptable.
5. Anatomic side marker is not evident.

Repeatable error(s): 2 (The foramen is well demonstrated, and this may not be a repeatable error by itself.)

D. Optic foramina, Rhese method (C13-138)
1. Optic foramen is distorted and totally obscured.
2. Skull appears to be overextended. (The AML was not perpendicular.) This projects the optic foramina into the infraorbital rim structure. Skull also appears to be underrotated, toward a lateral position. (If the skull is rotated less than 53° from the lateral position, the optic foramen will be projected into the lateral margin of the orbit.)
3. Collimation is evident and appears satisfactory. CR and IR placement are correct.
4. Exposure factors are acceptable.
5. Anatomic side marker is not evident.

Repeatable error(s): 1 and 2

E. Lateral facial bones (C13-139)
1. Very distal end of mandible is cut off. Probably would not justify repeat exposure unless this was a specific area of interest.
2. Skull is rotated. (Note the separation of rami of mandible, greater wings of sphenoid, and orbits).
3. Collimation is evident and acceptable (except for cutoff of lower tip of mandible). CR and IR placement are acceptable.
4. Exposure factors appear to be satisfactory.
5. Anatomic side marker is not evident.

Repeatable error(s): 2 (possibly 1)

## Review Exercise H: Critique Radiographs of the Paranasal Sinuses

A. Parietoacanthial transoral (open-mouth Waters) (C13-140)
1. Sphenoid and maxillary sinuses not well demonstrated. Petrous ridges are projected into lower aspect of maxillary sinuses. The base of skull is superimposed over sphenoid sinus.
2. Skull is underextended, leading to errors previously described. (Chin not elevated sufficiently.)
3. Collimation is not centered to film. CR is centered too low (inferior) according to circular collimation on top, but this is not a repeatable error by itself. Film appears centered high, not aligned with CR.
4. Exposure factors are acceptable.
5. Anatomical side marker is not evident.

Repeatable errors: 1 and 2

B. Parietoacanthial (Waters) (C13-141)
1. Maxillary sinuses not well demonstrated. Petrous ridges are projected into lower aspect of maxillary sinuses. Artifacts appear to be either surgical clips and devices or external hair pins or clips.
2. Skull is underextended and severely rotated.
3. Collimation is not evident. CR centering and film placement are slightly now.
4. Exposure factors are acceptable.
5. Anatomaical side marker is not evident.

Repeatable errors: 1 and 2

C. Submentovertex (SMV) (C13-142)
1. Maxillary and ethmoid sinuses not well demonstrated and partially cut off. Mandible is superimposed over sinuses.
2. Skull is grossly underextended and tilted. (Also some rotation.)
3. Collimation would have been OK if centering would have been correct. CR centering is off laterally. This led to cut-off of the anatomy.
4. Exposure factors are acceptable.
5. Anatomical side marker is not evident.

Repeatable errors: 1, 2, and 3 (CR centering)

D. Submentovertex (SMV) (C13-143)
1. Part of ethmoid and maxillary sinuses not well demonstrated due to superimposed mandible. Earrings were not removed.
2. Skull is underextended and slightly rotated to the right.
3. Collimation is acceptable. CR centering and film placement are acceptable but slightly anterior.
4. Exposure factors are acceptable for the sphenoid/ethmoid sinuses.
5. Anatomical side marker is not evident.

Repeatable errors: 1 and 2

**13**

# SELF-TEST

My Score = _____ %

Directions: This self-test should be taken only after completing all of the readings, review exercises, and laboratory activities for a particular section. The purpose of this test is not only to provide a good learning exercise but also to serve as a strong indicator of what your final evaluation exam will be. It is strongly suggested that if you do not get at least a 90% to 95% grade on each self-test, you review those areas in which you missed questions before going to your instructor for the final evaluation exam for this chapter. (There are a total of 82 questions or blanks—each is worth 1.2 points.)

1.  The majority of the hard palate is formed by:

   A. Maxilla            C. Zygomatic bone

   B. Palatine bones     D. Mandible

2.  Which of the following is *not* an aspect of the maxilla?

   A. Frontal process    C. Zygomatic process

   B. Body               D. Ramus

3.  Match each of the following definitions or characteristics to the correct facial bone (using each choice only once):

   _____ A. Mandible              1. Contains four processes

   _____ B. Lacrimal bones        2. Forms lower, outer aspect of orbit

   _____ C. Palatine bones        3. Lie just anterior and medial to the frontal process of maxilla

   _____ D. Inferior nasal conchae   4. Unpaired bone in the adult

   _____ E. Nasal bones           5. Located anteriorly in medial aspect of orbit

   _____ F. Maxilla               6. Help to mix air drawn into nasal cavity

   _____ G. Zygomatic bone        7. Possesses a vertical and horizontal portion

4.  Identify the seven (cranial and facial) bones that form the bony orbit (Fig.13-11):

   A. _____

   B. _____

   C. _____

   D. _____

   E. _____

   F. _____

   G. _____

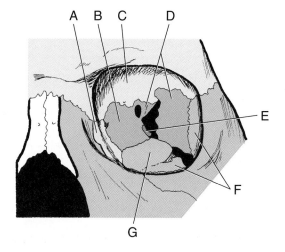

**Fig. 13-11.** Slightly oblique frontal view of orbit, A-G.

5.  On average, how many separate cavities make up the frontal sinus? _____

6.  True/False: All of the paranasal sinuses are contained within cranial bones, except the maxillary sinuses.

7.  True/False: All of the paranasal sinuses except the sphenoid communicate with the nasal cavity.

8.  True/False: In general, all the paranasal sinuses are fully developed by the age of 6 or 7 years.

9.  True/False: The frontal sinuses are usually larger in men than in women.

10. Identify the labeled structures on these radiographs of the paranasal sinuses (Figs. 13-12, 13-13, and 13-14)

A. _____    H. _____

B. _____    I. _____

C. _____    J. _____

D. _____    K. _____

E. _____    L. _____

F. _____    M. _____

G. _____

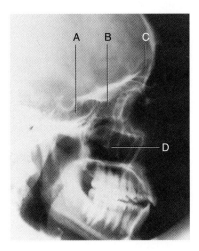

**Fig. 13-12.** Paranasal sinuses, A-D.

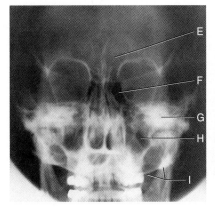

**Fig. 13-13.** Paranasal sinuses, E-I.

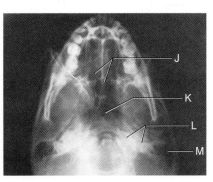

**Fig. 13-14.** Paranasal sinuses, J-M.

11. Which aspect of the ethmoid bone contains the ethmoid air cells? _____

12. The sphenoid sinus lies directly inferior to the _____

13. True/False: Ultrasound of the sphenoid sinus can be performed to rule out sinusitis.

14. Which one of the following imaging modalities would best demonstrate bony erosion of the maxillary sinus due to acute sinusitis?

A.  CT          C.  Ultrasound

B.  MRI         D.  Conventional radiography

15. True/False: Facial bone studies should be performed erect whenever possible.

16. True/False: A Le Fort fracture produces a "free-floating" zygomatic bone.

17. Which frontal projection of the facial bones best visualizes the region of the maxilla and orbits?

_____

18. For possible cranial trauma, which single projection of the facial bones best demonstrates any possible air-fluid levels in the sinuses if the patient can't stand or sit erect?

    _____

19. Which plane is placed parallel to the IR with a true lateral projection of the facial bones?

    _____

20. A. What is the angle between the OML and plane of image receptor with a parietoacanthial (Waters) projection?

    _____

    B. This will place the _____ positioning line perpendicular to the IR.

21. The CR is centered to exit at the level of the _____ for a well-positioned parietoacanthial projection.

    A. Nasion          C. Inner canthus

    B. Glabella        D. Acanthion

22. The CR is centered to exit at the level of the _____ for a well-positioned 15° PA axial projection of the facial bones.

    A. Nasion          C. Midorbits

    B. Glabella        D. Acanthion

23. Where are the petrous ridges projected for a properly positioned modified parietoacanthial projection?

    _____

24. True/False: The lateral projection of the nasal bones should be performed using a small focal spot, detail screens (IR), and close collimation.

25. True/False: The CR should be angled as needed to be parallel to the glabellomeatal line (GML) for the superoinferior projection of the nasal bones.

26. Which positioning line is placed perpendicular to the image receptor for a modified parietoacanthial projection?

    _____

27. Where is the CR centered for a lateral projection of the nasal bones?

    _____

28. Which positioning line, if placed parallel to the image receptor, will ensure adequate extension of the head for the submentovertex projection for zygomatic arches?

    _____

29. How much skull tilt and rotation are required for the oblique inferosuperior (tangential) projection for zygomatic

    arches? _____

30. How much CR angle is required for the AP axial projection of the zygomatic arches if the IOML is placed perpendicular to the IR? (HINT: This is the same as for an AP axial skull.)

    _____

31.  The proper method name for the "three-point landing" projection for the optic foramen is the

     _____

32.  Where should the optic foramen be located with a well-positioned parieto-orbital projection?

     _____

33.  What type of CR angulation should be used for an axiolateral projection of the mandible?

     _____

34.  Which one of the following factors will prevent superimposition of the ramus on the cervical spine for the axiolateral mandible projection?

     A.  Angle CR 10 to 15° cephalad              C.  Extend chin slightly

     B.  Have patient open mouth during exposure   D.  Rotate head toward IR

35.  How much skull rotation toward the image receptor is required for the axiolateral projection of the mentum?

     A.  10 to 15°        C.  45°

     B.  30°              D.  None; keep skull in true lateral position

36.  How much CR angulation should be used for a PA axial projection of the mandible?

     A.  None                    C.  20° to 25° cephalad

     B.  10° to 15° cephalad     D.  5° cephalad

37.  What structures are better defined when the CR angulation is increased from 35° to 40° caudad for the AP axial projection of the mandible?

     _____

38.  Where is the CR centered for an SMV projection of the mandible? _____

39.  The thyroid dose range for the SMV projection of the mandible is:

     A.  10-50 mrad        C.  200-300 mrad

     B.  50-100 mrad       D.  400-500 mrad

40.  During a Panorex procedure, it is important to keep the _____ positioning line parallel to the floor.

     A.  OML        C.  IOML

     B.  AML        D.  GAL

41.  What CR angulation is used for the AP axial projection of the TMJ with the OML perpendicular to the

     image receptor? _____

42.  True/False: The modified Law method requires a tube angulation of 25°.

43.  True/False: The Schuller method requires that the skull be placed in a true lateral position.

44.  True/False: A grid is not required for the oblique inferosuperior (tangential) projection for zygomatic arches.

45.  Where is the CR centered for a lateral projection of the paranasal sinuses? _____

**13**

46. Why should patients remain in an erect position for at least 5 minutes before sinus radiography?

    _____

47. Which projection is best for demonstrating the maxillary sinuses? _____

48. Why should a horizontal CR be used for the erect PA (Caldwell) projection for sinuses rather than the usual 15°

    caudad angle? _____

49. A radiograph of a 15° PA projection of the facial bones reveals that the petrous ridges are projected at the level of the midorbital rims. What specific positioning or CR angling error led to this radiographic outcome?

    _____

50. Which positioning line should be perpendicular to the image receptor for the Rhese method projections for optic foramina?

    A. Acanthomeatal line (AML)          C. Infraorbitomeatal line (IOML)

    B. Mentomeatal line (MML)            D. Glabellomeatal line (GML)

51. A radiograph of an SMV projection of the mandibular condyles reveals that the zygomatic arches are superimposed over the petrous pyramids. What adjustment to this position is needed to avoid this problem during the repeat exposure?

    _____

52. A radiograph of lateral position for sinuses reveals that the greater wings of the sphenoid bone are not superimposed. What specific positioning error is present?

    _____

53. **Situation:** A patient with severe facial bone injuries comes into the emergency room. The patient is wearing a cervical collar and cannot be moved. What type of positioning routine should be performed for this situation?

    _____

    _____

54. A superoinferior, tangential projection for the nasal bones was taken with the following factors: 8 × 10-inch (18 × 24 cm) IR crosswise, 85 kV, 13 mAs, 40-inch (102-cm) SID. The resultant radiograph was unsatisfactory because of poor visibility of the facial bones. Which technical factors should be changed for the repeat exposure?

    _____

55. **Situation:** A patient with possible facial fractures, including a possible "blowout" fracture to the right orbit, was brought from the emergency room to the radiology department. What special facial bone projection should be included with the basic facial bone routine of a lateral, parietoacanthial (Waters), and PA axial (Caldwell)?

    _____

    _____

56. **Situation:** A patient with a clinical history of secondary osteomyelitis comes to the radiology department. Which imaging modalities or procedures can be performed to demonstrate the extent of damage to the sinuses?

    _____

    _____

# Self-Test Answers

## Chapter 1
### General Anatomy, Terminology and Positioning Principles
Self-Test A: General, Systemic, and Skeletal Anatomy and Arthrology

1.
  A. Integumentary
  D. Osseous
2. C. 206
3. B. Circulatory
4. B. Urinary
5. D. Integumentary
6. B. Axial and appendicular
7. A. Spongy or cancellous
8. C. Hyaline or articular cartilage
9. D. Diploe
10. A. Diaphysis
11. C. Epiphyses
12. A. Fibrous
13. B. Cartilaginous
14. C. Distal tibiofibular joint
15.
  1. C
  2. A
  3. B
  4. D
  5. C
  6. A
  7. D
  8. C
16. D. Fibrous
17.
  1. E
  2. A
  3. F
  4. C
  5. B
  6. D
  7. B
  8. D
  9. A

Self-Test B: Positioning Terminology
1. C. Midcoronal
2. False
3. C. Sagittal plane
4.
  1. E
  2. I
  3. G
  4. J
  5. A
  6. K
  7. C
  8. H
  9. B
  10. F
  11. L
  12. D

5.
  1. L
  2. G
  3. F
  4. J
  5. A
  6. H
  7. D
  8. C
  9. B
  10. K
  11. I
  12. E
6. D. Projection
7. A. LAO
8. C. Ventral decubitus
9. D. Anteroposterior
10. C. RPO
11. D. AP oblique with lateral rotation
12. A. Dorsoplantar
13. D. Fowler's
14. C. PA oblique with medial rotation
15. A. Tangential
16. C. Transthoracic
17. D. Parietoacanthial
18.
  1. D
  2. H
  3. I
  4. F
  5. J
  6. C
  7. A
  8. G
  9. B
  10. E

Self-Test C: Positioning Principles
1. False
2. False
3. D. None of the x-ray equipment manufactured after 1994
4. True
5.
  1. B
  2. B
  3. A
  4. A
  5. B
  6. A
  7. A
  8. B
  9. A
  10. A
6. C. Two
7. B. 10 × 12
8. C. 100
9. A. Iliac crest
10. B. Jugular notch

11. A. T-9/10.
12. D. Hypersthenic

## Chapter 2
### Image Quality, Digital Technology, and Radiation Protection
Self-Test A: Image Quality in Film-Screen Imaging
1. C. Kilovoltage
2. A. Density
3. B. Milliamperage seconds (mAs)
4. False
5. B. Decrease to 5 mAs
6. B. Kilovoltage (kV)
7. C. 110 kV 2mAs
8. A. 60 kV, 30 mAs
9. True
10. False
11. C. 60 kV and 5 mAs
12. D. All of the above
13. False
14. D. Shortening the exposure time
15. D. 0.3 mm focal spot and 40-inch SID
16. B. Compensating filter
17. D. Distortion
18. C. 72-inch SID and 3-inch OID
19. False
20. B. Parallel

Self-Test B: Image Quality in Digital Radiography
1. A. Pixels
2. D. Algorithms
3. False
4. True
5. True
6. B. Brightness
7. C. Processing algorithms
8. A. Contrast resolution
9. B. Display pixel size
10. False
11. True
12. D. Exposure index
13. A. Noise
14. True
15. False
16. B. Scatter radiation
17. C. Post-processing
18. A. Smoothing
19. B. Contrast
20. False

Self-Test C: Applications of Digital Technology
1. False
2. True
3. D. Bar code reader

4. D. Photostimulable phosphor
5. A. Laser
6. False
7. C. 30
8. False
9. True
10. True
11. False
12. True
13. True, film-screen images can be scanned in
14. C. Radiology information system
15. A. A set of standards to ensure communication among digital imaging systems
16. D. Teleradiology
17. B. Penumbra
18. C. Display matrices
19. A. Computer-assisted detection
20. D. Detection quantum efficiency

Self-Test D: Radiation Protection
1. B. Gray
2. D. Roentgen
3. D. 5 rem or 50 mSv
4. A. 250 mSv
5. B. 0.1 rem or 1 mSv
6. D. 10 R/minute
7. C. 3 to 4 R/minute
8. A. Absorb lower energy x-rays
9. B. AP thoracic spine (14 × 17″ collimation)
10. C. 50 to 90%
11. C. Shadow shield
12. False
13. True
14. True
15. False (2%)
16. D. Collimation
17. C. Increase kV and lower mAs
18. D. Behind radiologist
19. A. Bucky slot shield
20. B. .05 rem (0.5 mSv)

## Chapter 3
## Chest
1.
  1. E
  2. C
  3. D
  4. B
  5. A
2. D. Vertebra prominens
3. C. Jugular notch
4. A. Right and left bronchi
5. B. Carina
6. D. Hilum
7. B. Alveoli
8. B. Hilar pleura
9. B. Hemothorax
10. A. Costophrenic angle
11. C. Epiglottis
12. D. Asthenic

13. D. 130 kVp, 600 mA, 1/60 sec, 72 in. SID
14.
  A. 8
  B. 10
  C. 1
  D. 5
  E. 4
  F. 11
  G. 9
  H. 13
  I. 7
  J. 3
  K. 6
  L. 12
  M. 2
15.
  A. Superior portion (apex) of left lung
  B. Jugular notch (superior margin of manubrium)
  C. Trachea
  D. Esophagus
16.
  A. Esophagus
  B. Descending aorta
  C. T4-T5 vertebra
  D. Trachea
  E. Superior vena cava
  F. Ascending aorta
  G. Sternum
  H. Left lung region
17. A. Pigg-O-Stat
18. C. 65 kVp, short exposure time
19. A. To reduce patient dose
20. D. To reduce chest rotation
21. A. Remove scapulae from lung fields
22. C. 3 to 4 inches (8 to 10 cm) below jugular notch
23. True. CT is replacing bronchography to study the bronchial tree.
24. A. Atelectasis
25. C. Pulmonary edema
26. B. Pulmonary emboli
27. D. Tuberculosis
28. A. Be Reduced
29. C. Rotation into an LAO position
30. Yes, 10 ribs showing is acceptable. (Some healthy patients can inhale deeper and show 11 ribs.)
31. Yes. The costophrenic angles must be visualized on both the PA and lateral projections.
32. D. Raise upper limbs higher
33. No. This separation is acceptable and is caused by the divergent x-ray beam.
34. B. Perform AP semi-axial projection
35. C. Yes. Decrease exposure factors
36. A. Left lateral decubitus
37. C. 60 degrees LAO
38. D. Left lateral decubitus

39.
  A. (a), (c), (f) (slight rotation is evident)
  B. Criterion (a)
  C. (a), (f), (g)
40.
  A. (b), (c), (f)
  B. Criteria (b) and (f)
  C. (a), (d), (e)

## Chapter 4
## Abdomen
1. D. Peritoneum
2. C. Psoas muscles
3. A. Duodenum
4. C. Ileocecal valve
5.
  1. D
  2. H
  3. G
  4. F
  5. C
  6. A
  7. I
  8. B
  9. E
6. D. Kidney
7. C. Ureter
8. D. Gallbladder
9. D. Mesentery
10.
  A. RLQ
  B. RUQ
  C. LUQ
  D. LUQ
  E. RUQ
  F. LLQ
  G. RLQ
  H. RUQ and LUQ
  I. RUQ
11. A
12.
  1. A
  2. A
  3. B
  4. A
  5. B
  6. A
  7. C
  8. B
  9. C
  10. B
13. A. T9-10
14.
  1. E
  2. A
  3. G
  4. B
  5. C
  6. F
  7. D
15. B. Greater trochanter
16. A. Iliac crest

17. A. Short exposure time
18. D. Ascites
19. B. Ileus
20. A. Intussusception
21. D. Ulcerative colitis
22. C. Pneumoperitoneum
23. B. Diaphragm
24. B. Ascites
25. D. Ileus
26.
    A. Iliac crest
    B. L4 lumbar spine
    C. Psoas muscles
    D. Coccyx
    E. Symphysis pubis
    F. Obturator foramen
27.
    A. Liver
    B. Gallbladder
    C. Duodenum
    D. Stomach
    E. Splenic flexure of colon
    F. Pancreas
    G. Spleen
    H. Left kidney
    I. Abdominal aorta
    J. Inferior vena cava
28. B. 78 kV, 600mA, $\frac{1}{30}$ sec, grid, 40 in. SID
29. C. Rotation toward the right
30. A. Expiration
31. B. Use two cassettes placed cross-wise
32. D. 5 minutes
33. B. Diaphragm
34. A. Left lateral decubitus
35. D. AP erect abdomen
36. B. Left lateral decubitus
37. C. Dorsal decubitus
38. B. AP erect abdomen
39. B. Left lateral decubitus
40. A. Sonography
41. D. Nuclear Medicine
42. D. Close collimation
43.
    A. True
    B. False (250 to 300 range)
    C. False (AP is about 35% greater than PA)
    D. True (testes are out of primary field)
44.
    A. (a), (b), (c), (g)
    B. Criteria (a) and (c)
    C. (b), (c), (g)
45.
    A. (a), (b)
    B. Criterion (a)
    C. (b)

# Chapter 5
# Upper Limb
1.
    A. A. 14
    B. B. 8
    C. B. 27
2.
    A. 7
    B. 4
    C. 2
    D. 5
    E. 1
    F. 6
3.
    A. 11
    B. 13
    C. 4
    D. 15
    E. 7
    F. 17
    G. 5
    H. 18
    I. 12
    J. 1
    K. 16
    L. 8
    M. 2
    N. 3
    O. 9
    P. 14
    Q. 6
    R. 10
4. C. Hamate
5. D. Trapezium
6. A. Scaphoid
7. D. Scaphoid and trapezium
8.
    A. 6
    B. 3
    C. 8
    D. 2
    E. 5
    F. 11
    G. 9
    H. 1
    I. 4
    J. 7
    K. 10
9. C. PA-Radial deviation
10. C. Scaphoid
11. A. PA–Ulnar deviation
12. B. Scaphoid
13. D. Ulna
14. A. Anterior aspect of distal humerus
15. C. Lateral and medial epicondyle
16. A. Medial aspect of coronoid process
17. A. Head of ulna
18.
    A. 4
    B. 3
    C. 2
    D. 1
    E. 4

19.
    A. 2
    B. 1
    C. 4
    D. 3
    E. 2
    F. 9
    G. 7
    H. 5
    I. 4
    J. 1
    K. 10
    L. 1
    M. 3
    N. 6
    O. 8
20.
    A. 5
    B. 3
    C. 8
    D. 7
    E. 11
    F. 1
    G. 2
    H. 4
    I. 10
    J. 9
    K. 6
21. True
22. False
23. B. Causes the proximal radius to cross over the ulna
24. A. Supinated
25. B. Pronated
26.
    A. 3
    B. 4
    C. 1
    D. 2
    E. 1
    F. 4
    G. 2
27. False
28. B. Parallel to long axis of the IR
29. D. Soft-tissue structures within certain synovial joints
30.
    1. F
    2. H
    3. G
    4. E
    5. B
    6. D
    7. A
    8. C
31. C. Osteoporosis
32. A. Affected PIP joint
33. D. All of the above
34. B. Third MCP joint
35. A. Increased OID
36. C. Bennett's fracture
37. True
38. False

39. D
40. True
41. C. Decrease obliquity of hand
42. A. Rotate upper limb medially
43. C. Rotate wrist laterally 5 to 10°
44. A. Insufficient medial rotation
45. B. Place humerus/forearm in same horizontal plane
46. B. Wrist
47. C. Wrist/forearm
48. D. 68 to 70 kV or 10 mAs
49. A. Coyle method
50.
    A. (a). Lateral rotation
    B. (c), (e), (g)
    C. Criteria (e) and (g)
Note: Insufficient lateral rotation may be considered a marginal repeatable error by itself. But with no anatomical marker visible, both of these errors make it repeatable.
    D. (a), (e), (g)
51.
    A. (b) Radial deviation
    B. (a), (b)
    C. Criteria (a) and (b)
    D. (b)

## Chapter 6
## Proximal Humerus and Shoulder Girdle

1. D. (While both terms are correct [B and G], scapulohumeral joint is the preferred term)
2. C. Acromioclavicular
3. B. Medial angle
4. D. Coracoid process
5. False
6. A. Scapular spine
7. C. Acromion
8. B. Spheroidal
9.
    A. 3
    B. 11
    C. 5
    D. 8
    E. 12
    F. 10
    G. 7
    H. 2
    I. 9
    J. 4
    K. B. External rotation
    L. 2
    M. 12
    N. 3
    O. 6
    P. 13 or 5
    Q. 1
    R. 8
    S. A. Inferosuperior axial projection—Lawrence method (transaxillary projection)

10. A. Center and right AEC chambers activated
11. True
12. True
13. D. Nuclear medicine
14. A. Ultrasound
15.
    1. D
    2. E
    3. C
    4. F
    5. G
    6. A
    7. B
16. D. Scapular Y or Neer method
17. A. Osteoarthritis
18. B. Rheumatoid arthritis
19. A. External rotation
20. C. 1 in (2.5 cm) inferior to coracoid process
21. C. Internal rotation
22. B. 25° to 30° medially
23. B. Use exaggerated, external rotation
24. A. 25° anterior and medial
25. D. Grashey method
26. C. 10° to 15°
27. B. Reduced OID
28. A. Neer method
29. B. Transthoracic lateral
30. A. 10 to 15° caudad
31. C. Scapulohumeral dislocations
32. True
33. True
34.
    1. B. (66 mrad)
    2. C. (3 to 8 mrad)
    3. C. (1 to 3 mrad)
    4. B. (45 mrad)
    5. A. (1005 mrad)
    6. C. (10 mrad)
    7. C. (1 mrad)
    8. C. (0 mrad)
35. D. Rotate body more toward affected side
36. C. Garth method
37. A. Increase CR angulation
38. A. AC joint series—non-weight and weight-bearing projections
39. D. Tangential projection-Fisk method
40. A. Wrong direction of CR angle
41. AP clavicle (C6-85)
    A. (b), (c), (e), (f)
    B. Criteria (b), (e), (f)
    C. (a), (b), (f)
42. AP scapula (C6-87)
    A. (a), (b), (d), (e)
    B. Criteria (a), (b), (d), (e)
    C. (a), (b), (d), (e)

## Chapter 7
## Lower Limb

1. B. Tail
2. False
3. A. Plantar surface near head of first metatarsal
4. D. Navicular
5. C. Intermediate cuneiform
6. B. Subtalar joint
7. B. Tibial plafond
8. False (not the lateral aspect of the ankle joint)
9.
    1. D
    2. G
    3. B
    4. F
    5. A
    6. E
    7. C
10.
    A. 3
    B. 4
    C. 5
    D. 1
    E. 2
    F. C. AP ankle
11.
    A. 6
    B. 8
    C. 5
    D. 2
    E. 3
    F. 1
    G. 7
    H. 4
    I. 9
    J. 2
    K. 5
12. A. Fig. 7-11
13. A. Affected MTP joint
14. B. 10 to 15° posterior
15. C. Tangential
16. D. 30 to 40°
17. D. Dorsoplantar projection
18. A. 10° posterior
19. C. AP oblique-medial rotation
20. D. Intercondylar tubercles
21. A. Intercondylar fossa
22. A. (5 to 7°)
23. True
24. B. Base
25. C. Cruciate
26. C. Menisci
27.
    A. 3
    B. 9
    C. 6
    D. 8
    E. 1
    F. 4
    G. 2
    H. 10

I. 5

J. 7

28. B. AP oblique-medial rotation

29.

    A. 3

    B. 5

    C. 1

    D. 6

    E. 2

    F. 3

    G. 5

    H. 1

    I. 4

    J. 7

30. B. Under rotation toward IR

31. True

32. C. Over rotation of knee toward IR

33. D. Osgood-Schlatter disease

34. D. Osteomalacia

35. A. Osteogenic sarcoma

36. B. Runner's knee

37. C. Base of third metatarsal

38. B. AP oblique (15-20° medial rotation)

39. D. Interepicondylar

40. B. Proximal tibiofibular

41. True

42. D. All of the above

43. D. Merchant

44. C. Requires overflexion of knee

45. B. Lateral rotation of lower limb

46. C. Increase central ray angle to 45°

47. A. Increase CR angulation to 40°

48. D. AP and horizontal beam lateral position

49.

    A. (a), (d), (e), (g)

    B. Criteria (a), (d), (e), (g)

    C. (d), (e), (g)

50.

    A. (a), (g), (c)

    B. Criteria (a) (anterior tubercle is obscured), (g)

    C. (a), (f)

## Chapter 8
## Proximal Femur and Pelvis

1.

    A. Left hip bone

    B. Right hip bone

    C. Sacrum

    D. Coccyx

2.

    A. Ilium

    B. Ischium

    C. Pubis

3. D. All of the above

4. Obturator foramen

5. B. Lesser trochanter

6.

    A. Body

    B. Ramus

7. Brim of the pelvis

8.

    1. B

    2. A

    3. A

    4. B

    5. A

    6. B

    7. B

9. Acute; less than

10.

    A. Greater trochanter

    B. Neck of femur

    C. Acetabulum

    D. Anterior superior iliac spine (ASIS)

    E. Crest of ilium

    F. Ischial spine

    G. Superior ramus of pubis

    H. Symphysis pubis

    I. Ischial tuberosity

    J. Female

    K. Neck of femur

    L. Lesser trochanter

    M. Greater trochanter

    N. Ischial tuberosity

    O. Axiolateral (inferosuperior axial projection) or (Danelius-Miller method)

    P. Ala (wing) of left ilium

    Q. Body of left ilium

    R. Body of left pubis

    S. Inferior ramus of left ischium

    T. Greater trochanter

    U. Lesser trochanter

    V. Neck of right femur

    W. AP bilateral frog-legs (modified Cleaves method)

11.

    1. M

    2. M

    3. F

    4. F

    5. F

    6. M

12. A. Ischial spines

13. Fovea capitis

14. C. Fractured proximal femur

15. D. Ankylosing spondylitis

16.

    1. F

    2. B

    3. A

    4. E

    5. D

    6. C

17. C. Limited view of the lesser trochanter in profile

18. B. 200 to 500

19. True

20. A. Bilateral frog-leg

21. D. 30-45° cephalad

22. True

23. False. (Midway between ASIS and symphysis pubis)

24. False. (Trauma projection)

25. Posterior oblique acetabulum Judet method

26. B. AP axial method

27. 1 inch (2.5 cm) medial from the upside ASIS

28. Less

29. Right (downside) joints

30. The AP axial outlet projection (Taylor method) will elongate the pubis and ischium and define this region more completely.

31. It is soft tissue from the unaffected thigh. This leg must be flexed and elevated high enough to keep it from superimposing the affected hip.

32. The primary positioning error is over rotation of the pelvis toward the patient's right. The ideal posterior oblique positions for SI joints require only 25° to 30° of the pelvis.

33. No. It is an acceptable image because the lesser trochanters should not be visible at all or only minimally on a well-positioned AP hip projection.

34. AP pelvis and bilateral "frog-leg"

35. B. Reverse central ray angle

36. Rotation of pelvis toward the patient's left. The elevated or upside obturator foramen will become more narrowed as compared to the opposite side.

37. Multiple answers are correct: Posterior oblique projections (Judet method) will demonstrate possible pelvic ring and acetabular fractures and AP axial "outlet" and AP axial "Inlet" projections will demonstrate possible fractures involving the ischium and pubis.

38. C. 40° caudad

39. Angle the CR 15 to 20° cephalad to open up the lower aspect of the SI joint

40.

    A. (a), (e)

    B. (a), (e)

    C. (e), (f)

41.

    A. (a), (b), (f), (h)

    B. (a), (b), (f), (h)

    C. (b), (g), (h)

## Chapter 9
## Cervical and Thoracic Spine

1. Lower border of first lumbar (L1) vertebrae

2. Five

3. A. Thoracic; D. Sacral

4. True
5. Kyphosis
6. Scoliosis
7. Herniated nucleus pulposus (HNP)
8. Intervertebral foramina
9. Zygapophyseal joints
10. B. Nucleus pulposus
11. False (vertebral artery and vein)
12. False (C-spine possesses bifid spinous processes)
13. 45°
14. Transverse atlantal ligament
15. Zygapophyseal joint
16. Demifacets
17. C. T11; D. T12
18. A. Each has three foramina (one in each transverse process plus the vertebral foramina).
    B. Bifid spinous processes
19. Presence of facets for articulation with ribs
20. Lateral position
21.
    A. Anterior arch (with anterior tubercle), C1 (atlas)
    B. Dens (odontoid process), C2
    C. Transverse atlantal ligament, C2
    D. Transverse foramen, C1
    E. Superior facets (atlanto-occipital articulation), C1
    F. Posterior arch, C1
    G. Dens (odontoid process), C2
    H. Transverse process, C1
    I. Articular pillar (lateral mass), C2
    J. Right zygapophyseal joint, C2 to C3
    K. Bifid, spinous process, C4
    L. Vertebra prominens (spinous process), C7
    M. Superior articular process, T10
    N. Intervertebral disk space, T10 to T11
    O. Facet for costovertebral joint, T11
    P. Right zygapophyseal joint, T11 to T12
    Q. Right intervertebral foramen, T12 to L1
    R. Facet of inferior articular process, L2
    S. Lower thoracic (T10, 11, and 12) and upper lumbar (L1 and 2).
    T. Evident by facets for articulation with ribs on upper three but not on lower two. (Note also that the last two thoracic vertebrae do not have facets on transverse processes for costotransverse joints, characteristic of T11 and T12.)
22.
    A. Lateral mass (articular pillar), C1
    B. Zygapophyseal joint, C1 to C2
    C. Body, C2

D. Spinous process (superimposed by body), C2
    E. Inferior articular process, C2
    F. Dens (odontoid process), C2
    G. Upper incisors (teeth)
23. Lateral position
24. Left zygapophyseal joints (downside joints)
25. 1. B
    2. A
    3. C
    4. D
    5. F
    6. E
26. D. Nuclear medicine
27. B. Clay shoveler's fracture
28. A. Scoliosis and/or kyphosis
29. False. Most common at the L4 to L5 level
30.
    A. Close side collimation
    B. Place a lead mat on tabletop behind patient
31. AP open-mouth projection
32.
    A. 15 to 20 degrees cephalad
    B. 15 degrees caudad
    C. 15 degrees cephalad
33. B. Left anterior oblique (LAO)
34.
    A. Suspend respiration on full expiration
    B. Have patient hold 5 to 10 lb. in each hand.
35. Cervicothoracic lateral or "swimmer's" projection
36.
    A. AP projection-Fuchs method
    B. PA projection-Judd method
37. Tilt and/or rotation of the spine
38. Not keeping spine parallel to the film and/or not aligning the CR perpendicular to spine
39. Yes. (The technologist needs to assume there may be a fracture present. A horizontal beam cross-table lateral projection should be taken for all suspected trauma to the cervical spine. A physician must examine the radiograph and clear the patient for the remaining projections.)
40. AP open-mouth projection. Note that a horizontal beam lateral projection must be taken and cleared first.
41. C. 100 to 200 mrad
42. D. 4 times greater
43. D. 900 to 1000 mrad
44. C. 10 to 15 times greater
45. Excessive flexion of skull
46. AP and lateral cervical spine projections

47. Hyperflexion and hyperextension lateral positions
48. D. Collimate as close as possible
49.
    A. (a), (c), (f)
    B. Criteria (a), (f)
    C. Criteria (a), (e), (f)
50.
    A. (a), (b), (c), (g)
    B. Criteria (a), (c), (g)
    C. Criteria (c), (d)

# Chapter 10
# Lumbar Spine, Sacrum, and Coccyx

1. C. Larger and more blunt
2. C. Promontory
3. B. 30
4. 45°
5. C. Between superior and inferior articular processes
6.
    A. Left ala superior articular process
    B. Left ala or wing of sacrum
    C. Pelvic (anterior) sacral foramina
    D. Apex of sacrum
    E. Right and left superior articular processes
    F. Sacral promontory (also seen on frontal view)
    G. Auricular surface (for sacroiliac joint)
    H. Coccyx
    I. Apex of coccyx
    J. Horn (cornu) of coccyx
    K. Horn (cornu) of sacrum
    L. Median sacral crest
7.
    A. Spinous process
    B. Lamina
    C. Transverse process
    D. Pedicle (also shown on lateral view)
    E. Vertebral foramen
    F. Body (also shown on lateral view)
    G. Superior articular process
    H. Inferior articular process
    I. Region of articular facets (R and L sides superimposed as seen on a lateral view)
    J. Intervertebral notch or foramen
8. Large vertebral body and large, blunt spinous process
9. Synovial, plane (gliding)
10.
    A. Superior articular process (ear)
    B. Transverse process (nose)
    C. Pedicle (eye)
    D. Inferior articular (leg)
    E. Pars interarticularis (neck)
    F. Zygapophyseal joint (between L-4/5)

11. Zygapophyseal
12. B. Lower costal margin
13. False (would obscure essential anatomy since the ovaries are located near the lower lumbar spine).
14. False (ovaries are slightly anterior, thus AP results in about 30% greater gonadal dose than PA).
15. Opens the intervertebral disk space by reducing the normal lumbar curvature of the spine.
16. False. The lead blocker should be used with digital imaging to prevent secondary scatter from reaching sensitive image receptor. Scatter radiation produces greater "noise" in the processed image.
17. True
18. C. Compression fracture
19. B. Spina bifida
20. A. Ankylosing spondylitis
21. 1 to 1.5 in. (3 to 4 cm) above the iliac crest
22. Right, or the upside joints
23. 50 degrees from plane of table
24. A patient with a wide pelvis and narrow thorax
25. B. 5° to 8°, caudad
26. A. 35°, cephalad
27. Level of ASIS at the midline of the body
28. True
29. PA (AP) projection, Ferguson method (with and without block under convex side of curve)
30. Hyperextension and hyperflexion lateral projections
31. Midway between the symphysis pubis and ASIS
32.
    A. Close collimation
    B. Use a lead blocker on tabletop behind patient
33. To reduce gonadal dose
34. C. 1000 to 1500 mrad
35. Rotation to the patient's right.
36. Decrease rotation of the spine
37. Insufficient cephalad CR angulation or the CR was angled in the wrong direction
38. A lateral projection (may include a coned down spot AP/PA and lateral of the L3 region)
39. AP, lateral, L5-S1 spot lateral and right and left 30 degree oblique positions
40.
    A. (a), (b), (c), (e), (f)
    B. (a), (b), (f)
    C. (a), (b), (e), (f)

## Chapter 11
## Bony Thorax—Sternum and Ribs

1.
    A. Manubrium
    B. Body
    C. Xiphoid process
2. Xiphoid process
3. Sternal angle
4. D. Manubrium
5. A. True rib attaches directly to the sternum with its own costocartilage.
6. D. Does not possess costocartilage
7. True rib
8. D. Sternal angle
9. D. All of the above
10.
    1. A
    2. A
    3. B
    4. A
    5. B
11.
    A. Left clavicle
    B. Left sternoclavicular (SC) joint
    C. First rib (sternal end)
    D. Manubrium
    E. Sternal angle
    F. Body
    G. Xiphoid process
    H. Jugular notch
    I. Manubrium
    J. Sternal angle
    K. Body
    L. Xiphoid process
12.
    A. Suspended inspiration
    B. Low to medium kV (65 to 75)
    C. Erect (if patient is able)
13. 40 in. (100 cm)
14. B. Breathing technique
15.
    A. Place the area of interest closest to IR.
    B. Rotate the spine away from the area of interest.
16.
    A. Pneumothorax
    B. Hemothorax
17.
    A. 15 to 20 degrees
    B. More
18. C. Patients with history of multiple myeloma
19. D. Blunt trauma
20.
    A. 66 mrad (50 to 100 range)
    B. 3 mrad (2 to 5 range)
21. C. (LPO)
22. B. Drawn back
23. The SC joints are equal distance from the midline of spine

24. 15 degrees
25. Midway between the xiphoid process and lower rib cage
26. B. 65 to 75 kV
27. A. LAO
28. Over-rotation of the sternum. A large-chested patient only requires approximately 15 degrees of rotation. Over-rotation will lead to foreshortening along the width of the sternum and will shift the sternum away excessively from the spine.
29. Rotation of the upper body from a true lateral will cause the ribs to be superimposed over the sternum.
30.
    A. AP and RPO performed recumbent
    B. Suspend upon expiration
31.
    A. PA and RAO performed recumbent
    B. Expose upon inspiration
32. 15 to 20 degrees LAO will rotate the right SC joint away from the spine. (A RAO with less obliquity of only 15 degrees would also demonstrate the left SC joint region by aligning it next to the spinal column).
33. LPO and horizontal beam lateral positions
34. PA and lateral chest study
35. False. (AEC is generally not recommended for rib routines due to the need for high-contrast, optimum detail exposures, which can generally be better achieved manually.)
36. False. Exposure is made with suspended respiration upon expiration.
37.
    A. (c), (e), (f)
    B. (f)
    C. (b), (c), (f)

## Chapter 12
## Skull and Cranial Bones

1. C. Occipital
2. C. Squamous
3.
    A. Right parietal
    B. Left parietal
    C. Sphenoid
    D. Ethmoid
4. Parietal tubercles or eminences
5. External occipital protuberance or inion
6.
    A. 5
    B. 6
    C. 3
    D. 7
    E. 2

7. Petrous portion or petrous pyramids
8. True
9. True
10. Clivus
11. Lateral labyrinth or masses
12. Crista galli
13. Left pterion
14. Squamosal suture
15. Sutural or wormian bones
16.
    1. C
    2. C
    3. B
    4. C
    5. D
    6. D
    7. A
    8. D
    9. E
    10. A
    11. B
    12. E
    13. A
    14. C
    15. E
17.
    A. Orbital or horizontal portion, frontal
    B. Supraorbital margin (SOM), frontal
    C. Crista galli, ethmoid
    D. Sagittal suture
    E. Midlateral orbital margin (zygoma)
    F. Petrous ridge, temporal
    G. Petrous portion, temporal
    H. Petrous ridge, temporal
    I. Dorsum sellae, sphenoid
    J. Posterior clinoid processes, sphenoid
    K. Orbital or horizontal portion, frontal
    L. Sella turcica (body), sphenoid
    M. Sphenoid sinus, sphenoid
18. C. Brachycephalic
19. A. Mesocephalic
20.
    A. External auditory meatus (EAM)
    B. Angle (gonion) of mandible
    C. Mental point (mentum)
    D. Acanthion
    E. Nasion
    F. Glabella
    G. Glabellomeatal line (GML)
    H. Orbitomeatal line (OML)
    I. Infraorbitomeatal line (IOML)
    J. Acanthomeatal line (AML)
    K. Lips-meatal line (LML)
    L. Mentomeatal line (MML)
21. Auricular point
22. A. Pinna
23. B. IOML
24. B. 7 to 8°
25. A. Rotation

26.
    A. 5
    B. 6
    C. 2
    D. 4
    E. 1
    F. 3
27. D. Multiple myeloma
28. A. Computed tomography (CT)
29. B. MRI
30. Squamous portion
31. Petrous portion
32. Tympanic membrane
33. A. Malleus
34. Eustachian or auditory tube
35. Auditory nerve and blood vessels
36. Epitympanic recess; mastoid
37. Encephalitis
38. C. Stapes
39. Membranous
40. Cochlea, vestibule, semicircular canals
41. A. Malleus
    B. Incus
    C. Stapes
    D. Internal acoustic meatus – for auditory nerve and blood vessels
    E. Cochlea
    F. Eustachian or auditory tube
    G. Tympanic cavity
    H. Tympanic membrane or ear drum
    I. External acoustic meatus (EAM)
42. C. Cholesteatoma
43. True
44.
    A. AP axial projection (Towne method)
    B. PA axial projection (Haas method)
45.
    A. 37 degrees caudad
    B. 30 degrees caudad
46. 2 in. (5 cm) superior to the EAM
47. Interpupillary
48. Superior to the mastoid processes and symmetrical
49. ³⁄₄ in. (2 cm) anterior to the level of the EAMs, midway between the angles of the mandible
50.
    A. 37 degrees caudad
    B. 30 degrees caudad
51. Increase CR angle approximately 7 degrees caudad
52. Rotation
53. Increase extension of the skull to place the OML perpendicular to the IR (this will project the petrous ridges into the lower one third of the orbits).
54. Horizontal beam lateral skull projection will demonstrate any possible air-fluid levels in the sphenoid sinus

55. Perform the AP projection with a 15 degree cephalad CR angle to the OML
56. Use the IOML instead of OML and increase CR angle an additional 7 degrees caudad for a total of 37 degrees.
57. Insufficient angulation of the CR will lead to superimposition of the upside mastoid upon the region of interest
58. Additional CR angulation will project the dorsum sellae into the foramen magnum and elongate the petrous pyramids
59. Approximately a 40 degree oblique will profile the downside petrous bone. 45 degrees of rotation is required for a mesocephalic skull. Since there is a wider angle between the petrous portion and the midsagittal plane with a brachy-cephalic skull, *less* rotation of the skull is required for the Stenvers projection
60.
    A. (a), (b), (c), (e), (f), (g)
    B. Criteria (a), (*b), (c), (e), (f), (g) (*Note: CR appears to be slightly high. Not a major error, though.)
    C. (a), (b), (e), (f)
61.
    A. (c), (e), (g), (i)
    B. (*c), (e), (g), (i) (*Note: Petrous ridges should be in the lower ¹⁄₃ of orbits.)
    C. (a), (e), (f), (g)

## Chapter 13
## Facial Bones and Paranasal Sinuses

1. A. Maxilla
2. D. Ramus
3.
    A. 4
    B. 5
    C. 7
    D. 6
    E. 3
    F. 1
    G. 2
4.
    A. Lacrimal
    B. Ethmoid
    C. Frontal
    D. Sphenoid
    E. Palatine
    F. Zygomatic
    G. Maxilla
5. 1 to 2 sinuses
6. True
7. False

8. False
9. True
10. A. Sphenoid sinuses
    B. Ethmoid sinuses
    C. Frontal sinuses
    D. Maxillary sinuses
    E. Frontal sinuses
    F. Ethmoid and sphenoid sinuses superimposed
    G. Petrous portion of temporal bone
    H. Maxillary sinuses
    I. Base of skull
    J. Ethmoid sinuses
    K. Sphenoid sinus
    L. Petrous portion of temporal bone
    M. Mastoid portion of temporal bone
11. Lateral masses or labyrinth
12. Sella turcica
13. True
14. A. CT
15. True
16. False (The tripod fracture does this.)
17. Parietoacanthial (Waters) projection (dense petrous pyramids are projected below the maxillary sinuses)
18. Horizontal beam (cross-table) lateral projection
19. Midsagittal plane
20.
    A. 37 degrees
    B. Mentomeatal line (MML)
21. D. Acanthion

22. A. Nasion
23. Lower half of the maxillary sinuses
24. True
25. False (glabelloalveolar, GAL)
26. Lips-meatal line (LML)
27. ½ in. (1.25 cm) inferior to nasion
28. Infraorbitomeatal line (IOML)
29. 15 degrees rotation and 15 degrees tilt toward the affected side
30. 37 degrees caudad
31. Parieto-orbital oblique projection or Rhese method
32. Lower outer quadrant of the orbit
33. 25 degrees cephalad
34. C. Extend chin slightly
35. C. 45°
36. C. 20 to 25° cephalad
37. Temporomandibular fossae
38. 1½ in. (4 cm) inferior to mandibular symphysis (or midway between angles of mandible)
39. C. 200 to 300 mrad
40. C. IOML
41. 35 degrees caudad
42. False (15 degrees caudad)
43. True
44. True
45. Midway between outer canthus and EAM
46. To allow any fluid in the sinuses to settle

47. Parietoacanthial (Waters) projection
48. To demonstrate any air-fluid levels without distortion
49. Excessive flexion of the head, or insufficient caudal CR angle
50. A. Acanthomeatal (AML)
51. Increase extension of the head and neck, or angle the CR. The IOML must be parallel to the film and perpendicular to the CR.
52. Rotation of the skull
53. Reverse parietoacanthial (Waters) projection with the use of cephalic CR angle to keep CR parallel to MML. In addition, horizontal beam lateral projection must be included as part of the positioning routine
54. Reduce kVp to 50 to 60 range and increase mAs accordingly
55. Modified parietoacanthial (modified Waters) or a PA axial projection with a 30 degree caudad angle will best demonstrate the floor of the orbit. Note that the modified Waters is more commonly performed for possible blowout fractures over the standard parietoacanthial (Waters) projection.
56. Routine radiographic sinus series can be performed but CT may demonstrate bony erosion better.